Fall 1991.

MEDICAL CARE IN THE NURSING HOME

NOTICE

Medicine is an ever-changing science. As new research and clinical experience broaden our knowledge, changes in treatment and drug therapy are required. The authors and the publisher of this work have checked with sources believed to be reliable in their efforts to provide information that is complete and generally in accord with the standards accepted at the time of publication. However, in view of the possibility of human error or changes in medical sciences, neither the editors nor the publisher nor any other party who has been involved in the preparation or publication of this work warrants that the information contained herein is in every respect accurate or complete. Readers are encouraged to confirm the information contained herein with other sources. For example and in particular, readers are advised to check the product information sheet included in the package of each drug they plan to administer to be certain that the information contained in this book is accurate and that changes have not been made in the recommended dose or in the contraindications for administration. This recommendation is of particular importance in connection with new or infrequently used drugs.

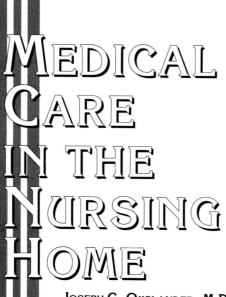

MEDICAL CARE IN THE NURSING HOME

JOSEPH G. OUSLANDER, M.D.
*Medical Director, Jewish Homes for the Aging
of Greater Los Angeles
Associate Professor, Multicampus Division
of Geriatric Medicine and Gerontology
UCLA School of Medicine, Los Angeles, California*

DAN OSTERWEIL, M.D.
*Medical Director, Jewish Homes for the Aging
of Greater Los Angeles
Associate Professor, Multicampus Division
of Geriatric Medicine and Gerontology
UCLA School of Medicine, Los Angeles, California*

JOHN MORLEY, M.D.
*Dammert Professor of Gerontology
Division of Geriatric Medicine
St. Louis University Medical Center
Director of GRECC
Veterans Administration Medical Center
St. Louis, Missouri*

Foreword by Robert L. Kane, M.D.

McGraw-Hill, Inc.
HEALTH PROFESSIONS DIVISION

New York   St. Louis   San Francisco   Bogotá   Caracas
Hamburg   Lisbon   London   Madrid   Mexico   Milan   Montreal
New Delhi   Panama   Paris   San Juan   São Paulo   Singapore
Sydney   Tokyo   Toronto

MEDICAL CARE IN THE NURSING HOME

Copyright © 1991 by McGraw-Hill, Inc. All rights reserved. Printed in the
United States of America. Except as permitted under the United States
Copyright Act of 1976, no part of this publication may be reproduced or
distributed in any form or by any means, or stored in a data or retrieval
system, without the prior written permission of the publisher.

1234567890   DOCDOC   9987654321

ISBN   0-07-047949-6

This book was set in Korinna by University Graphics, Inc.
The editors were J. Dereck Jeffers and Muza Navrozov;
the production supervisor was Richard Ruzycka;
the cover was designed by Judy Allan;
the index was prepared by Elizabeth Babcock-Atkinson.
The printer and binder was R.R. Donnelley & Sons Company.

Library of Congress Cataloging-in-Publication Data

Ouslander, Joseph G.
    Medical care in the nursing home / Joseph G. Ouslander, Dan
Osterweil, John Morley ; foreword by Robert L. Kane.
        p.   cm.
    Includes bibliographical references.
    Includes index.
    ISBN 0-07-047949-6
    1. Nursing home care.   I. Osterweil, Dan.   II. Morley, John E.
III. Title.
    [DNLM: 1. Homes for the Aged.   2. Long Term Care—in old age.
3. Nursing Homes.   4. Physician's Role.   WT 30 094m]
RC954.3.O87 1991
362.1'6—dc20
DNLM/DLC
for Library of Congress   90-13692
                                                                     CIP

CONTENTS

FOREWORD

Doctors do not like nursing homes. Many physicians go to great lengths to avoid them. They feel uncomfortable there. The lack of staff support and the advanced stages of the patients create a sense that little can be done to make a difference. This perception is both an irony and a tragedy. The establishment of geriatrics as a specialty, or at least an area of special competence, has done a great deal to redress some of this error, but much remains to be done.

Ironically, nursing home residents are probably one of the groups who can profit most from careful attention to both their medical problems and the way their care is rendered. Nursing homes are not fixed institutions incapable of change. Quite the contrary, they are at least as responsive to leadership and innovation as were hospitals a few decades ago.

What is missing is that leadership. Only a handful of physicians have chosen to invest their energies in improving nursing home care. A larger group of physicians are reluctant participants in such care, viewing it as unrewarding both medically and fiscally.

Nursing home care stands at a crossroads. External pressures are continually demanding higher standards. History is gradually repeating itself as the nursing home comes more and more to look like the extended care facility envisioned in the original Medicare legislation of 1965, with a more debilitated case-mix than ever before. Physician leadership is needed, but if it is not forthcoming, other professions stand ready to take up that role.

This volume is a welcome and timely addition to the sparse collection of practical manuals on how physicians can effectively function to improve the nursing home environment. It is intended primarily for the generalist physician who follows his patients into the nursing home, but it has useful advice too for the physician who is prepared to devote the extra effort needed to serve as a medical director, although other books cover this subject in greater detail.

This book is important because it is practical. Much of the physicians' reluctance to work with nursing homes likely stems from their sense that there is nothing effective they can do. This volume helps to debunk that perception of impotence by providing specific lists of critical steps to be taken for the variety of problems faced in such care. It is written by physicians who have direct experience delivering this kind of care and practical knowledge about how to improve it.

We have reached the stage where we can no longer simply curse the darkness of nursing home care. This book helps to light some useful candles.

Robert L. Kane, M.D.
Minnesota Chair of Long-Term Care and Aging
University of Minnesota School of Public Health

PREFACE

Two basic concerns stimulated us to write *Medical Care in the Nursing Home*. First, no matter how successful the disciplines of Geriatric Medicine and Gerontology become at helping people to age successfully and to live in their own homes as long as possible, the need and demand for nursing home care will continue to increase over the next several decades. Second, we believe that improvements in the medical care provided in most of this country's nursing homes are both necessary and possible and that these improvements will have positive effects on the quality of life of nursing home residents, their loved ones, and the staff that cares for them.

Medical Care in the Nursing Home is directed toward primary physicians and medical directors who provide care to nursing home residents. It presumes a sound knowledge of general and geriatric medicine and is meant to complement textbooks that focus on these areas.

Recognizing that the state of the art in medical care in the nursing home is not as well developed as in other settings and populations, we have tried to synthesize both data and opinion in order to provide clear and specific recommendations for clinical practice. Some may disagree with our recommendations, and we encourage you to communicate your thoughts to us, so that we can improve the next edition of this text.

As with any book, we have a number of people to thank for their assistance. Drs. Tom Yoshikawa, Robert Kane, Dean Norman, Mark Beers, Darlene Fujimoto, and Barbara Bates-Jensen provided valuable input by reviewing several of the chapters. Laura Hodson provided invaluable assistance in preparing the text and tables. Science Graphics (Santa Clarita, California) is responsible for the illustrations, and Steve Nelson for the photographs. We would also like to thank the editorial staff at McGraw-Hill for their encouragement and support as we developed and worked on the book.

Last but not least, we thank the nursing home residents and numerous health professionals who have taught us so much about nursing home care, and our families, who have tolerated numerous days and nights without our presence so that we could complete this text.

ONE

GENERAL AND ADMINISTRATIVE ASPECTS OF MEDICAL CARE IN THE NURSING HOME

Is Anybody Listening?

I am an 84-year-old woman, and the only crime which I have committed is that I have an illness which is called chronic. I have severe arthritis and about five years ago I broke my hip. While I was recuperating in the hospital, I realized that I would need extra help at home. But there was no one. . . . So I wound up at a convalescent hospital in the middle of Los Angeles.

All kinds of people are thrown together here. I sit and watch, day after day. As I look around this room, I see the pathetic ones (maybe the lucky ones—who knows?) who have lost their minds, and the poor souls who should be out but nobody comes to get them, and the sick ones who are in pain. We are all locked up together. . . .

For the last few years I have been reading about the changes in Medicare regulations. All I can see from these improvements is that nurses spend more time writing. For, after all, how do you regulate caring? Most of the nurses' aides who work here are from other countries. Even those who can speak English don't have much in common with us. So they hurry to get their work done as quickly as possible. There are a few caring people who work here, but there are so many of us who are needy for that kind of honest attention.

A doctor comes to see me once a month. He spends approximately three to five seconds with me and then a few more minutes writing in the chart or joking with the nurses. (My own doctor doesn't come to convalescent hospitals, so I had to take this one.). . . .

I noticed that most of the physicians who come here don't even pay attention to things like whether their patients' fingernails are trimmed or whether their bodies are foul-smelling. Last week when the doctor came to see me, I hadn't had a bath in 10 days because the nurse's aide took too long on her coffee break. She wrote in the chart that she gave me a shower—anyway, who would check or care? I would be labeled as a complainer or losing my memory, and that would be worse. . . .

I remember how I used to bake pies and cakes and cookies for friends and neighbors and their children. In the five years I have been here, I have had no choice—no choice of when I want to eat or what I want to eat. . . .

As I write this, I keep wishing I were exaggerating. . . .

I am writing this because many of you may live to be old like me, and by then it will be too late. You, too, will be stuck here and wonder why nothing is being done, and you, too, will wonder if there is any justice in life. Right now, I pray every night that I may die in my sleep and get this nightmare of what someone has called life over with, if it means living in this prison day after day.

(Abstracted from an anonymous letter published in the Los Angeles Times, September 23, 1979.)

DEMOGRAPHICS AND ECONOMICS
OF NURSING HOME CARE

INTRODUCTION

Nursing home care is a growing industry. Currently there are close to 19,000 nursing homes (NHs) and between 1.5 million and 2 million NH beds. This is almost triple the number of acute care hospitals and double the number of acute care hospital beds. Expenditures for NH care now exceed $30 billion, of which close to half comprises public monies.

Several sociodemographic factors are going to dramatically increase the demand for and cost of NH care over the next several decades.

The purpose of this chapter is to review, briefly and graphically, demographic and economic factors that are relevant to current and future NH care. An awareness of these factors is important for all physicians and health professionals who care for NH residents.

DEMOGRAPHICS AND THE DEMAND
FOR NURSING HOME CARE

Three basic factors contribute to the need for NH care: (1) the number of frail people with such severe functional disabilities that they cannot live independently or with mental, behavioral, or physical conditions that make management by a community caregiver difficult; (2) the social support system available for individuals who cannot live independently; and (3) the availability, accessibility, and financing of community long-term-care resources. Table 1-1 summarizes these factors.

The frail geriatric population is the most rapidly growing segment of our society. Figure 1-1 depicts this growth over the next several decades. By the year 2030, the number of Americans older than 65 will double, to over 60 million. Average life expectancy at age 65 now approaches 10 years; even at age 85, it is still close to 5 years (Fig. 1-2). This will result in more than doubling the number of those age 85 and older by the year 2030—a group currently numbering close to 3 million. With the dramatic growth of the "old old" population will come an increased number of people with the conditions listed in Table 1-1, which contribute to NH admission.

Table 1-1 Factors affecting the need for nursing home admission

Characteristics of the individual
    Age, sex, race
    Marital status
    Living arrangements
    Degree of mobility
    Ability to perform basic and instrumental activities of daily living
    Urinary incontinence
    Behavior problems
    Mental status
    Memory impairment
    Mood disturbance
    Tendency for falls
    Clinical prognosis
    Income
    Payment eligibility
    Need for special services

Characteristics of the support system
    Family capability
        Age of spouse (if married)
        Presence of responsible relative (usually adult child)
        Family structure of responsible relative
        Employment status of responsible relative
    Physician availability
    Amount of care currently received from family and others

Community Resources
    Formal community resources (see Table 1-2)
    Informal support systems
    Presence of long-term-care institutions
    Characteristics of long-term-care institutions

Source: After Kane RL, Ouslander JG, and Abrass IB: Essentials of Clinical Geriatrics, 2d ed. New York, McGraw-Hill, 1989.

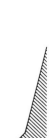

Figure 1-1 Actual and projected growth of the U.S. geriatric population. (After Kane RL, Ouslander JG, and Abrass IB: *Essentials of Clinical Geriatrics*, 2d ed. New York, McGraw-Hill, 1989.)

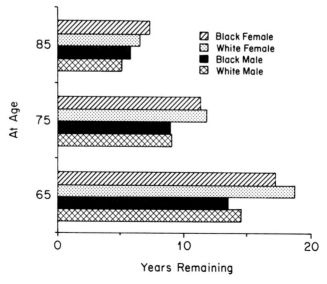

Figure 1-2 Life expectancy in the geriatric population. (After Kane RL, Ouslander JG, and Abrass IB: *Essentials of Clinical Geriatrics*, 2d ed. New York, McGraw-Hill, 1989.)

Recent data suggest that close to 40 percent of community-dwelling individuals aged 85 and older have some degree of dementia. Thus, as depicted in Fig. 1-3, the number of people with dementia and associated disorders will also rise dramatically.

At the same time, the social support system is unlikely to improve and may worsen. Among those of age 75 and above, about 20 percent of men and 50 percent of women live alone. Of the elderly who live alone, close to one-third have no children, and between 40 percent and 50 percent see their children once a week or more often (Fig. 1-4). Most formal and informal long-term-care services are currently arranged for or provided by daughters.

The cohort of people who are growing old at the present time have had fewer children and tend to be geographically separate from the children they do have. In addition, increasing numbers of women are working, which will make it more difficult and stressful for them to care for a frail parent or grandparent.

A growing number and variety of services are available for the frail elderly outside of NHs (Table 1-2). These services clearly delay or prevent NH admission in a subgroup of the frail geriatric population. On the other hand, these services are generally not well coordinated and are not reimbursed by most insurance and government programs (see below). Better coordination of these services is being fostered through case managers, hospital and community-based geriatric programs, and other strategies. The increasing number of such programs (e.g., home care) and the increasing number of elderly who, either themselves or through their children, can

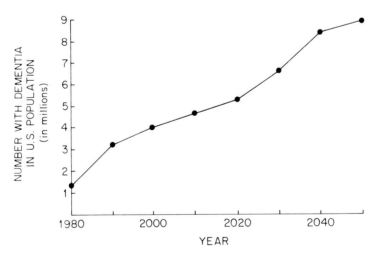

Figure 1-3 Projected number of persons with dementia in the U.S. population. *(Based on prevalence estimates and projections from the National Institute on Aging and U.S. Bureau of Census.)*

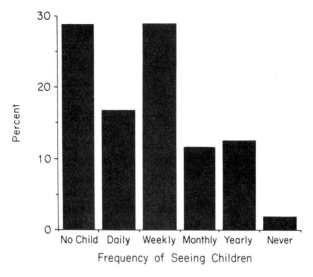

Figure 1-4 Frequency of seeing children among community-dwelling elderly who live alone. (After Kane RL, Ouslander JG, and Abrass IB: *Essentials of Clinical Geriatrics,* 2d ed. New York, McGraw-Hill, 1989.)

Table 1-2 Examples of formal community services available outside nursing homes

Housing	Outpatient clinics
Senior apartments	Geriatric
Assisted living	Psychosocial counseling
Foster care	Rehabilitation
Life care community	Adult day care
Health promotion activities	Day hospital
Wellness programs	Home health
Exercise classes	Home health agencies
Family and patient education	Medicare-certified
Nutrition consultation	Private
Meal programs	Visiting nurse association
Volunteer programs	Hospice
Outreach	Homemaker
Screening clinics	Part-time housekeeper
Mobile vans	Home infusion therapies
Discharge planning	Durable medical equipment
Case management	Acute inpatient units
Information and referral	Geriatric
Meals-on-Wheels	Rehabilitation
Transportation	Psychiatric
Emergency response system	Alcohol/substance abuse

afford these services will improve the accessibility of community-based long-term-care services for a subgroup of the growing frail geriatric population. But these factors will not be enough to dramatically reduce the growing need for NH care. Even among those who are able to live in the community despite severe functional impairments, many eventually come to a time when it is in their and their caregivers' best interests to consider entry into a NH.

Current rates of NH usage vary with age, sex, race, and NH bed availability. As can be seen in Fig. 1-5, the percentage of blacks in NHs is generally lower than that of whites; a greater proportion of white women than white men in each age group are in an NH; and the proportion in NHs increases dramatically with age to close to 25 percent among white women aged 85 and older. Table 1-3 lists NH beds and NH bed usage rates for those aged 85 and older; they vary substantially from state to state.

Even these statistics are, however, deceiving, because point prevalence rates underestimate the actual number of people who spend time in an NH. This number is much higher, because a subgroup of NH residents turns over rapidly. Data on length of NH stay are somewhat difficult to interpret because they will vary depending on whether they are calculated in a cohort of admissions, current NH residents, or discharges. Figure 1-6 depicts the median length of stay based on discharge status (alive versus dead). As can be seen, in either case median length of stay is less than 6 months. In fact, close to half of all NH admissions stay less than 6 months, although many are readmitted after a stay in an acute care hospital. Thus the prevalence of NH use depicted in Fig. 1-5 and Table 1-3 underestimates the lifetime risk of NH admission. Current estimates suggest that the risk of NH admission now approaches 25 percent to 40 percent.

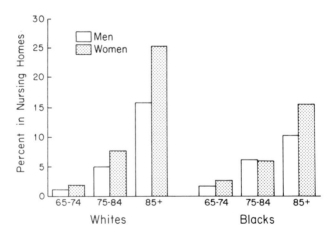

Figure 1-5 Percent of population age 65 and older in nursing homes by age, sex, and race. *(Based on 1985 data from the National Center for Health Statistics.)*

Table 1-3 State-specific data on nursing home beds

	NH beds	NH beds/1000 age 85+		NH beds	NH beds/1000 age 85+
Alabama	20,650	607	Montana	5,651	642
Alaska	1,028	1,715	Nebraska	18,989	801
Arizona	9,308	468	Nevada	2,021	562
Arkansas	19,237	731	New Hampshire	6,671	687
California	163,481	750	New Jersey	37,824	524
Colorado	17,309	712	New Mexico	3,074	349
Connecticut	21,243	595	New York	103,951	534
Delaware	2,529	477	North Carolina	32,172	713
District of Columbia	3,179	497	North Dakota	6,449	796
Florida	36,121	308	Ohio	76,279	703
Georgia	30,040	763	Oklahoma	27,100	797
Hawaii	2,804	501	Oregon	17,381	612
Idaho	4,354	512	Pennsylvania	75,906	584
Illinois	88,382	771	Rhode Island	8,652	721
Indiana	44,510	818	South Carolina	11,989	600
Iowa	34,640	772	South Dakota	8,646	824
Kansas	25,207	755	Tennessee	21,691	524
Kentucky	26,264	750	Texas	101,327	905
Louisiana	21,671	711	Utah	5,051	568
Maine	11,316	803	Vermont	4,705	784
Maryland	20,725	634	Virginia	27,376	666
Massachusetts	52,253	707	Washington	39,152	944
Michigan	80,081	981	West Virginia	6,422	331
Minnesota	41,930	794	Wisconsin	49,846	897
Mississippi	12,252	521	Wyoming	1,758	503
Missouri	46,690	764	U.S. total	1,537,288	684

Source: Based on usage rates in 1980 from the National Center on Health Statistics and population data from the U.S. Census Bureau.

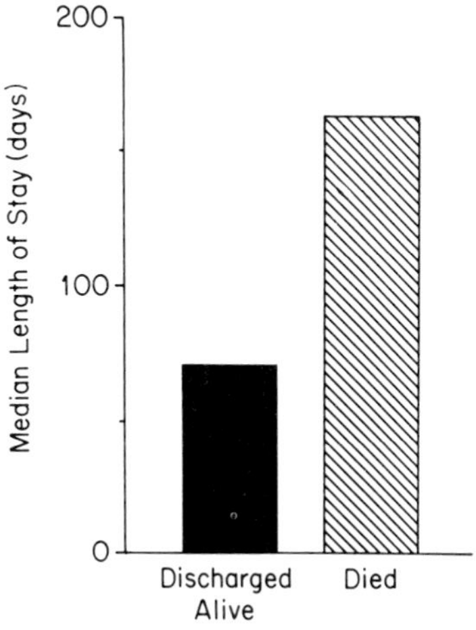

Figure 1-6 Median length of stay in nursing homes among residents who were discharged alive versus residents who died in the nursing home. (After Kane RL, Ouslander JG, and Abrass IB: *Essentials of Clinical Geriatrics,* 2d ed. New York, McGraw-Hill 1989.)

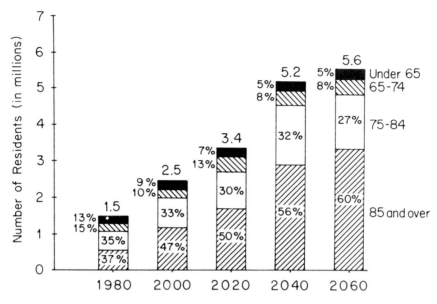

Figure 1-7 Projected growth in the nursing home population. *(Based on estimates from the National Center for Health Statistics, 1977.)*

All these factors will contribute to a growing demand for NH care over the next several decades. The number of NH residents is expected to more than double over the next 30 years and to exceed 5 million by the year 2040 (Fig. 1-7). This increased number of NH residents will be accompanied by dramatic—and, to many, frightening—increases in the cost of caring for this population.

ECONOMIC CONSIDERATIONS

NH care is expensive. In 1986, the United States spent $38 billion for NH care, and the expenditures are escalating rapidly. From the NH resident's perspective, care in a decent facility can cost anywhere from $20,000 to $45,000 per year.

Who pays for NH care? A recent survey of older people found that the majority thought the answer was Medicare. Table 1-4 summarizes major federal programs that support health and other types of care for the elderly. As shown, Medicare does provide for 150 days of skilled care in a nursing facility (after a 3-day acute care hospitalization) but through various mechanisms sharply restricts its expenditures on this type of care. Thus, while Medicare funds about half the per capita health expenditures of the elderly, it contributes very little to the cost of NH care (Fig. 1-8). Overall, Medicare

Table 1-4 Summary of major federal programs for the elderly

Program	Eligible population	Services covered	Deductibles and copayments
Medicare (Title XVII of the Social Security Act)			
Part A: Hospital insurance	All persons eligible for Social Security and others with chronic disabilities, such as end-stage renal disease, plus voluntary enrollees 65+	Per benefit period, "reasonable cost" for 90 days of hospital care plus 60 lifetime reservation days; 100 days of skilled nursing facility (SNF); home health visits including 80 h/year of respite care (if terminal)	Full coverage for hospital care after a deductible of about 1 day and for SNF days 21–29
Part B: Supplemental medical insurance	All those covered under Part A who elect coverage; participants pay a monthly premium	80% of "reasonable cost" for physicians' services; supplies and services related to physician services; outpatient, physical, and speech therapy; diagnostic tests and radiographs; mammogram; surgical dressings; prosthetics; ambulance	Deductible and 20% copayment (no copay after a limit reached)

11

Table 1-4 (*Continued*)   Summary of major federal programs for the elderly

Program	Eligible population	Services covered	Deductibles and copayments
Medicaid (Title XIX of the Social Security Act)	Eligibility criteria vary from state to state. Persons receiving Supplemental Security Income (SSI), such as welfare; receiving SSI and state supplement; meeting lower eligibility standards used for medical assistance criteria in 1972; eligible for SSI; or who were in institutions and eligible for Medicaid in 1973. Medically needy who do not qualify for SSI but have high medical expenses are eligible for Medicaid in some states	Mandatory services for categorically needy: inpatient hospital services, skilled nursing facility, limited home health care, laboratory tests and radiographs, family planning, early and periodic screening, diagnosis and treatment for children through age 20 Optional services vary from state to state: dental care, therapies, drugs, intermediate care facilities, extended home health care, private-duty nurse, eyeglasses, prostheses, personal care services, medical transportation, and home health care services (states can limit the amount and duration of services)	None, once patient spends down to eligibility level

Social Services Block Grant (Title XX of the Social Security Act)	All recipients of Aid to Families with Dependent Children (AFDC) and SSI; optionally, those earning up to 115% of state median income and residents of specific geographic areas	Day care; protective services; family counseling; home-based services; employment, education, and training; health-related services; information and referral; transportation; family planning; legal services; home-delivered and congregate meals	Fees are charged to those with incomes greater than 80% of state's median income
Title III of the Older Americans Act	All persons 60 years and older; low-income, minority, and isolated older persons are special targets	Homemaker; home-delivered meals; home health aides; transportation; legal services; counseling; information and referral plus 19 others (50% of funds must go to those listed)	Some payment may be required

Source: After Kane RL, Ouslander JG, and Abrass IB: *Essentials of Clinical Geriatrics*, 2d ed. New York, McGraw-Hill, 1989.

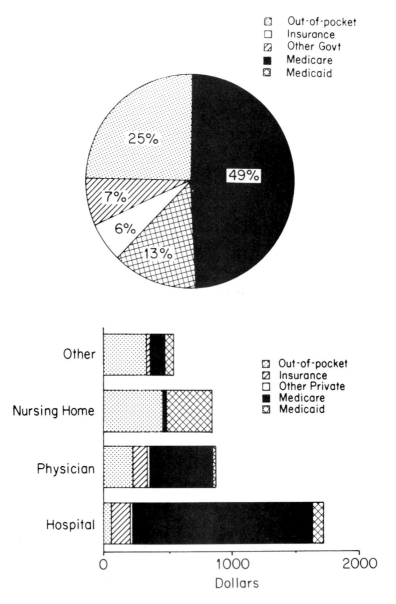

Figure 1-8 *Top:* Sources of overall health care expenditures for the geriatric population. *Bottom:* Per capita health care expenditures by type of care and source for the geriatric population. Based on 1984 data. (After Kane RL, Ouslander JG, and Abrass IB: *Essentials of Clinical Geriatrics,* 2d ed. New York, McGraw-Hill, 1989.)

supports less than 3 percent of this cost. As shown in Fig. 1-9, only 1 percent of Medicare dollars went to NH care in 1984, in contrast to 68 percent of Medicaid expenditures and 42 percent of out-of-pocket expenditures for health care by the elderly.

Medicare limits its expenditures for NH care by narrowly defining *skilled* (as opposed to *custodial*) care and by limiting the duration of the "skilled" benefit. The Health Care Financing Administration has made some recent attempts to standardize and modestly expand the definitions of skilled care (see Chap. 22). Still, decisions are made by local intermediaries, who too frequently do not precisely define their guidelines. As a result, deci-

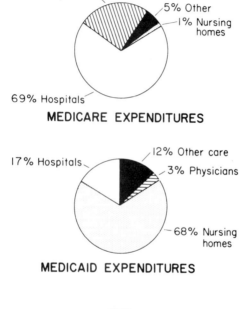

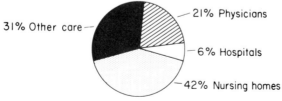

Figure 1-9 Proportions of Medicare, Medicaid, and out-of-pocket expenditures used for different types of care by the geriatric population. Based on data from the United States Special Committee on Aging, 1986. (After Kane RA and Kane RL: *Long Term Care: Principles, Programs, and Policies.* New York, Springer, 1987.)

sions about what constitutes skilled care vary considerably across the country. As a result, NHs and contracted providers (such as rehabilitation therapists) often become frustrated and develop adversarial relationships with their intermediaries. Medicare also limits its reimbursement for physician services in NHs. This creates several potentially negative incentives, which are discussed further in Chap. 5.

Limited Medicare reimbursement for NH care has important implications for the NH as well as the NH residents and their families. For the NH, Medicare guidelines result in time-consuming utilization review activities that attempt to maximize Medicare reimbursement. Medicare reimbursement is critical to fiscal viability in the predominantly proprietary NH industry because it is generally significantly higher than other types of reimbursement. In California, for example, the per diem Medicare rate is approximately double the per diem Medi Cal (Medicaid) rate; it is even higher for NHs that have "distinct part" Medicare units or that are hospital-based. For NH residents and their families, limited Medicare coverage can result in limited access to a NH or to certain services in the NH (such as physical therapy). It can also lead to financial ruin.

The fact that over 90 percent of NH care is paid for by either out-of-pocket expenditures or by Medicaid (Figs. 1-8 and 1-9) has led to a phenomenon known as "spend down." Individuals who need NH care and do not qualify for the Medicare skilled benefit, or whose Medicare coverage has been terminated through the facility-based utilization review process, must spend down their assets until they are impoverished and can pass the means test for Medicaid. Because of the high cost of NH care, the virtual lack of private insurance coverage for it and the prevalence of near poverty among the elderly (about 12 percent are below the poverty line and close to one-third are between the poverty line and double it), most elderly who require NH care for longer than a few weeks end up spending down to qualify for Medicaid. Medicaid reimbursement for NH care varies considerably; the per diem rate in some states is under $40, and in others it exceeds $80. In addition, not all services are covered by Medicaid. For example, in California, Medi Cal has a relatively restrictive formulary of drugs it will pay for in NHs. Although most classes of drugs are available, many recently released drugs and over-the-counter medications are not. Thus, the resident either has to use limited funds, has to have family who are willing to pay for these drugs, or does not get them.

Many government officials, providers, and consumers recognize the need to change the system of reimbursement for NH care. But change will not occur rapidly. In the meantime, physicians and other health professionals who provide care to NH residents should familiarize themselves with the reimbursement system and make a concerted effort to provide appropriate care in the most cost-effective manner possible. Whenever feasible, Medicare coverage of skilled nursing should be considered, even if for only brief periods of time. Strategies to provide desirable uncovered services should be explored with NH administrators, residents, and residents' families—recognizing that there will always be limitations.

THE FUTURE

Given the growing demand for NH care, the present reimbursement system, and the staggering federal deficit, what does the future hold? It is beyond the scope of this book to discuss health policy in any detail. Just a few issues relevant to the future of NH care will be covered briefly. First, it is clear that more reimbursement for long-term care, whether it be community-based or in an NH, will be necessary. This will require public and private input. From the government standpoint, some shifting of the focus from acute, expensive, high-technology care toward the care of frail functionally impaired elderly will be necessary. Current demonstration programs involving case management and social health maintenance organizations are efforts in this direction. The fostering of tax incentives for families caring for this population, for tax-deferred savings for long-term-care needs, and the use of reverse mortgages for paying for NH care are being considered. From the private perspective, the development of continuing care *(life care)* retirement communities that include NHs and the development of long-term-care insurance policies are examples of evolving strategies to deal with the costs of long-term care.

Whatever changes in the reimbursement system do occur over the next several years, one thing seems certain: some type of case-mix reimbursement will become national. Several states already do reimburse on the basis of their own measures of case mix. The Health Care Financing Administration is in the process of creating a "minimum data set" that will have become a mandatory component of the assessment process in all federally supported NHs by the time this book is in press and that will eventually be used in the case-mix reimbursement system. The minimum data set is discussed further in Chap. 22.

The most likely candidate for case-mix reimbursement is Resource Utilization Groups (RUGs). This system has been developed in New York and is in use in the Veterans Administration NHs. Figure 1-10 illustrates an example of a RUGs classification system. Each RUG category is reimbursed at a different level. The potential problem with the RUG system is the incentive it provides to keep NH residents sicker and more dependent so as to achieve higher reimbursement. Appropriate incentives for rehabilitation approaches must therefore be built in.

One appealing alternative to a case-mix reimbursement system has been developed by Dr. Robert Kane over the last several years: reimbursement based on NH performance in relation to projected outcomes for dif-

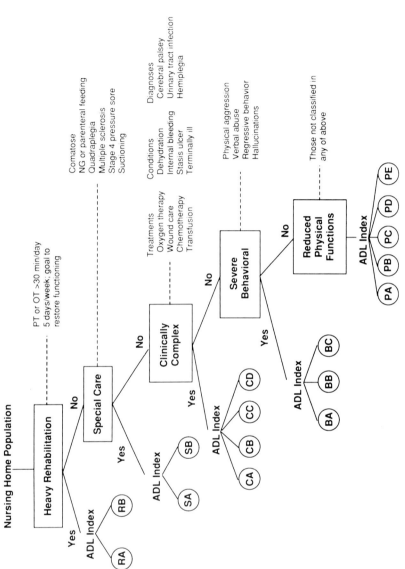

Figure 1-10 Example of case-mix Resource Utilization Group (RUG) categorization. Within each of the five major categories, further subgrouping is done based on an activities of daily living (ADL) index. The ADL index ranges from 3 to 10 based on ability to perform toileting, eating, and transferring. This figure depicts the RUG-11 system, but not all details are shown. RUG-11 is currently undergoing further testing and modification. (After Schneider DP, Fries BE, Foley WJ, Desmond M, and Gormley WJ: "Case mix for nursing home payment: Resource utilization groups, version II. *Health Care Financing Review* 1988, annual supplement, pp 39–51.)

ferent types of residents. This system requires a sophisticated ability to accurately predict the clinical course of NH residents (which has been done in a relatively large sample) but offers the advantage of providing an incentive to maintain or improve the resident's status—in contrast to the potentially negative incentive in the RUG system.

We would be remiss if we did not mention one other strategy to deal with the frightening projected growth in the costs of NH care: support for biomedical and health services research. This type of research would require only a minuscule fraction of the cost of NH care. Only through research will disorders such as Alzheimer's disease and osteoporosis—which account for so much morbidity and expenditure at the end of life—be prevented or cured and cost-effective methods of managing conditions affecting NH residents be developed.

SUGGESTED READINGS

American Health Care Administration: *Long Term Care Data Book.* Washington, DC, American Health Care Associates, 1988.

Kane RA and Kane RL: *Long Term Care: Principles, Programs, and Policies.* New York, Springer, 1987.

Schneider EL and Guralnik JM: The aging of America: Impact on health care costs. *JAMA* 263:2335–2340, 1990.

Vladeck BC: Long term care for the elderly: The future of nursing homes. *West J Med* 150:215–220, 1989.

THE NURSING HOME ENVIRONMENT AND THE GOALS OF NURSING HOME CARE

The nursing home (NH) is often pictured as a sterile one- or two-story building with a small reception area and business office near the entrance, long corridors with shiny waxed floors, 25 to 50 residents' rooms, each with two or three hospital-type beds crowded in it, and a few scattered, cramped nursing stations. Nursing home residents are generally thought of as old, female, wheelchair-bound, and demented.

Although these stereotypical images are common, NHs and their residents are much more heterogeneous than is often believed by physicians whose contact with them is limited. The purpose of this chapter is to provide a brief overview of NHs and NH residents nationwide and to outline the basic goals of NH care, so that physicians will have a broader context within which to view their own NH practice.

NURSING HOMES

Nursing homes in this country have evolved over the last century from publicly run facilities housing the indigent and chronically ill. Three major factors have lead to the development of today's NH: (1) legislation in the 1950s (Hill-Burton) that provided public funding for the construction of NHs, (2) the institution of Medicare and Medicaid in the 1960s, and (3) the strict federal and state regulations that currently control NH care.

Unfortunately for the physical environment of today's NH, all three of these factors have led to an emphasis on "nursing" rather than "home." As a result, relatively few facilities offer a homelike atmosphere for those chronically ill residents who may live several of the last years of their lives in an NH. Nursing homes are too commonly structured like small hospitals. Long corridors restrict many residents' access to social life. Rooms tend to be cramped, offering little privacy and little if any space for personal effects.

A growing number of architects have developed considerable interest and expertise in the design of NHs that combine homelike environments, creative space management, safety, accessibility, and color designs for physically and cognitively impaired residents while also meeting federal, state, and local requirements. Consultation from this type of expert should be sought whenever a NH is going to be renovated or rebuilt or when a new facility is in its initial planning phases.

At present there are close to 19,000 NHs in the United States, of which approximately three-quarters are certified as either skilled, intermediate, or both. Table 2-1 illustrates the distribution of NHs and NH beds by ownership, certification, and bed size. In the near future, new legislation will basically abolish the distinction between skilled and intermediate levels of care. Note that most facilities are small (over one-third have fewer than 100 beds, 80 percent fewer than 200 beds) and that a vast majority of NHs are run for profit.

Figure 2-1 illustrates the general organizational structure of a typical community-based NH, though there is considerable variability in this structure depending on ownership, facility size, and other factors. At the facility level, the two key individuals are the administrator and the director of nursing. As discussed in Chap. 6, the typical medical director is usually not based in the facility and has little influence on the process of care. Many NHs have full-time social workers and activities therapists, while others obtain these services by contractual, part-time arrangements. Rehabilitation therapists (physical, occupational, speech) and respiratory therapy as well as pharmacy, clinical laboratory, and radiology services are generally provided by contract with professionals, who often provide services to many NHs simultaneously. In hospital-based NHs, administrative oversight and health care services are generally provided by staff who are hired by and report to the acute hospital.

Several emerging trends are worthy of brief mention. First, many large, privately owned, for-profit chains of multiple NHs are developing. While there are potential disadvantages to this trend, it may offer a unique opportunity to implement many standardized medical care and quality assurance protocols. Second, the number of continuing-care retirement or life care communities, both private and nonprofit, is growing rapidly. Each of these communities has a NH. This structure affords the opportunity to develop an

Table 2-1 **Characteristics of nursing homes**

	Nursing homes		Nursing home beds
	Number	%	%
Total	19,100	100	100
Ownership			
Proprietary	14,300	75	69
Nonprofit	3,800	20	23
Government	1,000	5	8
Affiliation			
Chain	7,900	41	49
Independent	10,000	52	42
Government	1,000	5	8
Unknown	100	1	1
Certification			
Not certified	4,700	24	11
SNF Only	3,500	18	19
SNF/ICF	5,700	30	45
ICF Only	5,300	28	25
Bed Size			
<50	6,300	33	9
50–99	6,200	33	27
100–199	5,400	28	43
200+	1,200	6	20

Source: After Kane RA and Kane RL: *Long Term Care: Principles, Programs, and Policies.* New York, Springer, 1987.

efficient continuum of long-term-care services for a defined population and to maximize the quality of the NH because of the vested community oversight. Third, many hospitals are using unfilled beds to create hospital-based NHs. Although structurally even farther away from a "home" than the typical NH, these facilities can play an important role in providing optimal and efficient care to NH residents who are subacutely ill. Ready access to many of the ancillary services that are difficult to obtain in community NHs may be critical in these residents. (These issues are discussed further in Chap. 5.) Finally, some NHs are becoming affiliated with academic institutions. Multidisciplinary educational and research programs can provide a wealth of opportunity to modify the process and even the structure of NH care and can certainly contribute to improving and enlivening the NH environment. Education and research programs are discussed in Chap. 26.

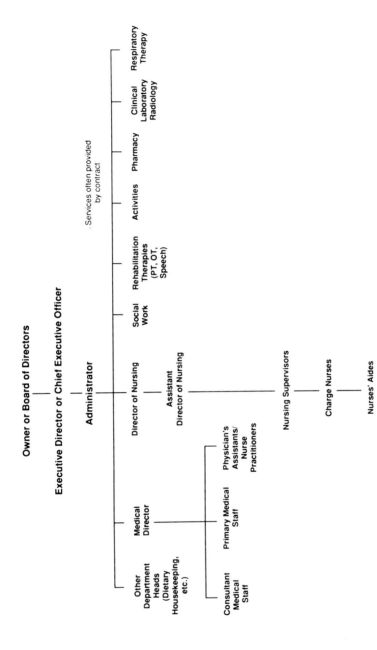

Figure 2-1 Organizational structure of a typical community-based nursing home.

NURSING HOME RESIDENTS

Table 2-2 shows some basic demographic characteristics of NH residents compared to the community-dwelling geriatric population. Figure 2-2 rather dramatically illustrates the degree of functional impairment of the NH population as opposed to elderly people in the community. In addition to these impairments in basic activities of daily living, the prevalence of dementia exceeds 50 percent in most NHs.

Despite the extremely high prevalence of functional disability and dementia, NH residents are actually quite a heterogeneous population. It is critical to recognize this heterogeneity if we are to develop appropriate goals and approaches to the care of individual residents. Nursing home residents can be broadly characterized on the basis of their length of stay: "short" (i.e., 1 to 6 months) versus "long." Short stayers can be subdivided into two groups: residents who enter the NH for short-term rehabilitation after an acute illness (e.g., hip fracture, stroke) and those who are medically unstable or terminally ill, who are either quickly discharged to an acute care hospital or die in the NH. Long stayers can be subdivided into three groups: those with primarily cognitive impairment (e.g., the ambulatory, wandering resident with Alzheimer's disease), residents with primarily physical impair-

Table 2-2   Demographic characteristics of nursing home residents versus community-dwelling residents, age 65 and older

	Nursing home residents	Community-dwelling residents
Age, years		
65–74	16	62
75–84	39	31
85+	45	8
Sex		
Male	25	41
Female	75	59
Race		
White (including Hispanic)	93	91
Black and other	7	9
Marital status		
Married	12	55
Widowed	69	34
Divorced or separated	5	6
Never married	14	4

Source: After Kane RL, Ouslander JG and Abrass IB: *Essentials of Clinical Geriatrics,* 2d ed. New York, McGraw-Hill, 1989.

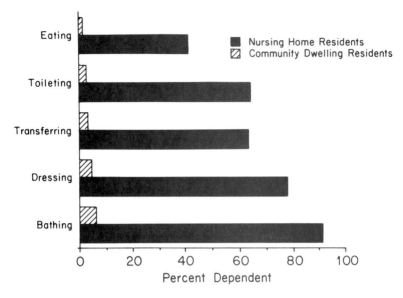

Figure 2-2 Ability to perform basic activities of daily living among nursing home residents versus community-dwelling elderly. (After Kane RL, Ouslander JG, and Abrass IB: *Essentials of Clinical Geriatrics,* 2d ed. New York, McGraw-Hill, 1989.)

ments (e.g., severe arthritis or end-stage heart or lung disease), and those with both cognitive and physical impairments.

Figure 2-3 illustrates this subgrouping of the NH population. Obviously residents may move from one subgroup to another when acute illnesses intervene, chronic illness develops or progresses, or cognitive function declines. Figures 2-4 to 2-8 illustrate case examples of each subgroup of residents.

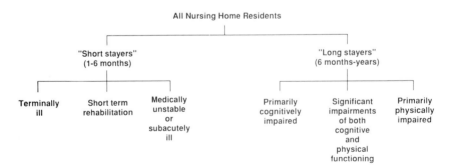

Figure 2-3 Basic types of nursing home residents. Residents frequently go from one subgroup to another. See text and Figs. 2-4 to 2-9 for examples. (After Kane RL, Ouslander JG, and Abrass IB: *Essentials of Clinical Geriatrics,* 2d ed. New York, McGraw-Hill, 1989.)

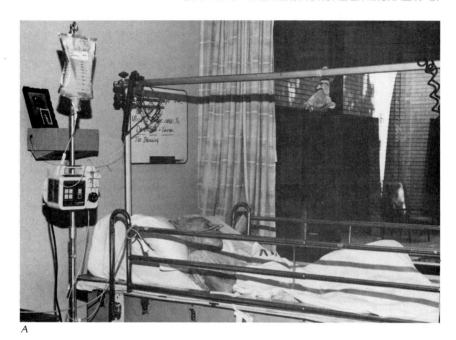

A

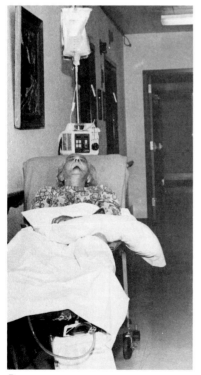

B

Figure 2-4 Examples of short-staying nursing home residents—terminally ill. *A.* A 93-year-old woman who suffered a massive stroke; she requires enteral feeding, oxygen, suctioning, and an air-fluidized mattress for the management of a deep pressure sore. *B.* An 88-year-old woman with end-stage renal failure (not on dialysis), severe multi-infarct dementia, and heart failure requiring enteral feeding, an indwelling catheter to monitor urinary output, and frequent doses of diuretics to manage respiratory distress.

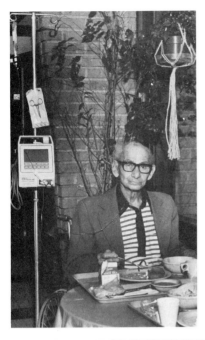

Figure 2-5 Example of a short-staying nursing home resident—subacutely ill. An 86-year-old man who developed subacute bacterial endocarditis and required 6 weeks of parenteral antibiotic therapy via a subclavian catheter.

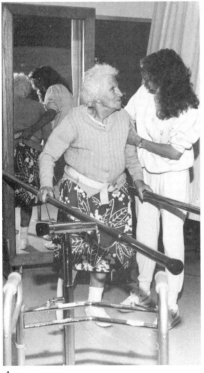

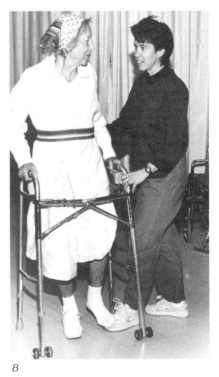

A

B

Figure 2-6 Examples of short-staying nursing home residents—short term rehabilitation. A. A 92-year-old woman undergoing gait retraining after a subcapital hip fracture and hemiarthroplasty. B. An 84-year-old woman getting physical therapy with partial weight bearing after an intertrochanteric hip fracture and surgical pinning of the fracture.

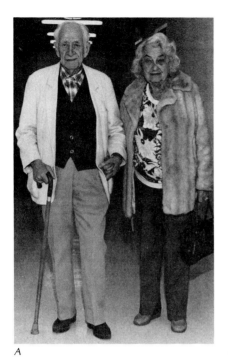

A

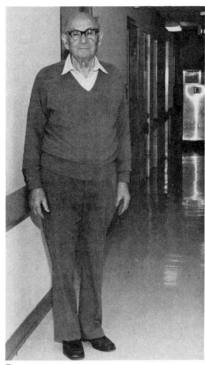

B

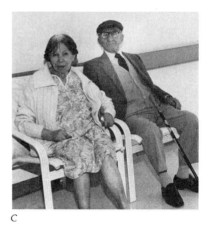

Figure 2-7 Examples of long-staying nursing home residents—primarily cognitively impaired. Five residents (A–C) in their mid- to upper eighties with moderate to severe primary dementia. They are ambulatory and generally healthy but require constant supervision in a special dementia unit.

C

The conceptualization of NH residents in this manner has important implications for the goals of NH care, quality assurance, and even the structure of the NH environment. The goals of caring for a previously healthy resident who is undergoing rehabilitation after a hip fracture are obviously very different from those of caring for one with advanced dementia and related behavioral disorders or another with a terminal malignancy. Simi-

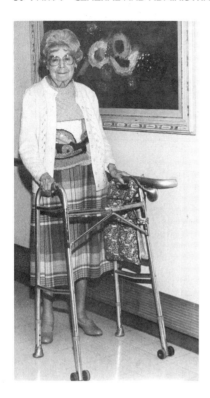

Figure 2-8 Example of a long-staying nursing home resident—primarily physically impaired. An 89-year-old woman with degenerative joint disease, osteoporosis, atherosclerotic cardiovascular disease, and recurrent syncope who requires periodic nursing observation and assistance with dressing and bathing.

larly, from the perspective of quality assurance, processes and outcomes of care that are relevant for one subgroup of residents may be inappropriate or irrelevant to another subgroup. From a structural standpoint, many NHs attempt to separate different subgroups of residents geographically. This approach, when it is feasible, offers many potential advantages: the physical environment can be modified for certain types of residents (e.g., wanderers), the staff can be trained and develop expertise in managing specific types of care (e.g., terminal or hospice-type care or rehabilitative care), and residents may be more comfortable when they are around others like themselves. This is especially true for cognitively intact residents who are often distressed by constant interaction, especially at mealtimes, with residents who have dementia and associated behavioral disorders.

GOALS OF NURSING HOME CARE

Table 2-3 outlines broad goals for the care of NH residents. Physicians who care for NH residents must recognize the importance of focusing on functional abilities, autonomy, quality of life, comfort, and safety as goals of

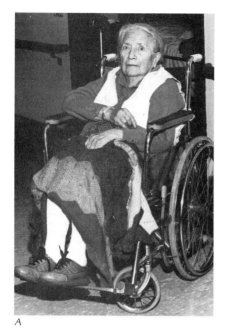
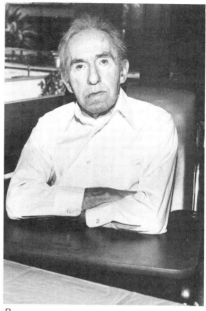

A   B

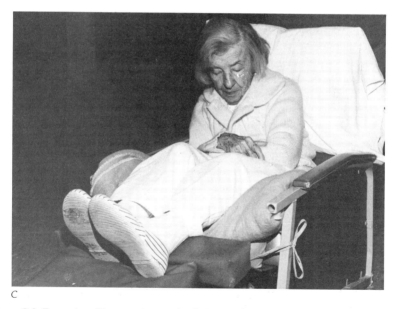

C

Figure 2-9 Examples of long-staying nursing home residents with impairments of both physical and cognitive functioning. *A.* A 92-year-old woman with severe congestive heart failure, degenerative joint disease of the lumbosacral spine, and moderately advanced Alzheimer's disease. *B.* An 87-year-old man with severe Parkinson's disease and dementia. *C.* A 79-year-old woman with a rapidly progressive dementia, depression, and frequent agitated and disruptive behaviors who is nonambulatory due to gait apraxia.

Table 2-3 Goals of nursing home care

Provide a safe and supportive environment for chronically ill and dependent people

Restore and maintain the highest possible level of functional independence

Preserve individual autonomy

Maximize quality of life, perceived well-being, and life satisfaction

Provide comfort and dignity for terminally ill residents and their loved ones

Stabilize and delay progression, whenever possible, of chronic medical conditions

Prevent acute medical and iatrogenic illnesses and identify and treat them rapidly when they do occur

---

Source: After Kane RL, Ouslander JG, and Abrass IB: *Essentials of Clinical Geriatrics,* 2d ed. New York, McGraw-Hill, 1989.

medical care. While optimal medical care is clearly essential to these types of outcomes, the vast majority of NH residents would rather be safe, comfortable, maximally independent, and able to participate in decisions about their lives and their health care than have the most advanced high-tech medical care available. This implies that primary care physicians must be sensitive to the nonmedical complaints of their residents (e.g., as to difficulties with roommates or other residents, the quality of their food, inability to leave the facility or to obtain clothing or other personal items). Although it may not be the primary physician's responsibility to deal in detail with these complaints, he/she should listen to them and try to communicate the expressed concerns to appropriate members of the interdisciplinary team as well as to help the medical director to change or create policies and procedures fostering an improved quality of life for the residents.

The goals of medical care per se are, insofar as is possible, to identify, stabilize, and delay progression of chronic medical conditions and to prevent acute medical and iatrogenic conditions—identifying and treating them rapidly when they do occur. The primary focus of most of this text is to provide physicians and health professionals with specific, practical, and—whenever possible—scientifically based strategies for managing these medical aspects of care among NH residents.

SUGGESTED READINGS

Kane RA and Kane RL. *Long Term Care: Principles, Programs, and Policies.* New York, Springer, 1987.

Ouslander JG: Medical care in the nursing home. *JAMA* 262:2582–2590, 1989.

PREADMISSION ASSESSMENT

The decisions involved in placing an individual in a long-term-care institution are complex and frequently associated with significant emotional distress. In this chapter, residential care (e.g., board and care, assisted living) and nursing homes (NHs) will be discussed as one continuum of long-term care. The purpose of this chapter is to review briefly the main reasons for institutionalization and the goals and objectives of preadmission assessment.

THE NEED FOR NURSING HOME CARE

A vast body of literature exists on the physical, psychological, social, and economic factors associated with the need for institutional care of the elderly and the disabled. It is commonly believed that disability and diminished social support are the predominant factors leading to institutionalization of the frail elderly. It is also recognized that relocation to a different environment, especially a NH, is associated with some adverse effects commonly referred to as relocation trauma.

Candidates for long-term care are generally dependent on the assistance of others for substantial periods of time. This assistance addresses the health, personal care, and social needs of individuals who lack some capacity for self-care (in Chap. 1, Table 1-1 describes in more detail characteristics of individuals who are in need of NH admission). Most long-term care in the United States is provided by a host of individuals referred to as "informal support." These persons may be family, friends, or neighbors. When this system fails to provide for the needs of persons with disability, a formal long-term-care system is needed. It is estimated that about 15 percent of the elderly have significant disability. For each person in a NH today, there are between one and three equally disabled persons living in the community. A variety of community-based long-term-care services are available, although they are generally not reimbursed by third-party payers and in many areas are fragmented and difficult to coordinate (in Chap. 1, Table 1-2 lists examples of community resources for long-term care). Nursing home placement becomes inevitable when community-based long-term-care alternatives fail, are inappropriate, not feasible, or not desired by the individual or the caregivers. Public demand for more NH beds is growing due to demographic and economic factors (see Chap. 1). The Prospective Payment System, implemented in 1983, has also placed pressure on acute care hospitals to shorten the average length of stay, resulting in a shift toward more skilled nursing placements.

Candidates for NH care need to be carefully assessed prior to admission in order to determine their needs and to advise them and their families on the most appropriate level of care. Studies in the United States and elsewhere have shown that careful assessment in community-based geriatric assessment clinics prevents inappropriate NH placement. In addition to determining care needs, a comprehensive geriatric assessment before NH admission can help prevent the underdiagnosis and underreporting of treatable illness and functional disabilities in elderly people. There is also a lack of emphasis on geriatric preventive measures such as vaccination against influenza and pneumococcal infection, screening for impaired vision and hearing, dental care, and assessment of ambulation. These, as well as more traditional preventive measures such as periodic screening for cancer, thyroid disease, and cognitive and affective disorders, can be accomplished when a preadmission assessment is being performed. New regulations [resulting from the Omnibus Budget Reconciliation Act (OBRA), 1987] also require screening for mental illness and/or mental retardation within 72 h of NH admission.

From the societal perspective, the preadmission assessment provides a gatekeeping function. In life care communities, the assessment is critical to ensure proper utilization of resources and cost-effectiveness of services, which, in turn, guarantee the financial viability of the institution. Table 3-1 summarizes the objectives of the preadmission assessment. The product of this assessment should be a multidisciplinary plan of care.

TIMING AND SITE OF ASSESSMENT

The timing of preadmission assessment is dictated by events that lead to increased dependence on services. This often occurs following a major illness that requires acute hospitalization. The site of the evaluation may vary.

Table 3-1   Objectives of preadmission geriatric assessment

Determine psychosocial and functional status
Identify active medical problems
Screen for cognitive impairment and mental health problems
Determine the appropriate level of care
Determine capacity to make decisions for health care
Determine program eligibility for third-party reimbursement
Act as a gatekeeper for appropriate use of long-term-care services
Develop a multidisciplinary approach to the individual's care needs

Patients awaiting discharge from the acute care hospital might be screened during their hospital stay by a registered nurse or geriatric nurse practitioner. In hospitals where a geriatrician is available, a gerontological consultation may be very helpful in the discharge planning.

Several states have developed specific preadmission assessment procedures, which are conducted by a registered nurse or a case manager and focus on the patient's functional and psychosocial needs. Such assessments are carried out in hospitals, rehabilitation units, clinics, and in the home setting.

THE PROCESS OF PREADMISSION ASSESSMENT

Depending on the setting, the assessment team may include only one person (a case manager, with social work or nursing background, for example) or as many as described in Table 3-2. It is our belief that an appropriate preadmission assessment can be performed only under the supervision of a physician interested and trained in geriatric medicine. For NHs or long-term-care programs that do not have geriatricians available, interested internists or family physicians may acquire the skills required for this kind of assessment through programs sponsored by universities or other geriatric educational centers.

It is important to assign specific tasks to each team member, to conduct the assessment efficiently, and to be sensitive to the patient's anxieties and potential to fatigue easily. Table 3-3 describes the team members and the

Table 3-2   Individuals involved with preadmission assessment

Clerical personnel
Social worker/case manager
Rehabilitation therapists (physical therapist, occupational therapist)
Geriatric nurse practitioner or registered nurse with geriatric assessment skills
Physician/geriatrician

Table 3-3   Examples of team assignments and instruments for preadmission assessment

Discipline	Tasks	Instrument/approach
Clerical worker	Determining financial eligibility for state or federal programs, information on methods of payment programs, identify responsible party and primary physician	Nonstructured or structured interview
Social worker	Interview for background, roommate compatibility, personal preferences Assess instrumental activities of daily living (IADL) Screen for affective disorders	Interview, Lawton IADL Scale Geriatric Depression Scale
Occupational therapist[a]	Assess basic activities of daily living	Katz ADL or direct observation (when applicable)
Physical therapist[a]	Gait and balance assessment	Tinetti Gait and Balance Scale or "Get up and walk and sit down" test
Nurse practitioner	Mental status exam Vision and hearing screen Review medical records	Folstein MMSE, Jaeger card, Welch Allyn Audioscope, or clinical method
Physician	History and physical exam	Systematic, focus on function Utilize structured forms

[a] If rehabilitation therapists are not available, these tasks may be performed by a trained nurse practitioner or registered nurse.

tasks they are responsible for. The sequence of the various assessments may vary, but geriatric medicine evaluation should be the last appointment, when information gathered by other team members is available. The administrative interview is critical for establishing eligibility for federal or state programs, determining availability of funds, and identifying the responsible party. The social worker may play a dual role in certain situations. Usually the social worker will gear the interview to leisure activities and social preferences. Social workers can also screen for cognitive and affective disorder by administering a depression scale and standardized mental status exam (examples are included in Chaps. 9 and 10).

Table 3-4 lists commonly used instruments and their characteristics. The choice of specific assessment tools is based on their validity, reliability, and the time it takes to administer them. Sometimes the choice is a compromise between the three characteristics. All assessment tools should be relevant to the patient and the environment he or she is going to live in.

Table 3-4 Instruments and procedures applicable to the preadmission assessment

	Function assessed	Administration	Strengths	Weaknesses	Comments
Katz ADL Scale	Basic self-care abilities	By patient or interviewer, based on judgment and report	Simple assessment of basic skills, useful in rehabilitation setting	Limited range of activities assessed, rating subjective	Not sensitive to small changes (see Chap. 22)
Instrumental ADL	More complex activities, food preparation, shopping, housekeeping, handling the phone, medications	By patient or interviewer, based on judgment and report	Assesses functions important for independent living	Rating subjective	Higher functions, not sensitive to small changes (see Table 3-5)
Tinetti Gait and Balance Scale	Performance-based testing of mobility	By observation of performance	Provides information about risk of falls; can identify specific abnormalities	No standard cutoff score	Sensitivity not determined (see Chap. 14)
Folstein Mini Mental State Examination (MMSE)	Memory, orientation, attention, constructional ability	By interviewer	Fairly quick and sensitive	Will not detect mild disability	Test score <24 considered abnormal but not necessarily indicative of dementia (see Chap. 9)
Geriatric Depression Scale (GDS)	Symptoms of depression	By patient	Quick, reliable, avoids an excess of somatic questions	Not evaluated for specificity among medically ill; use limited in presence of severe dementia	Score >14 on the long form or >5 on the short form indicates depression (see Chap. 10)
Cornell Scale	Symptoms of depression	By interviewer to patient and caregiver	Useful in patients with or without dementia; range of questions suited for elderly patients	Not widely tested, requires two interviewers	See Suggested Readings

The assessment instruments listed in Table 3-4 include both self-report and performance-based assessments. The time and economic advantage of using self-administered scales is counterbalanced by the fact that patients tend to rate their abilities higher than trained observers would. Family members tend to rate a patient's function lower. The cognitively intact elderly are, however, more accurate than family members and physicians. The rationale for administering an instrumental activities of daily living (IADL) scale is that some patients may be capable of living at home if most of these functions are preserved. Table 3-5 illustrates the Lawton IADL scale, which can be used for this purpose. Where it is clear from the beginning that a patient's NH placement is inevitable, a basic ADL assessment, such as the Katz ADL scale, is more relevant for determining the areas in which assistance is needed (see Chap. 22). The use of a performance-based gait and balance scale provides a description of function related to ambulation. It is useful in the sense that it helps describe any specific abnormalities and also yields a score that can be followed over time (see Chap. 14). The Folstein Mini Mental State Exam (MMSE) is useful because of its brevity, its relatively good sensitivity for significant abnormalities, and its excellent test-retest reliability (see Chap. 9). All depression scales have limitations. The Geriatric Depression Scale (GDS) was originally designed for self-administration; the validity of an interviewer-administered GDS has not yet been examined. In addition, the usefulness of the GDS in patients with moderate to severe dementia may be limited (see Chap. 10). The Cornell Scale has some promise, since it can be administered relatively easily and is suitable for the cognitively impaired as well. Other functional tests have been described—such as the timed hand-function test developed by Mark Williams—that correlate highly with the need for long-term-care services and institutionalization in particular.

These assessment tools are useful for establishing baseline characteristics, screening for undetected problems, and helping to set rehabilitational goals. In certain situations, such as life care communities, identifying persons at risk for needing more long-term-care services may be another goal of these assessments. Following administration of these assessments, a detailed history, review of any pertinent records, and a physical examination are necessary. Table 3-6 describes the focal points of the history and physical examination. Upper- and lower-extremity strength and performance, hand-grip strength, and mental status have been found to predict stability versus chronic deterioration in a cohort of frail older persons. The physical exam should particularly focus on factors that might impair functioning. Certain arm functions are important in performing activities; distal functions such as manual dexterity affect writing or using eating utensils. Proximal functions are involved in transfers from sitting to standing or lying to sitting, raising the arm to comb hair or brush teeth, and putting on a shirt. Falls and immobility often arise from the accumulated effects of multiple disabilities, which may include sensory and cognitive impairments as well as dysfunc-

Table 3-5 Instrumental activities of daily living (IADL) scale (self-rated version)[a]

Ability to use telephone		Laundry	
Operates telephone on own initiative, looks up and dials numbers, etc.	1	Does personal laundry completely	1
		Launders small items—rinses stockings, etc.	1
Dials a few well-known numbers	1	All laundry must be done by others	0
Answers telephone, but does not dial	1	Mode of transportation	
Does not use telephone at all	0	Travels independently on public transportation or drives own car	1
Shopping		Arranges own travel via taxi, but does not otherwise use public transportation	1
Takes care of all shopping needs independently	1		
Shops independently for small purchases	0	Travels on public transportation when accompanied by another	1
Needs to be accompanied on any shopping trip	0	Travel limited to taxi or automobile with assistance of another	0
Completely unable to shop	0	Responsibility for own medications	
Food preparation		Is responsible for taking medication in correct dosages at correct time	1
Plans, prepares, and serves adequate meals independently	1		
Prepares adequate meals if supplied with ingredients	0	Takes responsibility if medication is prepared in advance in separate dosages	0
Heats, serves, and prepares meals, or prepares meals, but does not maintain adequate diet	0		
		Is not capable of dispensing own medication	0
Needs to have meals prepared and served	0	Ability to handle finances	
Housekeeping		Manages financial matters independently (budgets, writes checks, pays rent, bills, goes to bank), collects and keeps track of income	1
Maintains household alone or with occasional assistance (e.g., "heavy work domestic help")	1		
Performs light daily tasks such as dishwashing, bedmaking	1		
Performs light daily tasks but cannot maintain acceptable level of cleanliness	1	Manages day-to-day purchases, but needs help with banking, major purchases, etc.	1
Needs help with all home maintenance tasks	1	Incapable of handling money	0
Does not particiapte in any housekeeping tasks	0	SCORE _____/8	

[a] This instrument is a component of the Philadelphia Geriatric Center Multilevel Assessment Instrument.

Source: Lawton MP, Moss M, Fulcomer M, Kleban MH: A research- and service-oriented multilevel assessment instrument. *J Gerontol* 37:91–99, 1982.

tion of the legs. A patient who has had recent trips or falls should be evaluated by being watched as he or she rises from a chair, walks about 10 ft, and returns and sits down as well as by a means of full neurological and musculoskeletal examination (see Chap. 14).

The score on the MMSE should be interpreted cautiously. It may be

Table 3-6 Key components of the preadmission geriatric evaluation

History
    Reasons for seeking admission
    Medical problems (active and chronic)
    Past medical history
    Preventive measures: vaccination, eye, dental, and foot care
    Medication history (including over-the-counter drugs)
    Review of symptoms

Physical Examination
    In addition to traditional system approach, focus on the following:
        Nutritional status (weight/height)
        Orthostatic changes in blood pressure
        Functional muscle strength
        Proximal and distal arm functions

Functional Assessment (see Tables 3-4 and 3-5)
    Corroborate responses with patient appearance, question family members if accuracy
        is uncertain

Mobility
    Ask patient to get out of chair, walk, turn around, and sit down
    Judgment based on direct observation
    Tinetti Gait and Balance Scale (see Table 3-4 and Chap. 14)

Cognitive Assessment
    Administer MMSE; if score < 24, search for causes of cognitive impairment (see Table 3-4
        and Chap. 9)
    Ask "Do you often feel sad or depressed?" If answer is yes, administer Geriatric
        Depression Scale (see Table 3-4 and Chap. 10)

Hearing
    Screen utilizing Welch Allyn Audioscope testing threshold of 20, 25, and 40 dB at 500,
        1000, 2000, 4000 Hz (see Chap. 15)
    Whisper a short easily answered question such as "What is your name?" in each ear while
        your face is out of direct view

Vision
    Utilize Jaeger card at 14 in. while patient wears his or her corrective lenses (inability to
        read greater than 20/40 is abnormal) or
    Have patient read something to test ability to see well enough to read

affected by level of education and, to a lesser degree, by impairments in hearing and vision. A score of less than 24 should lead to further investigation, but does not necessarily make the diagnosis of dementia. Patients with mental status scores at the borderline of normal may appear to function well because of assistance in daily activities that is being given by a spouse or other person. If this help is lost, the patient's functional disabilities related to mental impairment may become more prominent. This has significance in a board and care facility, where regulations require that resi-

Table 3-7   Format of preadmission consultation/evaluation

Patient identification	Recommendations/plans
Reason for consultation/evaluation	Limit to five focusing on management
Primary care physician	Data base following traditional format
	Present history
Referral source	Past medical history
Summary of assessments	Symptom review
Active medical problems	Results of functional status assessments
Functional problems	Physical examination
Rehabilitation potential	
Capacity to make health care decisions	
Psychosocial problems	

dents have the capacity to respond to emergencies. Thus, the discovery of mental impairment on the MMSE does not necessarily call for an immediate intervention but should alert the caregiver and prompt reevaluation if a source of support is lost. The Short Portable Mental State Questionnaire (SPMSQ) is a 10-item test that may serve as an alternative to the MMSE. This instrument is, however, less sensitive. Depression can be screened by a single, simple question: "Do you often feel sad or depressed?" However, this can also serve as an introduction to a more detailed investigation. Patients who respond affirmatively should be tested with the GDS (see Chap. 10).

A comprehensive preadmission assessment can become the cornerstone of the patient's care plan in the NH. The physician can summarize the multidisciplinary preadmission assessment in a dictated report. The report should be clear, summarizing the problems in a concise, organized manner, with no more than five recommendations. Recommendations should preferably focus on management rather than diagnostics. The report should include statements regarding the patient's prognosis, rehabilitation potential, and capacity for making health care decisions. Table 3-7 presents a suggested format for the report. The report is meant to serve the primary care physician as well as the NH staff.

It is always important to remember that even in cases where the assessment team is employed by the institution, the team is ethically obligated to provide any useful information to the patients and their caregivers in the event that the individual is not admitted to the institution.

SUGGESTED READINGS

Alexopoulos GS, Abrams RC, Young RC, Shamoian CA: Use of the Cornell Scale in nondemented patients. *J Am Geriatr Soc* 36:230–236, 1988.

Applegate WB, Blass JP, Williams TF: Instruments for the functional assessment of older patients. *N Engl J Med* 322:1207–1212, 1990.

Lachs MS, Feinstein AR, Cooney LM, et al: A simple procedure for general screening for functional disability in elderly patients. *Ann Intern Med* 112:699–706, 1990.

Munso-Ashman J: Geriatric assessment—An Australian idea. *Soc Sci Med* 29:939–942, 1989.

Williams ME, Hornberger JC: A quantitative method of identifying older persons at risk for increasing long term care services. *J Chronic Dis* 37:705–711, 1986.

FOUR

HEALTH MAINTENANCE, SCREENING, AND PREVENTIVE PRACTICES

This chapter provides several recommendations for practices related to health maintenance, screening, and prevention in the nursing home (NH) setting. These recommendations must be prefaced by several general comments. First, with few exceptions, the efficacy and cost-effectiveness of the recommendations presented herein have not been well studied. For the most part, they reflect the authors' opinions and judgments on the basis of current knowledge, best standards of care, practicality, and cost. Second, not all of the practices recommended are relevant for all NH residents. As discussed in Chap. 2 and depicted in Figs. 2-3 through 2-9, NH residents are heterogeneous. Thus, for example, recommendations for health maintenance and screening are generally not relevant to residents who are in the NH for short-term rehabilitation or terminal care. Third, while several of the practices recommended are mandated by federal and/or state guidelines, they are time-consuming and inadequately reimbursed. This is especially true when the practices must be carried out by primary care physicians. It is therefore critical that these practices be incorporated, to the extent possible, in the general context of medical practice in the NH and, where relevant, in the policies and procedures of the facility.

Before outlining the specific practices, we present a brief overview of the general context of medical care in the NH. It is within this context that the recommended medical practices should be implemented.

THE GENERAL CONTEXT OF MEDICAL PRACTICE IN THE NURSING HOME

Physicians whose practice is primarily in the NH are the exception rather than the rule. Most physicians visit NHs on a monthly basis—more often if they care for a substantial number of residents in a particular facility. Thus, if standard approaches to health maintenance, screening, and prevention are to be implemented consistently, the facility must develop appropriate policies, procedures, and documentation practices and convey them to the primary medical staff. This is one of the critical responsibilities of the medical director, as discussed in Chap. 6. Examples of specific policies and documentation formats are presented in the Appendix.

Table 4-1 outlines key aspects of the various types of medical assessments performed by primary care physicians in NHs. Physicians assess NH residents in four general contexts: (1) an initial assessment within the first few days of NH admission; (2) periodic assessments, generally performed monthly; (3) assessment of acute or subacute changes in status on an as-needed basis; and (4) a major reassessment of long-staying residents, generally done annually.

The initial assessment has several important objectives (Table 4-1). Because NH residents are frequently admitted and readmitted to the NH from an acute care hospital, previous hospital histories and physicals and/or discharge summaries are commonly used in the admission assessment. Because these hospital summaries too often omit data that are critical to the NH plan of care, we recommend that a separate assessment be documented, including such information as the resident's chronic medical conditions, psychosocial status and functional capabilities. In addition, we recommend that a Medical Face Sheet be completed (or revised in the case of a readmission), which summarizes critical information in an easily readable format. Examples of an admission assessment data base and Medical Face Sheet are included in the Appendix. As discussed in Chap. 24, these documents can be incorporated into a standard computer format for easy updating; they can also be linked to a data base for quality-assurance purposes. An extremely important component of the initial assessment process is the determination and documentation of treatment status decisions, including decisions about the intensity of care to be given should the resident become acutely ill. This is a complex yet important area that is discussed in detail in Chap. 25. The Appendix includes examples of policies, procedures, and documentation formats relevant to this process. The time necessary to complete the initial assessment will depend on the admitting physician's prior knowledge of the resident. If, as is often the case, there is a change in physician, information from prior physicians and acute care hospitalizations are critical and should be requested from appropriate sources. Since many NH residents cycle between an acute care hospital and the NH, it may not be

Table 4-1 Important aspects of various types of medical assessment in the nursing home

Type of assessment	Timing	Major objectives	Important aspects
Initial	Within 48 h of admission	Verify medical diagnoses Document baseline physical findings, mental and functional status, vital signs, and skin condition Attempt to identify potentially remediable, previously unrecognized medical conditions Get to know the resident and family (if this is a new resident) Establish goals for the admission and a medical treatment plan	A thorough review of medical records and physical examination are necessary Relevant medical diagnoses and baseline findings should be clearly and concisely documented in the medical record Medication lists should be carefully reviewed and only essential medications continued Requests for specific types of assessment and inputs from other disciplines should be made An initial medical problem list should be documented (see example of Medical Face Sheet in Appendix) Treatment status (i.e., no CPR, etc.) should be documented (see Chap. 25 and Appendix)
Periodic	Usually monthly	Monitor progress of active conditions Update medical orders Communicate with resident and NH staff	Progress notes should include clinical data relevant to active medical conditions and focus on changes in status (see Table 4-2) Unnecessary medications, orders for care, and laboratory tests should be discontinued Mental, functional, and psychosocial status should be reviewed with nursing staff and changes from baseline noted The medical problem list should be updated
As needed	When acute changes in status occur	Identify and treat causes of acute changes	On-site clinical assessment by the physician (or nurse practitioner or physician's assistant), as opposed to telephone consultation, will result in more accurate diagnoses, more appropriate treatment, and fewer unnecessary emergency room visits and hospitalizations

Table 4-1 *(Continued)* Important aspects of various types of medical assessment in the nursing home

Type of assessment	Timing	Major objectives	Important aspects
			Vital signs, food and fluid intake, and mental status often provide essential information
			Infection, dehydration, and adverse drug effects should be at the top of the differential diagnosis for acute changes in status
			Treatment status (i.e., no CPR, etc.) should be reviewed if appropriate
Major reassessment	Annual	Identify and document any significant changes in status and new, potentially remediable conditions	Targeted physical examination and assessment of mental, functional, and psychosocial status and selected laboratory tests should be done (see Table 4-4)

necessary to repeat the entire initial assessment data base at the time of readmission. A concise readmission note and updating of the Medical Face Sheet will generally suffice after a brief hospital stay. Strategies for communication and documentation between the hospital and the NH are discussed further in Chap. 5.

We recommend that NH residents generally be reassessed on a monthly basis. Table 4-2 suggests a format and outlines key data for routine medical progress notes on NH residents. If legibility is a problem, these notes can be dictated. Software is now available that can be used to format the progress notes and make the process more efficient for physicians who favor computers. Particular attention should be paid to the monitoring practices discussed below and to discontinuing or modifying outdated orders. Physicians' order sheets should be printed in an organized format to facilitate efficient but thorough review. An example of such a format is included in the Appendix. Routine rounds are best made with a nurse who knows the residents well. Nurse's notes and medication records should be reviewed. In our experience, monthly visits that encompass these recommended procedures on relatively stable residents take 10 to 15 min per resident. We also recommend that, on a periodic basis—quarterly, for example—interdisciplinary rounds be conducted with nursing, social service, and other staff to facilitate review of residents' progress. This will also enhance communication about residents with particularly difficult and complex problems.

Table 4-2 Format and key data for medical progress notes on nursing home residents

Subjective	New complaints
	Symptoms related to active medical conditions
	Reports from nursing staff
	Progress in rehabilitative therapy
	Reports of other interdisciplinary team members
Objective	General appearance
	Weight
	Vital signs
	Physical findings relevant to new complaints and active medical conditions
	Laboratory data
	Consultant reports
Assessment	Presumptive diagnoses of new complaints or changes in status
	Stability of active medical conditions
	Response to interventions, especially psychotropic medications and rehabilitative therapy
Plans	Changes in medications or diet
	Nursing interventions (e.g., monitoring of vital signs, skin care)
	Assessments by other disciplines
	Consultants
	Laboratory studies
	Discharge planning (if relevant)

Acute and subacute changes in status occur commonly among NH residents. They are relevant to the focus of this chapter in that many of these changes will result in new problems (which should be added to problem lists), new medications, a reevaluation of treatment status (i.e., CPR, etc.), and conditions that require monitoring, as described below. Since assessment of these acute or subacute changes is often done by telephone, it is important for the physician to document important events the next time they are in the facility. The management of acute and subacute conditions in the NH is discussed further in Chaps. 5 and 7.

The value of the annual history and physical examination in the NH population has been questioned. We suggest there are several important reasons to recommend some type of annual reassessment for long-staying NH residents. First, most of these residents do not undergo a thorough physical examination on routine visits. Thus, an annual physical examination is important to detect and document changes and conditions that may require intervention. Second, it affords an opportunity to thoroughly reassess the resident's functional status and to screen for changes in cognitive, affective, and social status that may require intervention. Third, an annual panel of screening tests is probably warranted in most NH residents and can be performed or ordered at the time of the annual reassessment. Recommendations for these screening practices are outlined below. A suggested format for documenting the annual review is included in the Appendix.

MONITORING

Table 4-3 lists examples of practices we recommend for periodic monitoring in selected residents. These practices focus on the management of common chronic medical conditions in the NH population, such as diabetes, cardiovascular disorders, arthritis, and anemia. Because many serious problems can develop insidiously and are commonly asymptomatic, we recommend these practices as an adjunct to the monthly visit. Examples of these problems include weight loss, dehydration, hyper- and hypoglycemia, hypo- or hypernatremia, azotemia, upper gastrointestinal bleeding from nonsteroidal anti-inflammatory drugs (NSAIDs), anemia, and drug toxicity. Appropriate policies on monitoring should help identify these conditions before serious consequences occur and can be a key component of a medical quality assurance program.

SCREENING

Recommendations for screening practices vary considerably among different patient populations and are highly debated in the medical literature. Very few studies have addressed the cost-effectiveness of screening in the NH population, and no specific recommendations for screening in the NH have been put forth by any organization.

Table 4-4 lists recommendations for what we believe to be reasonable screening practices in the NH setting. Obviously these recommendations apply only to the long-staying subgroup of NH residents. The assumptions underlying these recommendations are as follows: (1) even among very old NH residents with varying degrees of physical functional and cognitive impairments, remediable conditions can be identified, such as depression and incontinence; (2) screening for conditions such as weight loss, inadequate dentition, podiatric problems, and gait instability may lead to interventions that will prevent complications from malnutrition and falls; (3) the identification of depression, visual and auditory disturbances, and dental problems is critical for maximizing quality of life; (4) screening for tuberculosis may prevent outbreaks in a susceptible resident population and among staff who in many areas are immigrants from other countries; and (5) selected laboratory tests may be beneficial but should be limited to those tests whose abnormal results would lead to a specific intervention (e.g., fur-

Table 4-3   Examples of periodic monitoring practices in selected nursing home residents

Practice	Recommended frequency[a]	Comments
All residents		
Vital signs, including weight	Monthly	More often if unstable or subacutely ill
Diabetics		
Fasting and postprandial glucose, glycosylated hemoglobin	Monthly	More often if unstable Finger-stick tests may also be useful if staff can perform reliably
Residents on diuretics or with renal insufficiency (creatinine >2 or BUN >35) Electrolytes, BUN, creatinine	Every 2–3 months	Nursing home residents are more vulnerable to dehydration, azotemia, hyponatremia, and hypokalemia
Residents on nonsteroidal anti-inflammatory drugs (NSAIDs): Hemoglobin/ hematocrit, stool for occult blood	Every 1–2 months	Bleeding frequently asymptomatic
Anemic residents who are on iron replacement or who have hemoglobin <10 Hemoglobin/ hematocrit	Monthly until stable, then every 2–3 months	Iron replacement should be discontinued once hemoglobin value stabilizes
Blood level of drug for residents on specific drugs, e.g.: digoxin dilantin quinidine procainamide theophylline nortriptyline	Every 3–6 months	More frequently if drug treatment has just been initiated

[a] Data for the efficacy and timing of these practices are limited (see text).

ther evaluation of anemia, institution of thyroid replacement therapy). Note that annual chest radiographs and electrocardiograms are not recommended; there are no data to support their inclusion and they are very expensive, especially when the national costs of such recommendations are calculated.

Table 4-4   Examples of screening practices in the nursing home

Practice	Frequency[a]	Comments
History and physical examination	Yearly	Generally required, but yield of routine annual history and physical is debated Focused exam probably beneficial, including rectal, breast, and, in some women, pelvic exam
Weight	Monthly	Generally weight loss should prompt a search for treatable medical, psychiatric, and functional conditions (see Chap. 11)
Functional status assessment, including gait and mental status testing and screening for depression	Yearly	Functional status usually assessed periodically by nursing staff Systematic global functional assessment should be done at least yearly in order to document changes in status, detect potentially treatable conditions or prevent complications
Visual screening	Yearly	Assess acuity and intraocular pressure; identify correctable problems
Auditory	Yearly	Identify correctable problems
Dental	Yearly	Assess status of any remaining teeth and fit of dentures; identify any pathology
Podiatric	Yearly	More frequently in diabetics and residents with peripheral vascular disease
Tuberculosis	On admission and yearly	All residents and staff should be tested; control skin tests and booster testing are generally recommended for NH residents (see Chap. 17)

Laboratory tests
  Stool for occult blood
  Complete blood count
  Fasting glucose
  Electrolytes
  Renal function tests
  Albumin, calcium, phosphorus
  Thyroid function tests
	Yearly	These tests appear to have reasonable yield in the nursing home population

[a] Data for the efficacy and timing of these practices are limited (see text).

Table 4-5 Examples of preventive practices in the nursing home

Practice	Frequency[a]	Comments
Influenza vaccine	Yearly	All residents and staff with close resident contact should be vaccinated
Amantadine	Within 24–48 h of outbreak of suspected influenza A	Dose should be reduced to 100 mg/day in elderly; further reduction if renal failure present Unvaccinated residents and staff should be treated throughout outbreak (see Chap. 17)
Pneumococcal vaccine	Once	Efficacy in NH residents is debated
Tetanus booster	Every 10 years, or every 5 years with tetanus-prone wounds	Many elderly people have not received primary vaccinations; they require tetanus toxoid, 250 to 500 units of tetanus immune globulin, and completion of the immunization series with toxoid injection 4 to 6 weeks later and then 6 to 12 months after the second injection (see Chap. 17)
Tuberculosis prophylaxis (isoniazid 300 mg/day for 1 year)	Skin-test conversion in selected residents	Residents with abnormal chest film (more than granuloma), diabetes, end-stage renal disease, hematological malignancies, steroidal or immunosuppressive therapy, or malnutrition should be treated (see Chap. 17)
Antimicrobial prophylaxis for residents at risk	Generally recommended for dental procedures, genitourinary procedures, and most operative procedures	Chronically catheterized residents should not be treated with continuous prophylaxis (see Chap. 17)
Body positioning and range-of-motion exercises for immobile residents	Ongoing	Frequent turning of very immobile residents is necessary to prevent pressure sores Partially upright position is necessary for residents with swallowing disorders or enteral feeding to help prevent aspiration

Table 4-5 *(Continued)*   Examples of preventive practices in the nursing home

Practice	Frequency [a]	Comments
		Range-of-motion exercises for immobile limbs and joints are necessary to prevent contractures
Infection control procedures and surveillance (see Chap. 17)	Ongoing	Policies and protocols should be in effect in all nursing homes Surveillance of all infections should be continuous to identify outbreaks and patterns
Environmental safety	Ongoing	Appropriate lighting, colors, and the removal of hazards that could cause falls are essential in order to prevent accidents Routine monitoring of potential safety hazards and accidents may lead to alterations that can help to prevent further accidents

[a] Data for the efficacy and timing of these practices are limited (see text).

The Appendix contains a sample format for documenting the results of the annual review. Examples of commonly used assessments for functional and mental status, depression, and gait are included in relevant chapters throughout the text.

PREVENTION

While it may seem unusual to think of preventive practices in the NH, there are actually several that are relevant in this setting. Examples are listed in Table 4-5. Many preventive practices relate to infections and infection control, topics covered in more detail in Chap. 17. Because of the extreme immobility of many NH residents, body repositioning and range-of-motion exercises are important aspects of care to prevent pressure sores, contractures, and aspiration. The monitoring of environmental safety and the ongoing evaluation of accidents are critical quality assurance functions in every facility. This type of surveillance is designed to prevent, to the extent possible, unnecessary accidents and injuries among residents, staff, and visitors.

SUGGESTED READINGS

Domoto K, Ben R, Wei JY, et al: Yield of routine annual laboratory screening in the institutionalized elderly. *Am J Public Health* 75:243–245, 1985.

Gambert SR, Duthie EH, and Wiltzius F: The value of the yearly medical evaluation in a nursing home. *J Chronic Dis* 35:65–68, 1982.

Irvine PW, Carlson K, Adcock M, et al: The value of annual medical examinations in the nursing home. *J Am Geriatr Soc* 32:540–545, 1984.

Levenstein MR, Ouslander JG, Rubenstein LZ, et al: Yield of routine annual laboratory tests in a skilled nursing home population. *JAMA* 258:1909–1941, 1987.

Ouslander, JG: Medical care in the nursing home. *JAMA* 262:2582–2590, 1989.

Ouslander JG and Martin SE: Assessment in the nursing home. *Clin Geriatr Med* 3:155–174, 1987.

Patriarca PA, Arden NH, Koplan JP, and Goodman RA: Prevention and control of type A influenza infections in nursing homes. *Ann Intern Med* 107:732–740, 1987.

Wolf-Klein GP, Holt T, Silverstone FA, et al: Efficacy of routine annual studies in the care of elderly patients. *J Am Geriatr Soc* 33:325–329, 1985.

THE NURSING HOME–ACUTE CARE HOSPITAL INTERFACE

The interface between the nursing home (NH) and the acute care hospital is a dynamic one. Statistics are changing rapidly because of the Medicare prospective payment system and an increase in the severity of illness in the NH population. Data from some relatively recent studies of NH admissions and discharges are, however, illustrative of this dynamism.

The acute care hospital, in part because of Medicare's 3-day hospital requirement, is the source of many NH admissions. Viewed from the hospital's perspective, approximately 6 percent to 10 percent of hospitalized geriatric patients are discharged to a NH. The proportion is higher among women, those above age 80, patients with both physical and mental diagnoses, and patients who were admitted to the hospital from a NH. From the NH's perspective, approximately half of the residents admitted come from an acute care hospital. Once in the NH, approximately half stay just a few (1 to 6) months. Of those residents discharged alive, approximately half go to an acute care hospital. Many NH residents frequently bounce back and forth between one or more NHs and the acute care hospital. Reported hospitalization rates per NH bed per year during the 1980s varied from 0.21 to 0.55. Figure 5-1 illustrates this dynamism of the NH–acute care hospital interface by depicting the natural history of a cohort of NH residents discharged after their first NH admission.

Transfer of a NH resident to an acute care hospital is a costly process. The costs are high not only in terms of the dollars spent (on transporting the resident to the acute care hospital, emergency room evaluation, hospital

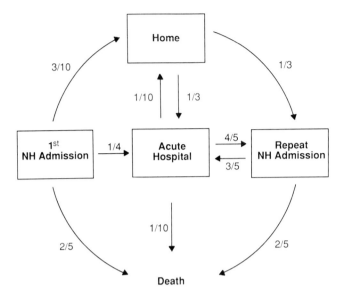

Figure 5-1 An example of the dynamic nature of the NH–acute hospital interface. The diagram represents the natural history of a cohort of NH residents after discharge from their first NH stay. Fractions represent approximate proportion moving from one status to another; not shown are about 5 percent of discharges that went from their first NH to another NH. (After Kane RL, Ouslander JG, and Abrass IB: *Essentials of Clinical Geriatrics*, 2d ed. New York, McGraw-Hill, 1989. Data source: Lewis MA, Cretin S, and Kane RL: The natural history of nursing home patients. *Gerontologist* 25:382–388, 1985.)

admission, and readmission to the NH) but also because hospitalization is often physically uncomfortable and emotionally traumatic for the NH resident and his or her loved ones. In addition, NH residents admitted to an acute care hospital are at relatively high risk for iatrogenic complications such as delirium (e.g., "sundowning"), adverse drug reactions, falls, pressure sores, and complications from diagnostic and surgical procedures.

The decision to hospitalize a NH resident is a complex one involving a myriad of considerations. The clinical status of the resident is, of course, paramount. Acute medical conditions must be treated unless an explicit decision has been made not to do so. Even in the latter instance, hospitalization may be necessary to provide optimal palliative and comfort care. Hospital-based NHs and many community facilities with "subacute" units are prepared to care for many of the common acute illnesses that frequently result in hospitalization, including infections, dehydration, gastrointestinal disorders, hip fractures, and decompensated chronic cardiac or pulmonary disease (Table 5-1). Most NHs, however, have limited capabilities in this regard. Factors such as financial incentives, the availability of ancillary ser-

Table 5-1   Conditions most commonly responsible for the hospitalization of nursing home residents[a]

	% of residents hospitalized
Infection	10–49
Dehydration	<17>
Cardiovascular	10–16
Gastrointestinal	13–17
Fracture	7–9
Behavioral disorders[b]	5–10

[a] Based on the results of several published studies.
[b] Includes depression, delirium, disruptive behaviors.

vices and trained nurses, the capability to provide on-site medical and mental health assessment and treatment, and ethical considerations all play a role in the hospitalization of NH residents. Table 5-2 summarizes these factors and their implications. The purpose of this chapter is to briefly discuss several of the key issues surrounding the NH–hospital interface. The extreme variability in the relationship between NHs and their affiliated acute care hospitals makes specific recommendations difficult to offer. Several general recommendations are presented that might improve the appropriateness, process, and outcomes of the hospitalization of NH residents.

ECONOMIC CONSIDERATIONS

For the most part, financial incentives strongly favor hospitalizing a NH resident who becomes acutely or subacutely ill. Reimbursement for adequate physician supervision and for the NH to provide subacute care is generally very limited. Hospital-based NHs get higher rates and can, to some extent, take advantage of economies of scale; community-based NHs with Medicare "distinct part" units can get higher reimbursement for subacute care. Such care within the NH may, however, result in logistically complex and emotionally disruptive movement of residents. At the same time, acute care hospitals with empty beds are more than willing to accept admissions from NHs, especially if the NH is willing and able to accept the patient back before he or she becomes a "DRG outlier." Physicians are also reimbursed much more adequately for providing hospital as opposed to NH care.

One pilot demonstration project in Monroe County, New York, tested a Medicare "sudden decline" benefit. The benefit was instituted rapidly and provided reimbursement to both the NH and the physician to manage acute

Table 5-2 Factors surrounding the hospitalization of nursing home residents

Factors	Implications	Potential strategies to reduce hospitalization	Caveats
Financial incentives	Physicians, NHs, and acute care hospitals each potentially benefit financially by hospitalizing NH residents	Reasonable reimbursement for NHs and physicians to care for selected acutely ill residents in the NH setting	Acute care hospitals with empty beds and substantial admissions from NHs may lose revenue The cost-effectiveness of such reimbursements has not been studied Criteria must be established so that residents who do require acute care are hospitalized
Availability of ancillary services	In order to effectively manage some acute illnesses in the NH, a variety of ancillary services—such as radiographs, blood drawing, and respiratory therapy—must be available	Contract arrangements with local providers or acute care hospitals for radiographs, blood drawing, laboratory testing, pharmacy supplies, respiratory therapy, etc.	These services may not be available locally to many NHs
Organization of medical staff	Physicians are rarely present and often unwilling to visit the NH regularly Medical directors frequently have only minimal involvement in the NH and supervise the medical care inadequately	Use nurse practitioners or physicians' assistants for the initial assessment and ongoing monitoring of acute problems (see Chap. 7) Establish a small, committed medical staff that visits the facility at least biweekly	Reimbursement is either unavailable or very limited for nurse practitioner services Few physicians are willing to commit a substantial amount of time to NH care

Problem	Description	Recommendation	Comment
		Hire and adequately reimburse a medical director with training and/or special interest in geriatrics and long-term-care administration	Relatively few physicians are committed to a career in geriatrics
Limitations in nursing care	Licensed nursing staff in many NHs are too few in number and/or inadequately trained to monitor acutely ill residents	Provide in-service training in the assessment and management of acute illnesses, especially parenteral fluid and antibiotic administration. Establish designated areas for "subacute" care with specially trained staff within larger NHs. Develop policies and procedures for notification of physicians for acute problems (see text and Appendix)	There are shortages of nursing staff in many areas, and qualified nurses often choose to work in other settings. Caring for the acutely ill may detract from the care of other residents. Criteria must be established so that residents who do require acute care are hospitalized
Lack of psychiatric care	Acute problems often involve psychological factors and psychiatric conditions	Provide adequate reimbursement for mental health services for NH residents. Develop a relationship with a psychiatrist, and/or psychologist with a special interest in geriatrics. Develop in-service programs for medical, nursing, and social service staff on the assessment and treatment of common psychiatric disturbances	There are very few psychiatrists and psychologists with training and/or interest in geriatric psychiatry. Current constraints in Medicare limit reimbursement for psychiatric care in NHs

Table 5-2 (*Continued*) Factors surrounding the hospitalization of nursing home residents

Factors	Implications	Potential strategies to reduce hospitalization	Caveats
Limited documentation	NH medical records are often superficial and inaccurate	Develop and monitor standards for medical documentation Carefully develop and utilize interfacility transfer forms (see text and Appendix) Consider the use of computers to maintain files of key medical information for use by on-call physicians	The NH record becomes discontinuous because of regulations on documentation Some NHs use more than one acute care hospital, making standardized documentation difficult Not all physicians are familiar with personal computers
Lack of protocols	Policies and procedures for preventing complications that could lead to acute illness are not well developed	Develop sound policies and procedures for infection control, catheter care, periodic screening and monitoring, and oral/enteral feeding to prevent aspiration (see Chaps. 4, 11, and 17)	The effectiveness of these types of protocols has not been proved in NH settings
Ethical dilemmas	Many severely ill NH residents and/or their loved ones do not want intensive treatment or any treatment at all that will prolong life	Encourage NH residents to complete advance directives Establish an ethics committee Develop, implement, and monitor policies for cardiopulmonary resuscitation, hospitalization, etc. (see Chap. 25 and Appendix)	Many NH residents do not have decision-making capacity or a suitable proxy Religious and cultural beliefs may make policy development and implementation difficult

illness in the NH. The results of this demonstration project were promising, but larger randomized trials of such strategies are necessary to clearly demonstrate their cost-effectiveness.

Until the reimbursement system is changed, financial incentives will continue to favor hospitalization. Thus, it is critically important for NHs to establish good working relationships with one or more acute care hospitals. The hospital can identify one discharge planner to oversee readmission to the NH, so that he or she can become familiar with the facility's staff and capabilities. Where feasible, NHs might arrange for acute care diagnostic and therapeutic services to be provided by the hospital facilities and staff (see section on "Ancillary Services, below"). As discussed later in this chapter, this type of relationship can also foster the development of better interfacility communication and documentation procedures.

ANCILLARY SERVICES

The ability of a NH to provide acute and subacute care is critically dependent on the availability of several ancillary services. These include a clinical laboratory and blood drawing service that can process tests rapidly, an onsite or portable radiology service as well as a radiologist to provide immediate interpretations, respiratory therapy for inhaled bronchodilator treatments and the monitoring of oxygen delivery, and a pharmacy that can provide medications (especially antibiotics) in a timely manner. Most facilities are too small to provide these services on site. In many areas, these types of services are readily available by contract. In Los Angeles, for example, there are services that will even provide on-site noninvasive vascular exams for deep vein thrombosis or abdominal ultrasonography. In many areas, however, these contracted services are difficult or impossible to find. Where they are available, they may be very costly. As already mentioned, it may be mutually beneficial for an NH to make arrangements with a local acute care hospital to provide some or all of these services. Making appropriate arrangements for the ancillary services listed above is a key responsibility of the NH medical director (see Chap. 6).

ORGANIZATION OF MEDICAL STAFF

The manner in which most medical care is provided to NH residents tends to foster the use of the emergency room and acute care hospital. Physicians are rarely based in NHs, and in most NHs a physician is available on site for very limited periods of time. Physicians who provide primary care to NH residents generally have busy office practices or other responsibilities at some distance from the NH. Thus, even if adequate reimbursement were available for the on-site assessment of an acute problem, logistical considerations often make it difficult for the physician to do so. In addition, medical directors, also, are generally not available on site and provide minimal supervision of medical staff activities. As a result, most acute problems are handled over the telephone and are often dealt with by transferring the patient to an emergency room for evaluation.

There are at least two alternatives to this approach. Some NHs are large enough and located in areas where there are enough physicians to organize a medical staff that can see the NH's residents more frequently or that may even be based in part at the facility. The second alternative is the use of physician's assistants (PAs) and/or nurse practitioners (NPs). Medicare now provides reimbursement for PAs in NHs. Recently proposed legislation will also provide reimbursement for NPs to work in NHs and, importantly, eliminate the requirement for on-site supervision. Reimbursement will still generally not be adequate to cover the full-time salary of an NP or PA, and when direct reimbursement to the NP or PA is requested, the physician is not reimbursed for the visit. Thus, creative strategies to supplement direct reimbursement—by shared funding by the NH and a physician group and/or an acute care hospital—are necessary in order to make this a viable option. The role of PAs and NPs in the NH is discussed further in Chap. 7.

NURSING CARE

The shortage of licensed nurses over recent years has been a major barrier to providing high quality care in NHs. Even before this shortage, the number of licensed nurses in NHs was limited. Typically there is one licensed vocational nurse for every 30 or so residents and one registered nurse for every 50 to 100 residents providing direct care during daytime hours. The vast majority of hands-on care is provided by nurses' aides, who are neither trained nor skilled in the assessment of acute or subacute illnesses. Training for nurses' aides is, in fact, an important provision of new federal regulations related to NH care. With the nursing shortage, nurse registries have begun to play an increasing role in the NH. The use of registry nurses poses several problems. In addition to the fact that they do not have a vested interest in the NH, registry nurses do not generally get to know the NH residents over time. Unlike the situation in an acute care hospital, this lack of familiarity with the chronically ill may make it more difficult for the registry nurse to recognize the subtle changes that often indicate the onset of an acute illness. Further, registry nurses are generally not familiar with the NH's policies and procedures, which may interfere with their ability to assess and manage acute illnesses in the NH setting.

Even when a NH is blessed with a stable group of licensed nurses, the management of acute illnesses may be problematic. Nurses who work in

NHs choose to do so in preference to working in acute care hospitals. They may, therefore, be less likely to be interested and skilled in the management of acute illnesses than they are in rehabilitation and chronic care. When acutely or subacutely ill NH residents are managed in the NH, it takes limited licensed staff time away from the care of the majority of residents who are chronically ill. Thus, it may be difficult to monitor vital signs frequently and to oversee the parenteral administration of fluids and medications without cutting back on other nursing care activities for less seriously ill residents.

Nursing homes that choose to manage some acute and subacute illnesses may assist their nursing staff in several ways. First, as already mentioned, PAs and NPs are extremely helpful in the assessment and treatment of acute and subacute illnesses in the NH. Second, NHs that are large enough may choose to create a "distinct part" unit in which all subacutely ill residents are managed. This may create some logistical complexities because of intrafacility room changes, but it can facilitate the training of selected nursing staff members to provide this type of care and offers the possibility of gaining higher per diem rates for Medicare bed days. Third, specific policies and procedures focusing on the assessment and management of acute and subacute conditions should be developed. One example is a policy and procedure for physician notification and physician responsiveness. We have developed such a policy, which is shown in the Appendix. It details the conditions that require immediate versus nonimmediate notification of the primary care physician; this provides the nursing staff with reasonable guidelines and assurance that their calls will be responded to appropriately. It also eliminates the need for many unnecessary telephone communications.

PSYCHIATRIC CARE

The high prevalence of psychiatric disorders among NH residents is being increasingly recognized. Behavioral disorders associated with dementia and/or depression are very common (see Chaps. 9 and 10). Psychiatric disorders may account for as many as 10 percent of transfers to acute care hospitals and probably contribute to many more. At the same time, psychiatric care in the NH is quite limited. Mental health professionals must become more involved with NH care, and reimbursement for their services should be set at an adequate level. We recommend that all NHs arrange for consultations and follow-ups with a psychiatrist and/or clinical psychologist who is interested and skilled in the management of common psychiatric disorders in the geriatric population. In addition, some social workers and nurses have special training in geriatric psychiatry and can provide valuable clinical skills as well as assistance in the development and implementation of appropriate policies and procedures related to psychiatric conditions. There is also a need to improve the prescription and monitoring of psychotropic medications. At present, this is handled largely by primary care physicians with limited knowledge of psychopharmacology. The use of psychotropic medications is discussed in detail in Chap. 21.

DOCUMENTATION

The frequent transfer of NH residents to acute care hospitals and back creates many problems with documentation and information transfer. Even when a NH has an ongoing relationship with only one such hospital, medical records become discontinuous and often omit information on chronic problems that are essential to the resident's care. Hospital discharge and NH admission or readmission frequently result in an inefficient transfer of critical information. Physicians orders, for example, are frequently written on a transfer form, retranscribed by a NH nurse, then reverified by telephone with the primary care physician.

Several documentation procedures can improve the efficiency and accuracy of information transfer at the NH–acute hospital interface. These include (1) a standard packet of information that accompanies the resident when transferred from NH to acute care hospital, including medical and administrative face sheets, recent orders, and medical/nursing progress notes and laboratory results; (2) a standard nursing assessment focusing on activities of daily living and nursing needs that accompanies the resident when transferred from acute hospital to NH; (3) an abbreviated hospital discharge summary (which can also serve as the required NH admission documentation) that contains information critical to the immediate care plans (a standard discharge summary that includes the necessary information can also serve this purpose if it can be transcribed *before* hospital discharge); and (4) physician's orders for the NH that are written by the physician and transferred to the NH at the time of acute hospital discharge. Examples of forms for these documentation practices are included in the Appendix. Some physicians and NHs are beginning to use FAX transmissions to handle some of these communications. The practical, administrative, and economic aspects of using FAX machines in the NH setting should be explored over the next several years.

ETHICS

A chapter on the NH–acute hospital interface would not be complete without at least brief mention of ethical issues that frequently arise at the time of interfacility transfer. A more complete overview of ethical issues is provided in Chap. 25.

Ethical concerns are common both at transfer from hospital to NH as well as at transfer from NH to hospital. In the former situation, the patient's decision-making capacity and autonomy become critical. Is it the individual's desire to be transferred to a NH? Is he or she capable of making independent decisions in this regard? Are family members acting in the patient's best interest? Are viable alternatives to NH admission available? With regard to a transfer from the NH to the acute care hospital, the resident's desires for intensive medical treatment are a critical concern. Situations clearly arise in which the best interests of the resident are not served by transferring him or her to a hospital for specific and/or intensive treatment (e.g., surgery, intravenous antibiotics, etc.). Instead, palliative and comfort care in familiar surroundings may be a more desirable option for all concerned. Unfortunately, prospective decision making and the use of advance directives is not yet a common practice. Because many NH residents are already incapable of making decisions at the time of NH admission, the use of advance directives must also be incorporated into the practice of geriatric medicine in ambulatory care settings. We recommend that all NHs develop policies and procedures for the use of advance directives and standardized documentation practices that will help ensure that the resident's desires for intensive treatment under specific conditions are honored. Examples of such policies and procedures and documentation formats are included in the Appendix.

SUGGESTED READINGS

Campion EW, Bang A, and May MI: Why acute care hospitals must undertake long-term care. *N Engl J Med* 308:71–75, 1983.

Gordon WZ, Kane RL, and Rothenberg R: Acute hospitalization in a home for the aged. *J Am Geriatr Soc* 33:519–523, 1985.

Irvine PW, Van Buren N, and Crossley K: Causes for hospitalization for nursing home residents: The role of infection. *J Am Geriatr Soc* 32:103–107, 1984.

Kane RL, Matthias R, and Sampson S: The risk of placement in a nursing home after acute hospitalization. *Med Care* 21:1055, 1983.

Kayser-Jones JS, Wiener CL, and Barbaccia JC: Factors contributing to the hospitalization of nursing home residents. *Gerontologist* 29:502–510, 1989.

Lewis MA, Cretin S, and Kane RL: The natural history of nursing home patients. *Gerontologist* 25:382–388, 1985.

Lewis MA, Kane RL, Cretin S, et al: The immediate and subsequent outcomes of nursing home care. *Am J Public Health* 75:758–762, 1985.

Rubenstein LZ, Ouslander JG, and Wieland D: Dynamics and clinical implications of the nursing home–hospital interface. *Clin Geriatr Med* 4:471–491, 1988.

Sager MA, Leventhal EA, and Easterling DV: The impact of Medicare's prospective payment system on Wisconsin nursing homes. *JAMA* 257:1762–1766, 1987.

Tresch DD, Simpson WM, and Burton JR: Relationship of long-term and acute care facilities: The problem of patient transfer and continuity of care. *J Am Geriatr Soc* 33:819–826, 1985.

Zimmer JG, Eggert GM, Treat A, et al: Nursing homes as acute care providers: A pilot study of incentives to reduce hospitalizations. *J Am Geriatr Soc* 35:124–129, 1987.

THE ROLE OF THE MEDICAL DIRECTOR

The importance of the medical director to the quality of medical care in the nursing home (NH) cannot be overemphasized. Until recently, very little has been written about the role and responsibilities of the NH medical director. Medical directorship in most NHs has largely been relegated to physicians with little if any training in geriatrics, long-term care, or administration; unfortunately, this responsibility has often been carried out in a perfunctory manner meeting only minimal requirements and standards.

Better defining the role of the medical director as well as strengthening and setting high standards for it is critical to improving NH care. The purpose of this chapter is to provide a brief overview of the role of the NH medical director. Those interested in more detailed information should read the books of Steven Levenson listed in the suggested readings. Many of the ideas set forth in this chapter are derived from his work and are included with his kind permission. In addition, NH medical directors should be encouraged to join the national association as well as such state or local organizations as may exist. The current address of the American Medical Directors Association (AMDA) is 10480 Little Patuxent Parkway, Suite 760, Columbia, Maryland 21044 [(301)740-9743 or (800)321-AMDA].

OVERVIEW OF THE ROLE

The specific role, responsibilities, and authority of the medical director will vary depending on a number of factors, such as those listed in Table 6-1. Politics are local, and the ratio of responsibility to authority will depend on

Table 6-1   Factors influencing the role of the medical director

Facility ownership
  (Private, nonprofit, government)

Location
  (Freestanding, hospital-based, component of a life care community)

Facility size

Administrative structure

Relationship of facility to other health care providers

Local demand for NH beds

Medical staff organization and structure
  (Formal hospital-like staff; full time versus part time; open versus closed)

Availability of primary and consultant physicians

Availability of ancillary services
  (Laboratory, radiology, etc.)

a number of these factors. The medical director of a nonproprietary facility in an area of high bed demand—with readily accessible ancillary services, an adequate supply of primary and consultant physicians, and an organized medical staff structure—will have considerable authority and leverage with respect to the medical staff. On the other hand, the medical director of a small proprietary facility in a rural community—with limited demand for NH beds, a relatively sparse physician population, and poor access to ancillary services—will have considerable responsibility but limited authority and leverage over the medical staff.

Whatever the local politics, medical directors should arrange for explicit terms of agreement with the NH owners or board of directors. Important aspects of such terms are listed in Table 6-2. The amount of time to be committed will vary depending on the size of the facility and whether or not the medical director also serves as a primary care physician. Even in the smallest facilities, the medical director should be present at least twice a month to meet with facility staff, solve problems, and carry out mandatory activities such as utilization review and quality assurance. Facilities of 100 to 200 beds should probably have a quarter-time medical director; those with more than 200 beds should have at least a half-time medical director. There are advantages and disadvantages to being a medical director who also serves as a primary care physician. The advantages are that he or she will be present in the facility more often and will get to know the staff, process, and quality of care well. The disadvantage is a potential conflict of interest between the roles of medical director and primary care physician. As discussed below, one of the key responsibilities of the medical director

Table 6-2   Important aspects of a medical director's agreement with the nursing home

Date and term of agreement

Terms of relationship (employee, contractor, etc.)

Line of reporting and authority

Job description (including privileges, rights, responsibilities, duties)

Hours per week, including a description of what is included in compensable time

Terms of compensation, including:

    Fringe benefits
    Professional liability coverage
    Rights to retain income from patient care and other revenues

Terms of renewal and termination of agreement

Source: After Levenson S (ed): *Medical Direction in Long Term Care: A Clinical and Administrative Guide.* Owings Mills, Maryland, National Health Publishing, 1988, p. 69.

is to ensure the quality of medical care; if the medical director provides primary care to a substantial proportion of the residents, a "fox guarding the chicken coop" situation can arise. The best strategy may be for the medical director to serve as primary care physician to a modest proportion of the facility's residents (e.g., 25 percent or less). Compensation for medical directors varies considerably; hourly rates range from $25 to $100 per hour and annual salaries for half- to full-time range from $45,000 to over $100,000.

Table 6-3 outlines the key responsibilities of the medical director. Each of these responsibilities is briefly discussed in the sections that follow.

Table 6-3   Key responsibilities of the nursing home medical director

Organize comprehensive medical services

Ensure that primary and consultant physicians and other health professionals fulfill their obligations to residents and the facility

Collaborate with administrators and other department heads to develop and implement appropriate policies and procedures

Monitor and attempt to continually improve the quality of medical services

Act as a spokesperson for the facility to other health care agencies and the community

Oversee an employee health program

Assist in the development, organization and presentation of educational activities for staff, residents, and families

Facilitate appropriate research

ORGANIZATION OF MEDICAL SERVICES

The diversity and complexities of medical conditions among NH residents as well as requirements for certain types of care (e.g., dental, podiatric) demand that a wide variety of medical services be available. Table 6-4 lists the types of services that NH residents should have access to. It is a fundamental responsibility of the medical director to ensure that the NH can provide or arrange for these types of services. The precise nature of these arrangements will vary considerably depending on the size and resources of the NH and the availability and accessibility of these services in the surrounding community.

With respect to primary care physicians, NHs are generally not large enough to have a full-time medical staff. Most NHs have a loosely organized panel of primary-care physicians who admit and care for residents in the facility. Frequently there are dozens of physicians involved in a single NH. This situation can create significant communication problems for the nursing staff and makes the oversight role of the medical director very difficult. In many areas there is no easy solution; there are not enough primary care physicians who have the time or interest to care for large numbers of NH residents. In addition, the NH may be dependent upon many physicians to

Table 6-4   Types of medical services needed for nursing home residents

Primary physicians	Dentistry
Consultant physicians, e.g.:	Podiatry
Cardiology	Audiology
Dermatology	Optometry
Gastroenterology	
Geriatric medicine	Pharmacy/consultant pharmacist
Gynecology	Diagnostic services
Nephrology	
Neurology	Clinical laboratory
Neurosurgery	Radiology
Oncology/hematology	Other
Ophthalmology	Ultrasonography
Otolaryngology	Noninvasive cardiovascular studies
Proctology	(Holter monitor, vascular Doppler, etc.)
Psychiatry	Pulmonary function
Pulmonary	
Radiology	Rehabilitation therapies
Rheumatology	Physical
Surgery (general)	Occupational
Urology	Speech
Vascular surgery	Prosthetics
	Respiratory therapy

admit their patients in order to fill the beds. The result is a large number of primary care physicians. Each of these cares for only a small proportion of the facility's residents, is physically present in the NH for very short periods of time, and is busy elsewhere with other activities when not in the NH. Whenever practical, NHs and medical directors should attempt to minimize the number of primary care physicians involved. While it is neither legal nor ethical to not allow NH residents their choice of a primary care physician, it may be both feasible and in the best interests of all concerned to strive to limit the number of primary care physicians involved in a particular NH. In some areas, this can be accomplished by arranging for a small group of physicians to provide most of the primary care and, if acceptable to all concerned, transferring the care of residents to this group at the time of NH admission. In some areas this type of arrangement has evolved naturally. The fewer physicians involved, the easier it will be to develop and adhere to policies, procedures, and high standards of care and the easier it will be for NH staff to develop a good rapport with the medical staff. Whatever specific arrangements are developed, the NH should have some type of written agreement from the primary care physicians that acknowledges their responsibilities to their residents as well as to the facility.

In most communities, consultant physicians in the various subspecialties—as well as dentistry, podiatry, audiology, and optometry—are available. Large NHs, especially those associated with other levels of care (e.g., life care communities), have developed subspecialty clinics that are held at the NH site. Though this requires space, some equipment, and NH staff time to assist with the clinics, it can save all the time and energy that would be required to transport residents to and from offices outside the NH. The medical director is responsible not only for ensuring that residents have access to these subspecialists but also for assuring the quality of care such consultants provide, developing appropriate documentation and communication practices, and assisting the consultants in adhering to the NHs policies and procedures with respect to resident care.

The medical director is also responsible for helping the NH to obtain and assure the quality of other resident care services. A well-organized pharmacy and experienced pharmacy consultants are critical to high-quality medical care in the NH. Many pharmacies have developed a NH specialty or are totally dedicated to providing services for NHs. The medical director must work closely with the pharmacy as well as the nursing staff to ensure the appropriate prescription and delivery of drugs. This is generally accomplished through the pharmacy committee (see below, under "Quality Assurance," and Chap. 21). The ready availability of several types of diagnostic services (listed in Table 6-4) is also critical to high-quality medical care. Some bioclinical laboratories, like pharmacies, have developed a specialty in providing services to NHs. These types of laboratories can be especially helpful because of their familiarity with the process of care in the NH, and many provide both in-service training and assistance with infection control. Portable radiology services are generally available in most areas. In some cities, services that perform other diagnostic testing, such as ultrasonography and noninvasive cardiovascular studies, will come to the NH. As discussed in Chap. 5, these services are essential for the NH's ability to assess and manage acute and subacute conditions. It may be practical and administratively and financially advantageous in some settings for the NH to contract for these services with a local acute care hospital that looks after the NH's residents when they become acutely ill. Whatever specific arrangements are made, the medical director is responsible for developing policies and procedures relating to the communication and documentation of results of diagnostic tests and for monitoring the utilization of the diagnostic services. Ancillary services that are critical for the quality of life of NH residents, such as dentistry, podiatry, and optometry, must be provided. Finally, several types of therapies are essential for NH residents. In addition to the traditional physical, occupational, and speech therapies and the related prosthetic services (e.g., braces, splints, special shoes, prostheses, etc.), respiratory therapy can be extremely valuable in managing subacutely ill residents. Respiratory therapists can help the nursing staff to oversee oxygen therapy, provide respiratory treatments (e.g., nebulized bronchodilators), monitor oxygenation, perform pulmonary function tests and test arterial blood gases, and assist in obtaining sputum specimens. Although the medical director may not be responsible for overseeing these therapeutic services, he or she must work with the director of nurses and administrator to assure their availability, quality, and appropriate utilization.

POLICY AND PROCEDURE DEVELOPMENT

The medical director must work collaboratively with the administrator, director of nursing, and other NH staff to develop, implement, and oversee adherence to appropriate policies and procedures. Obviously, just because policies and procedures exist does not ensure that they will be followed or that a high quality of care is being provided. But written policies and procedures offer several important advantages. First, they help to establish and communicate the medical director's and NH's expectations of the medical staff and services. Second, they assist in the development of specific standards of care. Third, they document these expectations and standards in writing, making it difficult for medical or other staff to evade responsibility for knowing what is expected of them. Finally, written policies and procedures are helpful in demonstrating to regulatory bodies that the facility has thought through specific approaches to various areas of care.

A wide variety of policies and procedures relating to medical care and the role of the medical director should be developed. Table 6-5 lists several

Table 6-5   Examples of policies and procedures

General policies
    Medical department and staff organization
    Job descriptions (e.g., physician's assistants,
       nurse practitioners, assistant medical director)

Admissions, discharges, transfers

Standards for primary and consultant physicians

Communications with nursing and other staff
    Physician notification for acute and subacute
      changes in resident status
    Physician responsiveness

Documentation
    Admission data base
    Periodic progress notes
    Medical record organization
    Physician orders
    Incident reports

Laboratory services and other diagnostic testing

Health maintenance (see Chap. 4)
    Screening
    Monitoring
    Preventive practices

Infection control and the use of antimicrobials
  (see Chap. 17)

Medication prescribing (see Chap. 21)
    General
    Psychotropics
    Antimicrobials

Specific medical care issues, e.g.:
    Pressure sores
    Incontinence management
    Indwelling catheter use and care
    Assessment of cognitive and affective status
    Rehabilitation, including gait and mobility
      assessment
    Nutrition and hydration
    Enteral feeding

Ethical issues (see Chap. 25)
    Assessment of decision-making capacity
    Determination of treatment status (i.e., DNR
      orders, etc.)

Employee health
    Preemployment examinations
    Annual examinations
    Accidents, injuries, workmen's compensation

specific examples. As indicated in the table, many of these policies and procedures are discussed in other chapters. New federal rules related to NH care (OBRA, 1987) will make the development of many such policies an essential role for the medical director. A summary of OBRA and specific examples of policies and procedures are included in the Appendix.

QUALITY ASSURANCE

The medical director is responsible for monitoring and continually attempting to improve the quality of medical services. Quality assurance is a complex activity, and quality assurance programs in NHs are generally not well developed. The OBRA legislation mandates that there be an active quality assurance program in every NH. In this chapter, we will provide a brief overview of quality assurance as it relates to medical care in the NH. More detailed descriptions of quality assurance programs can be found in the suggested readings at the end of the chapter.

Quality assurance in general focuses on three aspects of care: structure, process, and outcome. In a NH, this requires a multidisciplinary and interdisciplinary approach; all levels of staff—including the administrator, the directors of the medical and nursing departments, social services, pharmacy, dietary, housekeeping, and maintenance—must be involved. Structural considerations target the adequacy and safety of the physical environment. Most quality assurance activities tend to focus on the process of care. Assessing process is tedious and, in fact, sometimes boring; it has been overemphasized to the point of creating a lot of unnecessary paperwork that probably detracts from rather than enhances the quality of care. But some focus on process is necessary, especially in the NH, where standards of care are generally low and many procedures, such as simple medical documentation, are done poorly. Recent federal regulations have begun to emphasize the importance of assessing outcomes of care. In general, outcomes relevant to medical care include physiologic status, ability to perform the activities of daily living, pain, cognition, affect, social activities and interactions, satisfaction with care and environment, and quality of life. The technology to assess some of these outcomes (e.g., physiologic status, cognition) is reasonably well developed, but for others (e.g., pain, quality of life) is far from adequate. Although some research is in progress, much more is needed to develop valid and reliable measures of outcomes that are important for NH residents. In addition, because of the heterogeneity of the NH population, "good" outcomes must be viewed in the context of the overall goals of care for individual residents. For example, a good outcome for a resident admitted to the NH for rehabilitation after a hip fracture (independent ambulation and discharge home) may be inappropriate and irrelevant to a resident admitted to the NH with a terminal malignancy or end-stage dementia whose family can no longer care for him or her at home.

Table 6-6 presents a basic approach to quality assurance. In general, quality assurance involves selecting areas of interest to assess, developing standards for performance on outcomes, designing methods of measurement, collecting and analyzing data, identifying problems and solutions, and monitoring. In the NH, these activities are usually carried out through various committees. Most facilities have several committees that address quality assurance issues, including utilization review, pharmacy, and infection control. Utilization review committees are charged with evaluating the use of medical services, reviewing hospitalizations and admissions, and certifying residents for Medicare coverage. Periodic (usually annual) medical care evaluation studies are mandated in most areas and are generally presented in the utilization review committee. The scope of these studies is very broad, but they should focus on some aspects of care relevant to quality assurance. The pharmacy committee oversees the prescription, administration, documentation, and monitoring of drug therapy in the facility. Many strategies can be helpful in improving drug therapy in the NH; they are discussed further in Chap. 21. The infection control committee is responsible for reviewing surveillance data on infections that occur in the facility and for developing, implementing, and monitoring policies and procedures related to infectious diseases. Infections and infection control are discussed in detail in Chap. 17. Some examples of quality assurance activities include (1) identifying residents with low hemoglobin levels and determining if they have been evaluated appropriately; (2) determining if depression has been iden-

Table 6-6   Basic approaches to quality assurance

Develop, approve, and adopt broad principles, goals, and objectives for a quality-assurance program

Select areas of interest, including process and outcomes

Develop standards, criteria, and measuring tools

Collect data

Analyze and summarize the data

Identify problems and trends

Develop strategies to deal with problems and trends

Provide feedback to staff

Implement policies and procedures to correct problems

Reevaluate and provide feedback on problem resolution

tified and treated; (3) examining the appropriateness of drug prescription (e.g., antimicrobials, psychotropics); and (4) determining if recurrent fallers receive appropriate evaluation.

COMMUNITY RELATIONS

The medical director should act as a spokesperson for the NH to the community. Nursing homes often have a bad reputation both within and outside the medical community. The medical director has a responsibility to attempt to improve the image of the NH through informal and formal discussions with colleagues, health care agencies, and the general public. The NH's essential role in society and families' appropriate expections for care in the NH should be emphasized. Invitations to visit the facility might be extended to interested parties so that they can get a better understanding of the type and quality of care provided in the NH.

The medical director should also represent the facility to other health care providers in the community. This involves not only those listed in Table 6-4 but also local acute care hospitals, home care agencies, and other providers of long-term health care services. Appropriate policies and procedures for resident care should be mutually agreed upon (see Table 6-5), and strategies for effective communication and documentation should be developed. Some relevant examples that may be helpful to medical directors are provided in the Appendix.

EMPLOYEE HEALTH

The medical director is generally responsible for overseeing an employee health program for the NH. This basically involves three activities: (1) an initial health assessment (i.e., a preemployment history and physical examination), (2) periodic reassessment (usually an annual one is required), and (3) evaluation of injuries and in some cases workmen's compensation claims. Some medical directors incorporate the NH's employee health program into their own general practice, while others arrange for other physicians to do the examinations. Nurse practitioners and physician's assistants can play an important role in the employee health program (see Chap. 7). Workmen's compensation issues are often handled by outside entities, either through a union or other arrangements made by the facility. One consideration about employee health in the NH setting is worthy of further discussion. In many areas of the country, a large proportion of NH staff, especially nurses' aides, comprises recent immigrants and/or individuals of relatively low socioeconomic status. In addition, many licensed nurses are now being recruited from abroad. These characteristics of NH staff give rise to a whole set of health issues of which the medical director must be aware. These range from immunization status to the potential for communicable disease to alcohol and drug abuse. If the medical director is not familiar with these areas, he or she should seek consultation from others who can help in setting policies and procedures for the facility's employee health program.

EDUCATION AND RESEARCH

Teaching programs and research are critical to improving NH care. An increasing number of schools for health professionals are establishing affiliations with local NHs for teaching and research purposes. The medical director should facilitate the development of such affiliations and, where appropriate, become a faculty member at the school. In addition to teaching programs related to academic institutions, the medical director should be involved in the education of all levels of NH staff as well as that of residents and their families. The nature of research in the NH will increasingly involve more NHs in order to obtain adequate sample sizes, especially for clinical studies addressing issues important to typical community NHs. The support of medical directors will therefore become increasingly important to the success of NH research. Specific strategies to enhance the success of academic programs in the NH setting are discussed further in Chap. 26. The medical director must also continually educate himself or herself to keep current in geriatric medicine and administrative and regulatory issues related to long-term care.

SUGGESTED READINGS

Chambers LW: Promoting long term care quality assurance: Strategies used in Europe and North America. Danish Med Bull No. 5:21–28, 1987 (Special Supplement Series).

Donabedian A: The quality of care JAMA 260:1743–1748, 1988.

Fanale JE: The nursing home medical director. J Am Geriatr Soc 37:369–375, 1989.

Institute of Medicine. Improving the Quality of Care in Nursing Homes. Washington, DC, National Academy Press, 1986.

Joint Commission of Accreditation of Healthcare Organizations: Quality Assurance in Long Term Care. Chicago, Illinois, JCAHO, 1986.

Levenson S (ed): Medical Direction in Long Term Care. Baltimore, Maryland, National Health Publishing, 1988.

Levenson SA and Tarnove L (eds): Medical Director's Policy and Procedure Manual. Baltimore, Maryland, National Health Publishing, 1990.

Mohide EA, Tugwell P, Caulfield PA, et al: A randomized trial of quality assurance in nursing homes. Med Care 26:554–565, 1988.

Zimmer JG: Quality assurance, in Katz P, Calkins E (eds): Principles and Practice of Nursing Home Care. New York, Springer, pp. 91–112, 1989.

SEVEN

THE ROLE OF THE NURSE PRACTITIONER
AND PHYSICIAN'S ASSISTANT

Nurse practitioners (NPs) and physician's assistants (PAs) should play an increasing role in nursing home (NH) care over the next several years. Recent federal legislation allows for both types of providers to bill Medicare for services they provide in the NH and, importantly, allows services to be provided without on-site physician supervision. Although clinical service, especially the initial assessment of acute conditions, will probably be the predominant activity, NPs and PAs can potentially play a number of roles in the NH setting that will lead to improvements in medical care as well as interdisciplinary communication. At least three studies have documented that NPs can play an important role in improving the outcomes of NH residents. No studies have specially examined the impact of PAs in the NH, but their clinical training is clearly compatible with the role of a clinician in the NH setting. Our experience in NHs has been predominantly with NPs. NPs appear to us to have one important advantage: their background in nursing. Many of the day-to-day issues that arise in the care of NH residents are nursing-oriented, and much of the care depends on effective communication between the nursing staff and primary-care physicians. In our experience, the NPs' nursing background has been critical in their roles in the NH and has enabled them to act as effective liaisons between the nursing and medical staffs. Whether NPs or PAs are employed, their success is critically dependent on their ability to interact in a nonthreatening manner with the nursing staff and other members of the interdisciplinary team and on clearly defined roles, responsibilities, clinical privileges, and place within the organizational structure of the facility.

ROLES AND RESPONSIBILITIES

The NPs and PAs on a NH's staff can participate in a number of different clinical, administrative, educational, and research activities (Table 7-1). The extent of their participation will depend on a number of factors, including their qualifications and experience, who hires them, how they fit into the organizational structure of the facility, and the policies and extent of activities (e.g., educational, research) within the facility.

Clinical activities will be the basis of the NP's or PA's role and responsibilities in the vast majority of settings. These responsibilities can range from serving as a primary care provider in conjunction with the physician, to the assessment and management of acute and subacute conditions, to serving as a consultant to the interdisciplinary team and family members. With respect to primary care, the NP or PA can perform admission and readmission assessments, carefully documenting baseline findings, problems, and goals. He or she can also perform some of the required periodic visits as well as annual reassessments in conjunction with the primary-care physician. With respect to consultant activities, the NP or PA can play an integral role in establishing and participating in clinics for the evaluation of specific conditions (such as dementia, incontinence, and recurrent falls) or others that oversee the management of common chronic problems such as diabetes and hypertension. The NP or PA can also serve as a valuable consultant to the interdisciplinary team and family members, especially since most primary care physicians spend limited time at the facility. The NP or PA can explain the medical regimen and the rationale for it; discuss the results of diagnostic tests and their implications; and assist the team, the resident, and the family in developing realistic expectations and goals of care. Most primary care physicians do not have enough time to spend on these important discussions. The NP or PA can therefore play a critical role in enhancing communication and establishing the medical care plan.

Perhaps the most important clinical role and responsibility of the NP or PA is to assess acute changes in status and oversee the management of subacute problems in the NH. In the absence of NPs and PAs, the vast majority of acute problems are evaluated over the telephone, frequently result in an emergency room visit, and too often lead to a costly and unnecessary hospitalization. Although many factors influence decisions as to whether or not to hospitalize a NH resident (see Chap. 5), the availability of an on-site NP or PA will clearly decrease the likelihood that an unnecessary and expensive emergency room visit will occur. Many acute and subacute conditions can be assessed and managed in a typical community NH by a NP or PA. Protocols are available and others can be developed that are mutually acceptable to the medical director, medical staff, nursing staff, and NH administration. These protocols are discussed further under "Clinical Privileges and Protocols," below.

Table 7-1 Potential roles and responsibilities for nurse practitioners and physicians' assistants

Clinical
    Primary care (in conjunction with primary physician)
    Admission and readmission assessments
    Periodic (e.g., annual) medical and functional assessments
    Assessment of acute changes in status
    Management of subacute illness
    Participation in discharge planning at acute care hospital
    Consultant
    1. Organize and participate in special clinics

        Dementia
        Incontinence
        Falls
        Other (e.g., diabetes, hypertension)

    2. Serve as consultant to interdisciplinary team and family members

        Explain medical care regimens and diagnostic test results
        Discuss ethical issues
        Assist in the development of mutually acceptable, realistic expectations and goals of care

Administrative

    Participate in interdisciplinary team meetings

    Participate in medical and nursing staff committees and meetings

    Assist in the development of policies, procedures, and protocols

    Assist the medical director in administering an employee health program

    Participate in quality assurance activities

        Review and ensure appropriate documentation in progress notes and problem lists
        Assist in the implementation and completion of screening, health maintenance, and preventive protocols (see Chap. 4)
        Perform selected quality assurance audits
        Serve on institutional committees (e.g., infection control, pharmacy)

Educational

    Participate in the in-service education program for nursing staff

    Make presentations to residents and families

    Participate in undergraduate education programs for medical and nursing students

    Participate in graduate education programs for medical residents, geriatric medicine fellows, master's nursing students, and nurse practitioner trainees

    Represent the facility at community educational programs

Research

    Consult with investigators on the design of protocols to be implemented in the facility

    Facilitate the implementation of approved studies

    Assist with data collection (time should be supported by research funds if appropriate)

    Design and conduct independent clinical research projects

NPs and PAs can also play an important role in a variety of administrative activities (Table 7-1). They may be especially valuable in working with nursing staff to develop and implement policies and procedures related to medical and nursing care, such as "Immediate versus Nonimmediate Physician Notification" (see Appendix). The NP and PA staff can also play a critical role in the employee health program by performing on-site initial assessments of illness and injury. This may save the facility's compensation plan a considerable amount of money by reducing the number of emergency room and physician visits made by employees. The NPs and PAs can also play an important role in a variety of medical quality assurance activities (Table 7-1).

In facilities with active educational and research programs, appropriately qualified and experienced NPs and PAs can be active participants in enhancing these programs. All facilities have in-service programs for staff, and the NP or PA can assist in the development of curricula and in making selected presentations. The NP and PA can also make valuable contributions to the undergraduate and graduate education of physicians and nurses in facilities with university affiliations. Many NPs and PAs may qualify for appointments at the university's nursing or medical school. If the facility serves as a site for clinical research, the NP or PA can assist investigators in the development of appropriate protocols for the NH setting and facilitate the implementation of the research, especially by serving as a liaison between the investigators and the medical and nursing staff. Some NPs and PAs may want to design and conduct their own research projects or participate actively in projects being implemented at the facility. Whenever appropriate, time spent by NPs and PAs on funded research projects should be supported by research funds.

CLINICAL PRIVILEGES AND PROTOCOLS

No matter what the precise roles and responsibilities of the NP or PA in a particular NH may be, a specific set of clinical privileges and protocols should be developed, in addition to a complete job description.

Whether or not state laws require the NP or PA to have an explicit written agreement with a supervising physician, a list of clinical privileges should be developed and agreed upon by the NP or PA, the medical director, members of the medical staff who work collaboratively with the NP or PA, the director of nursing, and the facility administrator. This list of privileges serves to clarify for everyone involved what the NP or PA is qualified to do independently and what activities require consultation with the medical director or supervising physician. An example of a list of clinical privileges is included in the Appendix.

Clinical protocols are also a valuable tool in clearly defining the general approach that NPs or PAs will take toward their clinical care activities. As discussed in Chap. 4, the medical director and primary medical staff should develop standardized approaches to admission, readmission, and periodic (e.g., monthly, annual) assessments, which the NP or PA can use as guidelines in carrying out these activities. Examples of such data bases are illustrated in Table 4-2 for the monthly progress note and in the Appendix for admission and annual assessments. Examples of clinical protocols for the evaluation of five common acute conditions—fever, change in mental status, dyspnea, abdominal pain, and gastrointestinal bleeding—are illustrated in Figs. 7-1 through 7-5.

PLACE WITHIN THE FACILITY'S ORGANIZATIONAL STRUCTURE

In order for NPs or PAs to function effectively in a NH setting, their place within the facility's organizational structure must be clearly defined. There

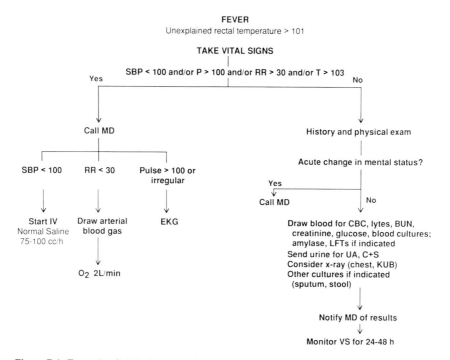

Figure 7-1 Example of clinical protocol for use by NPs or PAs in the assessment and management of fever in the NH.

ACUTE ABDOMINAL PAIN

Symptoms: Sudden onset of diffuse or localized abdominal pain with or
without nausea/vomiting/diarrhea

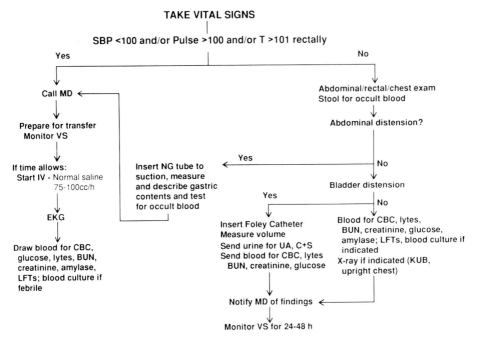

Figure 7-2 Example of clinical protocol for use by NPs or PAs in the assessment and management of acute abdominal pain in the NH.

are a number of different possibilities, but some general principles should be adhered to. First, irrespective of who the employer is, NPs or PAs should have a written job description that clearly defines their roles and responsibilities and refers to the clinical privileges and protocols discussed above. Second, the job description should be reviewed and approved by the medical director, director of nursing, and administrator of the facility. Third, the clinical supervision and performance evaluations must be done by an appropriately qualified individual; administrators and directors of nursing should be responsible for supervision and performance evaluation only if they themselves are qualified and experienced NPs, PAs, or MDs. Finally, it is very important to clearly separate the role and responsibilities of the NP or PA from those of the licensed nursing staff. This is especially critical in facilities where there is a shortage of licensed nurses.

In our experience, NPs have functioned most effectively when they are

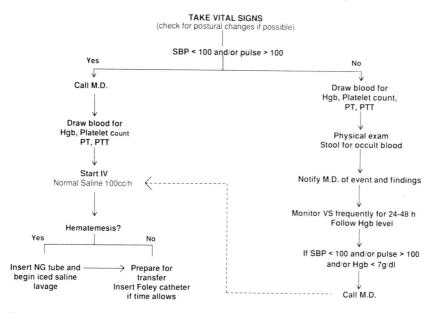

GASTROINTESTINAL BLEEDING
Symptoms: Resident or staff report hematemesis, tarry stool and/or red blood per rectum

TAKE VITAL SIGNS
(check for postural changes if possible)

SBP < 100 and/or pulse > 100

Figure 7-3 Example of clinical protocol for use by NPs or PAs in the assessment and management of gastrointestinal bleeding in the NH.

basically considered active members of the primary medical staff, limited only by their clinical privilege statement. Figure 7-6 illustrates the way in which the NP or PA fits into the facility's organizational structure under two different employment conditions—employed by the facility or employed by a physician or group of physicians.

EMPLOYMENT AND SALARY CONSIDERATIONS

The employer of the NP or PA is generally a facility, a physician, or a group of physicians. Joint employment by the facility and a physician or physician group is possible but would probably make things unnecessarily complicated. As mentioned earlier, recent legislation enables NPs and PAs to bill Medicare directly for services they provide in NHs at 85 percent of the rate for physicians. When NPs or PAs bill, however, the physician cannot also request reimbursement for the same activity. Whether NPs or PAs bill Medicare directly or their services are billed for by the facility or a physician or physician group, net clinical revenues are unlikely to support their entire

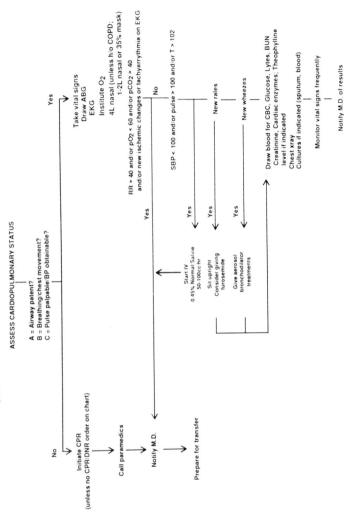

Figure 7-4 Example of clinical protocol for use by NPs or PAs in the assessment and management of acute dyspnea in the NH.

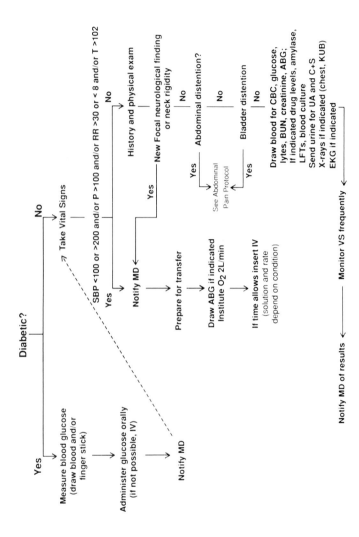

ACUTE MENTAL STATUS CHANGE

Symptoms: Delirium, lethargy, disorientation, psychomotor agitation, psychosis (delusions, hallucinations)

Diabetic?

Yes — Measure blood glucose (draw blood and/or finger stick) → Administer glucose orally (if not possible, IV) → Notify MD

No — Take Vital Signs

SBP <100 or >200 and/or P >100 and/or RR >30 or < 8 and/or T >102

Yes — Notify MD → Prepare for transfer → Draw ABG if indicated / Institute O₂ 2L/min → If time allows insert IV (solution and rate depend on condition)

No — History and physical exam

New Focal neurological finding or neck rigidity

Yes — Notify MD

No — Abdominal distention?

Yes — See Abdominal Pain Protocol

No — Bladder distention

Yes — Draw blood for CBC, glucose, lytes, BUN, creatinine, ABG; If indicated drug levels, amylase, LFTs, blood culture / Send urine for UA and C+S / X-rays if indicated (chest, KUB) / EKG if indicated

No —

Notify MD of results ← Monitor VS frequently

Figure 7-5 Example of clinical protocol for use by NPs or PAs in the assessment and management of an acute change in mental status in the NH.

87

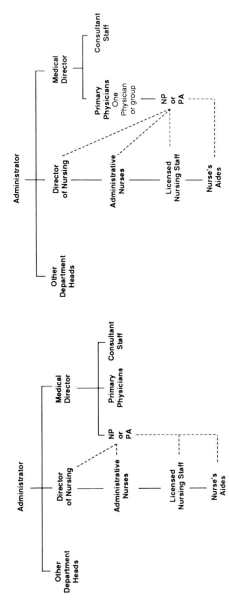

Figure 7-6 The place of the NP or PA in the organizational structure of an NH. Solid lines imply direct supervision and lines of reporting. Dotted lines refer to frequent interaction on clinical and administrative issues. In the diagram on the left, the NP or PA is employed by the facility; in the diagram on the right, she/he is employed by a physician or group of physicians who provide primary care at the facility.

salary and benefits. In the Los Angeles area, NPs are earning in the area of $35,000 and up at the entry level to close to $50,000 if they are highly qualified and experienced. Thus, creative methods of supplementing clinical revenues from the NH must be developed. In some cases, the NH will support part of the salary through its nursing and/or administrative budget. Similarly, a physician or physician group may support part of the salary from other income. If NPs or PAs do not spend full time at the NH, they may engage in other revenue-generating activities (e.g., clinical practice in a geriatric clinic or other geriatric program). Other possibilities are partial support from an affiliated acute care hospital for participating in discharge planning and quality assurance activities related to geriatric care or from a funded research project.

SUGGESTED READINGS

Garrard J, Kane RL, Radosevich DM, et al: Impact of geriatric nurse practitioners on nursing-home residents' functional status, satisfaction, and discharge outcomes. *Med Care* 28:271–283, 1990.

Kane RL, Garrard J, Skay CL, et al: Effects of a geriatric nurse practitioner on process and outcome of nursing home care. *Am J Pub Health* 79:1271, 1989.

Kane RL, Garrard J, Buchanan J, et al: The geriatric nurse practitioner as a nursing home employee: Conceptual and methodological issues in assessing quality of care and cost effectiveness, in Mezey MD, Lynaugh JE, and Cartier MM (eds): *Nursing Homes and Nursing Care: Lessons from the Teaching Nursing Homes.* New York, Springer, 1989.

Kane RA, Kane RL, Arnold S, et al: Geriatric nurse practitioners as nursing home employees: Implementing the role. *Gerontologist* 28:469–477, 1988.

Martin SE, Turner CL, Mendelsohn SE, et al: Assessment and initial management of acute medical problems in a nursing home, in Bosker G (ed): *Principles and Practice of Acute Geriatric Medicine*, 2d ed. St. Louis, Mosby, 1990.

Wieland D, Rubenstein LZ, Ouslander JG, et al: Organizing an academic nursing home. *JAMA* 255:2622–2627, 1986.

INTERDISCIPLINARY TEAMS

The use of the team approach has become part of the essence of geriatrics. Interdisciplinary teams were originally developed in missionary hospitals in the 1920s and were academized by the team developed by physiatrists at Montefiore Hospital in New York in the 1940s. Interdisciplinary teams represent a coordinated effort by a number of health professionals to develop a shared treatment plan for a given patient. They differ from the classical multidisciplinary approach of health care delivery where a physician makes all decisions for the patient, utilizing the services of others as consultants. Central to the interdisciplinary team approach is the concept that the sharing of information by all the health professionals caring for the patient will lead to better management decisions.

When interdisciplinary teams originally developed in missionary hospitals, there was a shortage of available physician time, forcing other members of the health care team to shoulder more responsibilities. Similarly, in America, the greatest cohesiveness and success of interdisciplinary teams have been in situations where there is less physician availability, such as in the nursing home (NH). Despite the general acceptance of the importance of the interdisciplinary team approach, there is no objective study demonstrating that formal interdisciplinary teams either improve the care of NH residents or are cost-effective.

POTENTIAL FUNCTIONS OF INTERDISCIPLINARY TEAMS

Interdisciplinary teams serve several purposes and can have multiple functions (Table 8-1). The first purpose of the interdisciplinary team is to allow the sharing of specialized information between health professionals of differing backgrounds. Thus, for example, the team allows the physical therapist to communicate the importance of the nursing staff's active involvement in ongoing physical therapy programs. The dietician may be able to highlight the severity of malnutrition in a resident and stress the need for encouraging her or him to complete all meals. The occupational therapist can work with the nursing staff to develop a program designed to assess and improve activities of daily living. The physician or pharmacist may share with other members of the team information about the specific potential side effects of a drug.

The second purpose of the interdisciplinary team is the sharing of different viewpoints of the resident experienced by different members of the team. This can be particularly useful in assessing the resident's motivation. It can also help to ensure that a quiet resident is not ignored.

The third purpose of the interdisciplinary team is to facilitate a unified approach to residents with behavioral problems. It is essential that team members agree to not allow a resident to play one team member against another. In these cases it is also important that all team members impart the same information to the resident on key issues, such as an impending discharge, setting limits on behavioral disorders, and the prognosis and management of a specific clinical condition.

A fourth purpose of the interdisciplinary team is to evaluate the rehabilitation potential of the resident. Coupled with this is the fifth purpose, which is to evaluate the discharge potential and make discharge plans for residents when appropriate. Clearly, multiple inputs including the social workers' assessment of the resident's social situation, the knowledge derived from a home visit by the occupational therapist, and the input of

Table 8-1   Functions of interdisciplinary teams

Sharing of specialized knowledge between team members from different backgrounds
Obtaining a composite view of the resident
Development of a unified approach to residents with behavioral problems
Evaluation of rehabilitation potential
Evaluation of the potential for the resident to return to noninstitutional living
Resolution of interpersonal conflicts
Formal and mutual education
Discussion of administrative issues
Acting as part of the facility's quality assurance program
Alleviation of caregiver stress
Development of a comprehensive individualized plan of care (see Tables 8-2 and 8-3)

those who see the resident's functioning throughout the 24-h period are all essential in order to determine whether the resident is capable of returning home.

The sixth purpose of the interdisciplinary team is to give the team members an opportunity to resolve interpersonal conflicts. This is an extremely important part of teamwork, and time should always be allocated to explore perceived and potential conflicts at team meetings.

The seventh purpose of the interdisciplinary team is to provide an opportunity for formal education for the group as a whole. The team meeting is a time when new information about management of nursing home (NH) residents with interdisciplinary implications can be shared by the group. An example might be data indicating that blood pressure can drop after meals and cause falls. The team meeting is also an excellent time to share articles or recent data on specific management problems with the group as a whole.

The eighth purpose of the interdisciplinary team is to share thoughts on administrative policies and procedures and also to help enforce old ones. The team meeting can also be a time when problems with administration can be fully explored.

The ninth purpose of the interdisciplinary team is to provide a part of the quality assurance program of the facility. For this reason, careful and accurate recording of both the team's plans and also the outcome of these plans is essential.

The final purpose of the team is to help alleviate caregiver stress. If the team is carrying out the first nine functions adequately, this goes a long way toward alleviating caregiver stress. In some cases the expertise of a psychologist may be necessary to diffuse stress among the members of the team.

In summary, the major functions of an interdisciplinary team involve improved communication and development of specific management plans as well as mutual education and a method of alleviating caregiver stress. An example of an individualized plan of care developed by an interdisciplinary team is given in Table 8-2.

COMPOSITION OF INTERDISCIPLINARY TEAMS

The development of the appropriate composition of the interdisciplinary team depends on the needs of the resident population to be served and the goals the team wishes to achieve. The core team always includes members of the nursing staff. Beyond this, there is no agreement on the optimal composition of the interdisciplinary team. A review of 200 health care teams suggests that almost as many disciplines can be involved as there are teams. While most texts include the physician as part of the core team, the physician is not an essential member of all interdisciplinary teams in the NH

Table 8-2 Example of an interdisciplinary care plan

Original date	Problem	Goals	Target date	Approaches	Discussion[a]	Assessments
8/20/90	Incontinent of urine	Resident will be continent during the day	9/20/90	Toilet every 2–4 h	NSG	
				Place resident on bedpan every 4 h at night or place bedpan in bed with resident		
				Rearrange room to provide access to bathroom	NSG	
					Hskp	
					NSG	
					NP	
				Assess urine for infection	MD	
					NSG	
				Catheterize for residual to rule out urinary retention	MD	
					NP	
8/20/90	Inability to dress and groom self	Resident will have clothing on correctly with snaps, buttons, etc., in place	9/20/90	Refer to therapies	MD	
					NP	
					OT	
				Assess ADL skills		
				Provide easy access to toilet articles	NSG	
				Teach resident techniques for self-help	OT	
					PT	
				Provide resident with assistive devices as necessary	OT	
					PT	
					NSG	
8/15/90	Edema, both feet	Edema will decrease in one month	9/20/90	Elevate feet while sitting	NSG	
				Limit intake of high sodium foods	MD	
					RD	
		Resident will not develop venous stasis ulcers		Monitor weekly weights	NSG	
				Diuretics if indicated		
				ROM exercises, every shift	NSG	

8/1/90	Does not attend recreational group programs	Resident will attend two programs every month	Ongoing	Investigate possibility of volunteer to visit once a week	ACT
				Staff visitation once a week to help develop hobbies, interests	ACT NP ACT NSG
				Encourage family visitation	SW
8/1/90	Poor hygiene	Resident will have showers twice a week and bed bath three times a week	Ongoing	Assess ability to perform independently	NSG
				Maintain privacy	NSG
				Assist resident as necessary with bath using mild soap and warm water	NSG
8/1/90	Tendency toward constipation	Resident will have normal bowel movements at least four times a week	Ongoing	Provide high fiber diet, include prune juice, bran cereal, wheat breads, and fresh vegetables daily	RD NP
				1 tablespoon bran in orange juice or applesauce daily	NP NSG
				Promote exercise if feasible	OT PT MD
				Encourage fluids	NSG
				Meds as ordered	MD
8/1/91	Inability to transfer	Resident will be able to transfer self and be independent in wheelchair mobility	10/30/90	Exercises three times a week for balance and muscle strengthening	PT MD
				Passive and active ROM all extremities every shift	NSG
				Assist with transfers and use of wheelchair twice daily	PT NSG

[a] NSG = nursing; Hskp = housekeeping; NP = nurse practitioner; MD = physician; OT = occupational therapy; PT = physical therapy; RD = dietition; ACT = activities director; SW = social worker.

setting. The major focus of an interdisciplinary team should be on the functional, social, dietary, and psychological needs of the resident. In this case, the nurse, or—ideally, if available—the nurse practitioner or physician's assistant can substitute for the physician. This often results in an appropriately less medicalized care plan. It is essential, however, that the physician review this care plan.

In the nursing home the key members of the interdisciplinary team are the nurses and/or nurse's aides, dietician, physical and occupational therapists, social worker, and recreation therapist. The physician can act as a consultant to this team. The golden rule of teams should be remembered: The smaller the team, the more functional it is likely to be. Larger teams often have increased interpersonal conflicts.

A team meeting that we have found particularly useful for handling the medical problems of residents includes the physician, registered nurse, nurse specialist (e.g., mental health nurse) and nurse practitioner and/or physician assistant. In a large NH (150 or more beds), a weekly meeting of this team can rapidly review medical problems of residents and make appropriate management decisions. This team format is also an excellent educational vehicle. Another advantage of utilizing this team is it separates the discussions of medical problems from the recreational, rehabilitation, and psychological needs of the resident. This prevents the medicalization of the regular NH interdisciplinary team meeting.

A number of other professionals such as pharmacists, medical specialists, and dentists can act as consultants to the team.

Team leadership is often a problem. In traditional teams, the physician uses the authority of his or her position to be the leader. However, many teams function much better when another member of the team assumes the leadership role. The concept of allowing all team members equal opportunity for participation and thus to spread responsibility for decisions to all team members can lead to a healthy work situation. Leadership can be shifted depending on which team member has the most knowledge in a particular situation. In all team meetings, a team recorder should be designated; he or she should be responsible for maintaining a record of all team decisions. The recorder should not be the team leader, as this can result in incomplete and in some cases biased recording.

RESIDENTS, FAMILY MEMBERS, AND THE TEAM

It can be very useful for a NH resident (or a designated family member if the resident is not capable) to be invited to be part of the nonmedical interdisciplinary team meeting. To prevent this becoming a situation of "misplaced hospitality," the resident and/or family member needs to be aware of and adhere to certain rules, such as the following: (1) the discussion will be time-limited; (2) negative comments may be made about the resident, which may be upsetting; (3) the resident and/or family member is a guest and will act predominantly as an observer; and (4) explanations of the discussion will be given to the resident and/or family member by individual team members after the meeting and should not be expected to be provided during the meeting. Some feel strongly that residents and family members should not be included in team meetings. Many staff members find the inclusion of residents or relatives threatening and find it difficult to have a frank discussion under these circumstances. Careful education, which is sensitive to the staff's feelings, can often overcome this problem. Teams that include the resident and family may, in fact, fail to reduce caregiver stress because they do not allow the staff to vent their feelings fully.

TEAM DEVELOPMENT AND MAINTENANCE

The first task of an interdisciplinary team is to develop rules of procedure and define the areas over which the team has authority. It is important to realize that decisions can be made unanimously, by consensus, through majority vote, by unilateral decision of the person with the authority (e.g., administrator, director of nursing, or medical director), or through failure of the group to form an adequate response. In certain circumstances each of these processes may be appropriate.

When conflict occurs in the team, it must be recognized and openly discussed. The team should not take sides but rather attempt to find an acceptable compromise. When this is not possible, there should at least be a full discussion of the confrontation, with a review of both the facts and feelings involved. It is important that conflicts be resolved without compromising the major functions of the team.

Table 8-3 lists the major dynamic techniques involved in allowing an interdisciplinary team to complete its functions. Numerous different behav-

Table 8-3 Dynamic techniques necessary for successful functioning of interdisciplinary teams

1. Informative questions and reports
2. Opinions solicited and opinions given
3. Elaborations on 1 and 2
4. Coordination to see that all are given an opportunity to participate in 1 through 3
5. Enumeration of all problems
6. Evaluation and criticism of information and problems
7. Development of solutions to problems
8. Encouragement of team members
9. Maintenance of time schedule
10. Recognition and solution of conflict
11. Distribution of specific tasks
12. Recording of problems and team decisions

iors can help to facilitate these roles. When team functions are being completed, minor disagreements should be ignored. It is important to see that one member of the team is not isolated from the rest of the team because of personality conflicts. When teams become truly dysfunctional, it may be helpful to obtain consultation from a team facilitator. Such a consultant can assess the dynamics of the team and attempt to solve problems by meeting with both individual team members and the whole team. When caregiver stress is particularly high, the services of a psychologist to provide group therapy may be extremely useful.

SUGGESTED READINGS

Cole KD, Jones FA: Interdisciplinary teams for the solution of nutritional problems, in Morley JE, Glick Z, Rubenstein LZ (eds): *Geriatric Nutrition: A Comprehensive Review*. New York, Raven Press, 1990, pp 457–470.

Evans MK: Multidisciplinary teams in geriatric wards: Myth or reality. *J Adv Nurs* 6:205, 1981.

Foley CJ, Libow LS, Charatan FB: The team approach to geriatric care, in Hazzard WR, Andres R, Bierman EL, Blass JP (eds): *Principles of Geriatric Medicine and Gerontology*. New York, McGraw-Hill, 1990, pp 184–191.

Tsukuda RA: Interdisciplinary collaboration: Teamwork in geriatrics, in Cassel CK, Riesenberg DE, Sorensen LB, Walsh JR (eds): *Geriatric Medicine* 2d ed, New York, Springer-Verlag, 1990, pp 668–676.

CLINICAL CONDITIONS

What Do You See?

What do you see nurses. What do you see.
Are you thinking. When you are looking at me?
A crabbit old woman, not very wise,
Uncertain of habit, faraway eyes,
Who dribbles her food, and makes no reply,
When you say in a loud voice, "I do wish you'd try."
Who seems not to notice, the things that you do,
And forever is losing, a stocking or shoe.
Who unresisting or not lets you do as you will,
When bathing and feeding, the long day to fill.
Is that what you are thinking, is that what you see?
Then open your eyes nurse, you are not looking at me.

I'll tell you who I am, as I sit here so still.
As I use at your bidding, as I eat at your will.
I'm a small child of ten, with a father and mother,
Brothers and sisters, who love one another.
A young girl of sixteen, with wings on her feet,
Dreaming that soon now a lover she'll meet.
A bride soon at twenty, my heart gives a leap,
Remembering the vows, that I promised to keep.
At twenty-five now, I have young of my own.

Who need me to build a secure happy home.
A woman of thirty, my young now grow fast.
Bound to each other, with ties that should last.
At forty my young sons now grow and will be gone,
But my man stays beside me to see, I don't mourn.
At fifty, once more babies play round my knee,
Again we know children, my loved ones and me.

Dark days are upon me, my husband is dead.
I look at the future I shudder with dread.
For my young are all busy, rearing young of their own.
And I think of the years, and the Love that I've known.
I'm an old woman now, and nature is cruel.
It's her jest, to make old age look like a fool.
The body it crumbles, grace and vigor depart,
There is now a stone, where I once had a heart.
But inside this old carcass, a young girl still dwells,
And now and again, my battered heart swells,
I remember the joys, I remember the pain,
And I'm loving and living, life all over again.
I think of the years, all too few—gone too fast,
And accept the stark fact, that nothing can last.
So open your eyes, nurses, open and see,
Not a crabbit old woman. Look closer—see me.

Anonymous

DELIRIUM AND DEMENTIA

Dementia is one of the causes, if not the leading cause, for nursing home (NH) placement. The prevalence of dementia in NHs ranges from 30 to over 50 percent, accounting for a substantial proportion of the cost of NH care. The incidence of delirium in the NH setting is unknown, but is commonly superimposed on dementia when a NH resident becomes acutely ill. Delirium is especially important to recognize because of the many potentially reversible underlying causes. This chapter will review the common causes and evaluation of dementia and delirium in the NH, discuss the significance of diagnosing these conditions in NH residents, and briefly review innovative approaches to the care of NH residents with dementia. Dementia is commonly complicated by depression, other psychiatric symptoms, and behavioral disorders. These conditions are discussed in Chap. 10.

DELIRIUM

Delirium is an acute confusional state involving a global disorder of cognition and attention associated with a decreased level of consciousness. Table 9-1 outlines the diagnostic criteria for delirium. Individuals with delirium usually have sleep disturbances, with wakefulness at night and drowsiness during the day. The onset is generally acute. Symptoms tend to fluctuate and are often worse at night. Delirium may be either of the agitated or apathetic type. Almost any medical disorder and a variety of drugs can precip-

Table 9-1 Diagnostic criteria for delirium

A. Reduced ability to maintain attention to external stimuli (e.g., questions must be repeated because attention wanders) and to appropriately shift attention to new external stimuli (e.g., perseverates in answering a previous question)

B. Disorganized thinking, as indicated by rambling, irrelevant, or incoherent speech

C. At least two of the following:
   1. Reduced level of consciousness (e.g., difficulty keeping awake during examination)
   2. Perceptual disturbances: misinterpretations, illusions, or hallucinations
   3. Disturbance of sleep-wake cycle with insomnia or daytime sleepiness
   4. Increased or decreased psychomotor activity
   5. Disorientation to time, place, or person
   6. Memory impairment (e.g., inability to learn new material, such as the names of several unrelated objects after 5 min, or to remember past events, such as history of current episode of illness)

D. Clinical features develop over a short period of time (usually hours to days) and tend to fluctuate over the course of a day

E. Either 1 or 2:
   1. Evidence from the history, physical examination, or laboratory tests of a specific organic factor (or factors) judged to be etiologically related to the disturbance
   2. In the absence of such evidence, an etiologic organic factor can be presumed if the disturbance cannot be accounted for by any nonorganic mental disorder (e.g., manic episode accounting for agitation and sleep disturbance)

Source: American Psychiatric Association, *DSM III Revised,* 1987.

itate delirium in a NH resident (Table 9–2). The cornerstone of treating delirium is the identification and treatment of the underlying cause. This basically requires a thorough physical and laboratory evaluation. In NHs, the most common cause of delirium is infection. Thus, acutely altered mental status should initially be treated as an infection until other potential causes are excluded. The medication list of any NH resident who becomes delirious should be reviewed and, where possible, any medications that may be responsible for the delirium should be discontinued. Silent myocardial infarction can also cause acute delirium in older persons; therefore, if the cause of the delirium is unclear, an electrocardiogram should be done. A delirious resident should be kept in a well-lit environment with minimal disturbances. Physical restraints are contraindicated, as they can make the symptoms of delirium worse. If the delirious resident is severely agitated or assaultive, the use of low-dose haloperidol (0.5 to 1 mg two or three times per day) may be helpful until the delirium clears. This drug should be discontinued as rapidly as possible to avoid side effects. More sedating drugs should be avoided because they can cause disturbances of consciousness that can mask recovery from the underlying delirium.

Table 9-2   Common causes of delirium in the nursing home

Metabolic disorders
  Hyponatremia
  Acid-base disturbances
  Hypoxia
  Hypercarbia
  Hypercalcemia
  Azotemia

Infections

Decreased cardiac output
  Dehydration
  Acute blood loss
  Acute myocardial infarction
  Congestive heart failure

Stroke (small cortical)

Drugs
  Anticholinergics
  Cimetidine
  Digoxin
  Narcotics
  Psychotropics

Intoxication or withdrawal (alcohol, other)

Hypo- or hyperthermia

Acute psychoses

Transfer to unfamiliar surroundings (especially when sensory input is diminished)

Other
  Fecal impaction
  Urinary retention

DEMENTIA

Dementia is defined as a loss of intellectual abilities of sufficient severity to interfere with an individual's ability to function. Dementia is a syndrome that can involve several distinct types of impaired intellectual functioning. Demented individuals generally have impaired memory and orientation; they may also exhibit impaired abstract thinking and judgment, apraxia (inability to carry out motor activities), agnosia (inability to recognize common objects), visuospatial disturbances, and alterations in personality. An underlying delirium must be ruled out before dementia can be diagnosed. Table 9–3 summarizes the diagnostic criteria for dementia and offers some caveats about these criteria in NH residents. Table 9–4 lists features that help distinguish delirium from dementia.

Table 9-3   Diagnostic criteria for primary dementia

Criteria	Caveats
Loss of intellectual ability of sufficient severity to interfere with social or occupational functioning	Demented individuals may appear to function reasonably well in the structured environment of a NH
Memory impairment	Not all impairment of memory implies dementia There are many causes of memory impairment other than dementia
One of the following four symptoms:	
Impairment of abstract thinking (e.g., when a person thinks that a statement like "people who live in glass houses shouldn't throw stones" pertains only to breaking glass)	
Impaired judgment (e.g., when a person with a severe gait and balance disorder continually ambulates without assistance and falls repeatedly)	History from relative or others who knew resident before admission to the NH may be helpful in identifying impaired judgment
Personality change (e.g., a person who is usually trusting becomes very suspicious)	Good history of personality traits is important
State of consciousness not clouded (i.e., individual is alert and aware of the surroundings)	When consciousness is clouded, then *delirium* rather than dementia is present Reversible causes of delirium should be identified (see Table 9-2)

The most common cause of dementia is Alzheimer's disease, and the next most common is multiple infarcts within the brain. There are a number of less common causes of nonreversible dementia such as Parkinson's disease, Pick's disease, Creutzfeld-Jakob disease, AIDS, Huntington's disease, and cerebellar degeneration. In the NH it is important to distinguish these predominantly untreatable dementias from those that are treatable. Although completely reversible dementias are rare, the causes of such dementias should be kept in mind. Table 9–5 lists the causes of reversible dementia. Among these, depression and medications are the most common. Withdrawal of suspect medications and/or a trial of antidepressant therapy for possible depression should always be attempted before labeling a demented NH resident as untreatable, because depression and Alzheimer's disease often coexist. A careful assessment should be undertaken to identify a potentially treatable depression. Clinical clues to depression in a NH resident with dementia include (1) the abrupt onset and rapid progression of

Table 9-4   Key features differentiating delirium from dementia

Feature	Delirium	Dementia
Onset	Acute, often at night	Insidious
Course	Fluctuating, with lucid intervals, during day; worse at night	Generally stable over course of day
Duration	Hours to weeks	Month to years
Awareness	Reduced	Clear
Alertness	Abnormally low or high	Usually normal
Attention	Hypoalert or hyperalert, distractible; fluctuates over course of day	Usually normal
Orientation	Usually impaired for time, tendency to mistake unfamiliar place and persons	Often impaired
Memory	Immediate and recent impaired	Recent and remote impaired
Thinking	Disorganized	Impoverished
Perception	Illusions and hallucinations (usually visual) relatively common	Usually normal
Speech	Incoherent, hesitant, slow, or rapid	Difficulty in finding words
Sleep-wake cycle	Always disrupted	Often fragmented sleep
Physical illness or drug toxicity	Either or both present	Often absent, especially in Alzheimer's disease

Source: Lipkowski, 1987 (see Suggested Readings).

Table 9-5   Causes of treatable or potentially reversible dementias[a]

D—Drugs
E—Emotional (depression)
M—Metabolic (e.g., hypothyroidism, vitamin B_{12} deficiency)
E—Ear and eye impairment (sensory deprivation)
N—Normal-pressure hydrocephalus
T—Tumors and masses (e.g., subdural hematoma)
I—Infection
A—Anemia

[a] Completely reversible dementias are rare in the NH population. Management of these conditions may, however, improve or delay progression of cognitive function.
Source: Lamy PP: *Prescribing for the Elderly.* Littleton, Mass. PSG Publishing, 1980.

cognitive deficits, (2) recognition of the deficits by the resident, (3) a tendency to answer questions with "I don't know" or to make no attempt to answer, and (4) an apathetic or agitated affect. If depression is suspected, a therapeutic trial should be undertaken (see Chap. 10). The dementia may not reverse completely, but the resident's functioning and quality of life may improve.

Other causes of reversible dementia are much less common. Normal-pressure hydrocephalus is distinguished by dementia coexisting with acute-onset incontinence and an ataxic gait disturbance. Residents with normal-pressure hydrocephalus who will respond to treatment usually show an improved gait after the removal of substantial amounts of cerebrospinal fluid. Vitamin B_{12} deficiency may be a cause of dementia. However, it is now recognized that individuals with dementia may develop low vitamin B_{12} levels, perhaps related to coexistent malnutrition. It is possible that dementia in these individuals may be improved by treatment with vitamin B_{12} as well as by adequate nutritional intake.

Assessment

The goals of assessing cognitive dysfunction in a NH resident are to (1) define the nature and extent of the cognitive deficits, (2) rule out delirium and potentially reversible causes of dementia, (3) determine the etiology of the dementia, and (4) identify behavioral disturbances that require management. The assessment is generally multidisciplinary, involving input from the physician, nursing staff, and social worker. When appropriate, an evaluation by occupational therapists may assist in objectively assessing functional capabilities, and an evaluation by an experienced psychiatrist or psychologist may provide very valuable input on the nature of cognitive deficits and behavioral disturbances.

Table 9–6 outlines the basic components of the assessment process. A careful history obtained by an experienced social worker is extremely valuable in providing essential background information. The medical evaluation should include a thorough physical examination (to identify treatable conditions) and selected laboratory studies. Table 9–7 lists the diagnostic studies recommended by an NIH Consensus Conference panel. The routine use of neuroimaging techniques remains controversial. We recommend that all NH residents with cognitive impairment of unclear etiology have either a computed tomography (CT) or magnetic resonance imaging (MRI) scan to rule out tumors and subdural hematomas. Although these conditions are unusual, it is impossible to exclude them on the basis of clinical examination alone, and they are treatable. Table 9–8 describes currently available neuroimaging techniques.

The cornerstone of the assessment of cognitive impairment is the mental status examination. This should include several components (Table 9–

Table 9-6 Basic components of assessing cognitive impairment in nursing home residents

History from family or significant others[a]
  Personal background
  Educational level
  Occupational history
  Onset of cognitive impairment
  Progression of cognitive impairment
  Evidence of impaired judgment
  Behavioral disturbances (e.g., wandering, agitation)
  Ability to carry out activities of daily living

Medical evaluation
  Physical examination to rule out treatable disorders
  Laboratory studies (see Tables 9-7 and 9-8)

Functional capabilities
  Nursing assessment
  Occupational therapy evaluation

Mental status examination
  General (see Table 9-9)
  Standardized test[b]
  Behavioral assessment[c]
  Psychiatric or psychological evaluation if indicated

---

[a] Especially important for newly admitted residents. Best obtained by experienced social worker.

[b] Several standardized tests are available and are useful in documenting cognitive impairments and following progress over time. An example of a commonly used mental status scale is illustrated in Fig. 9-1.

[c] See Chap. 10 for an example of an "agitation scale" that may be helpful in this assessment.

9). In addition to a general mental status exam, a standardized mental status test is useful in documenting deficits and following their progression over time. Figure 9–1 illustrates the Mini Mental State Examination, a commonly used scale for this purpose. Many other similar scales are also available. For some residents with dementia and psychiatric symptoms, an assessment by an experienced psychiatrist or psychologist, when available, can be valuable. Because of the high prevalence of behavioral disturbances in NH residents with dementia, an assessment of behavior should be carried out by nursing and/or social work staff. An example of such an assessment is included in Chap. 10.

The vast majority of demented NH residents have either Alzheimer's disease, multi-infarct dementia, or a combination of both. Table 9–10 lists the general criteria for the diagnosis of Alzheimer's disease developed by the National Institute of Neurologic and Communicative Disorders and

Table 9-7   Evaluating dementia: diagnostic studies

Blood studies
   Complete blood count
   Glucose
   Urea nitrogen
   Electrolytes
   Calcium and phosphorus
   Liver function tests
   Vitamin B_{12} and folate
   Antibodies to human immunodeficiency virus (HIV)[a]
   VDRL

Radiographic studies
   Chest films
   Computed axial tomography (or magnetic resonance imaging) of the head[a]

Other studies
   Electrocardiogram (possibly Holter monitor)
   Urinalysis
   Electroencephalogram[a]
   Neuropsychological testing[a]
   Lumbar puncture[a]

[a] These studies are not recommended for routine screening but may be helpful in some instances.

Source: NIH Consensus Conference, 1987 (see Suggested Readings).

Table 9-8   Imaging techniques in the diagnosis of dementia

Technique	Common findings
Computed tomography (CT)	Shows cortical atrophy with enlargement of the venticula and sulci. Not very different from findings in cognitively intact individuals.
Magnetic resonance imaging (MRI)	In Alzheimer's disease, will show same as above. Some will show high-intensity signals in the white matter, which are also seen in nonimpaired elderly. More sensitive than CT in detecting multiple infarcts.
Positron-emission tomography (PET)	A new technique, not widely available. Involves injecting radioactively labeled dioxyglucose which, when metabolized, permits visualization of active parts of the brain. Scans of patients with Alzheimer's are dark, indicating less activity than the bright images produced by the active brains of normal individuals. Early in the disease, the temporal and parietal cortex show the most prominent deficits. Diagnostic value not yet known.
Single-photon-emission computed tomography (SPECT)	Shows the blood flow through the brain rather than the rate of brain metabolism. Not yet widely available. Diagnostic value not yet known.

Table 9-9 Key components of mental status examinations

State of consciousness
General appearance and behavior
Orientation
Memory (short- and long-term)
Language
Intelligence, perception, and other cognitive functions (e.g., calculations)
Insight and problem-solving ability
Judgment
Thought content
Mood and affect

Stroke and the Alzheimer's Disease and Related Disorders Association. Features that suggest multi-infarct dementia include (1) history of hypertension, stroke or transient ischemic attack; (2) focal neurological symptoms or signs; (3) an abrupt onset with stepwise deterioration; and (4) emotional lability. In the NH, from a practical standpoint, the management of Alzheimer's disease and multi-infarct dementia is the same, with the possible exception of treating the latter with low-dose daily aspirin to prevent further infarcts and deterioration of cognitive function.

Management of Residents with Dementia

The basic principles of managing residents with dementia are not different from those that govern the management of other NH residents described throughout this text. The focus is on providing a safe environment that will compensate for cognitive impairments and appropriate management for behavioral disturbances, such as wandering and agitation, while minimizing the use of physical or chemical restraints. The findings from the multidisciplinary assessment should be incorporated into the resident's care plan. The care plan should address issues such as wandering and other behavioral disturbances, sleep disorders, nutrition, potential for falling, and functional capabilities (see Chap. 8). The treatment of underlying medical conditions should be optimized. Because small infarcts may worsen cognitive function, significant hypertension (i.e., systolic above 160; diastolic above 95) should be controlled to the extent possible without causing side effects. Many residents with dementia gradually develop malnutrition, which should be managed aggressively to prevent complications (see Chap. 11). Residents with dementia who are capable of carrying out their activities of daily living but who tend to require cuing for eating and toileting and/or who tend to get lost require a structured environment with appropriate staffing to supervise them. It is usually not until a resident reaches an advanced stage of dementia that he or she loses the ability to perform ADLs. Other significant man-

I. ORIENTATION (Maximum score 10)

Ask "What is today's date?" Then ask specifically
for parts omitted; eg, "Can you also tell me
what season it is?"

Ask "Can you tell me the name of this hospital?"
"What floor are we on?"
"What town (or city) are we in?"
"What county are we in?"
"What state are we in?"

Date (eg,Jan.21) ___
Year ___
Month ___
Day (eg, Monday) ___
Season ___
Hospital ___
Floor ___
Town/City ___
County ___
State ___

II. REGISTRATION (Maximum score 3)

Ask the subject if you may test his/her memory, then say "ball", "flag", "tree"
clearly and slowly, about one second for each. After you have said all 3 words,
ask subject to repeat them. This first repetition determines the score (0—3) but
keep saying them (up to 6 trials) until the subject can repeat all 3 words. If
(s)he does not eventually learn all three, recall cannot be meaningfully tested

"ball" ___
"flag" ___
"tree" ___

III. ATTENTION & CALCULATION (Maximum score 5)

Ask the subject to begin at 100 and count backward by 7. Stop after
5 subtractions (93, 86, 79, 72, 65). Score one point for each
correct number.

"93" ___
"86" ___
"79" ___
"72" ___
"65" ___
or

If the subject cannot or will not perform this task, ask him/her to
spell the word "world" backwards (D,L,R,O,W). The score is one point
for each correctly placed letter, eg, DLROW=5, DLORW=3. Record how
the subject spelled "world" backwards: _____
D L R O W

\# of correctly—
placed letters ... ___

IV. RECALL (Maximum score 3)

Ask the subject to recall the three words you previously asked him/her
to remember (learned in Registration)

"ball" ___
"flag" ___
"tree" ___

V. LANGUAGE (Maximum score 9)

Naming: Show the subject a wrist watch and ask "What is this?"
Repeat for pencil. Score one point for each item named correctly

Watch ___
Pencil ___

Repetition: Ask the subject to repeat, "No ifs, ands, or buts."
Score one point for correct repetition

Repetition ___

3—Stage Command: Give the subject a piece of blank paper and say,
"Take the paper in your right hand, fold it in half and put it
on the floor," Score one point for each action performed correctly

Takes in rt. hand ___
Folds in half ___
Puts on floor ___

Reading: On a blank piece of paper, print the sentence "Close your eyes."
in letters large enough for the subject to see clearly. Ask subject
to read it and do what it says. Score correct only if (s)he
actually closes his/her eyes

Closes eyes ___

Writing: Give the subject a blank piece of paper and ask him/her
to write a sentence. It is to be written spontaneously. It must
contain a subject and verb and make sense. Correct grammer and
punctuation are not necessary

Writes sentence ___

Copying: On a clean piece of paper, draw intersecting pentagons,
each side about 1 inch, and ask subject to copy it exactly as
it is. All 10 angles must be present and two must intersect
to score 1 point. Tremor and rotation are ignored
Eg,

Draws pentagons ___

TOTAL SCORE _____

Table 9-10 Clinical criteria for diagnosis of Alzheimer's disease[a]

Probable Alzheimer's disease	Dementia established by clinical examination with documented mental-status and neuropsychological test confirmation
	Deficits in two or more areas of cognition
	Progressive worsening of memory and other cognitive functions
	No disturbance of consciousness
	Onset between ages 40 and 90, usually after 65
	Absence of other identifiable causes
Possible Alzheimer's disease	Other significant disease present but, on clinical judgment, Alzheimer's disease is considered the most likely cause of the dementia (or the presentation of disease course is somewhat unusual)
Definite Alzheimer's disease	Histopathological confirmation, based on postmortem examination of brain tissues

[a] Summary of the criteria developed by the National Institute of Neurologic and Communicative Disorders and Stroke, and the Alzheimer's Disease and Related Disorders Association.

agement problems include behavioral disturbances and feeding problems, which are discussed in Chaps. 10 and 11. The Suggested Readings include articles and texts that also provide more detailed discussions of managing dementia.

Caregivers

Caring for a demented loved one, even if he or she is in a NH, is associated with tremendous emotional strain and disruption of normal personal, household, and work activities. These stresses place family caregivers at high risk for developing health problems of their own. The process that families undergo when they turn care over to others is painful and may have significant consequences, including depression, guilt, anger, and other psychological problems. Assisting and supporting a caregiver through this process should be part of NH admission. Many family caregivers continue to engage in invisible caregiving by managing their relative's finances and legal matters, and they must cope with a range of social and psychological problems after NH admission. In addition, family caregivers play an important role in medical decision making for demented NH residents who are no longer capable of making their own decisions. This aspect is discussed in Chap.

◄───

Figure 9-1. The Mini Mental State Examination. (Source: Folstein M, Folstein S, and McHuth P: Mini Mental State: A practical method for grading the cognitive state of patients for the clinician. *J Psychiatr Res* 12:189–198, 1975.)

25, on ethical and legal issues. Family caregivers may be helpful by participating in some aspects of care (feeding, for example) in conjunction with NH staff. Many family caregivers benefit from this participation and learn how to interpret the eating behaviors of their relative. Such participation may help family members develop a more positive attitude to their relative as well as a better appreciation of the care their relative is receiving. Family members should also be encouraged to contact the local Alzheimer's and Associated Diseases Association. This association provides much useful information on dementia at a level aimed at the lay public; it also offers a variety of support groups.

Special Care Units for Residents with Dementia

Special care units (SCUs) for NH residents with dementia have become increasingly popular. SCUs are intended to provide a safe therapeutic environment that will compensate for cognitive deficits and resultant disabilities. Table 9–11 describes some of the characteristics of SCUs. SCUs should be preferably limited in size and have stable, well-trained staff that takes pride in this unique working environment. A well-organized unit should provide effective staff and family support so as to reduce "burnout." Preventing burnout is critical in maintaining stable, competent staff, which is so important in the management of residents with dementia. A support group for staff, with parties or other tokens of appreciation, may be helpful in this regard.

Although the concept of the SCU may be sound, current data have not documented a significant impact on the course of dementia or on secondary complications. Most studies suffer from methodological limitations that limit generalization of their findings. Many SCUs simply segregate demented residents rather than offer alternative approaches to their care. One of the primary reasons for placement in a SCU is, in fact, to prevent demented residents from wandering and injuring themselves. This objective is likely to be met if the environment is designed appropriately. Whether health status and/or longevity are affected is still to be determined. The authors speculate that SCUs may have a measurable impact on caregivers (staff and families) and possibly on the quality of life of demented NH residents. It may be possible to create SCUs at a lower level of care, such as assisted living, and still maintain a safe level of care at a lower cost. The potential benefits may include improved quality of life, minimization of the use of chemical and physical restraints, improved nutrition, and a reduction in the frequency of falls and other accidents. It is important that SCUs have special programs (e.g., music therapy, exercise programs); otherwise there is a marked possibility that they will become areas that segregate the unwanted resident

Table 9-11   Characteristics of special care units (SCU) for demented nursing home residents

Staffing

Staff ratios on SCUs are higher than other units

Staff are specially trained in the causes and manifestation of dementia

Team approach is used, involving social worker, nurse, medical and psychiatry/
psychology input

Meetings held regularly to review and modify programs

Programs

More emphasis on reality orientation

More emphasis on music programs (may facilitate reminiscence more than other activities)

More textural materials used in enriched arts-and-crafts programs

Special feeding programs

Finger foods provided to encourage independent eating

Frequent snacks available

Environmental

Special exit doors with alarms

Furniture with rounded edges

More space for recreational activity

Quiet rooms provided for small gatherings or behaviorally disturbed residents

The dining room set up for optimal feeding of residents (some have single-seat-size serving
tables)

Nursing station located near elevators or exits to facilitate monitoring of wandering
residents

Pets sometimes permanent "residents" of unit[a]

Pictures and other designs used to cue residents to finding proper locations of rooms, etc

[a] Note that pet therapy may be a two-edged sword. Not everyone likes animals, and frail older persons are often afraid that they will be knocked over by a running pet.

and provide below-average care. A prospective randomized controlled study with a long follow-up in these areas still needs to be done.

SCUs can certainly provide an appropriate milieu for education and research. SCUs with specific admission criteria may become teaching sites for nurses' aides, nursing staff, medical and other health professional students, and geriatric fellows. Units that accept residents with particular diagnoses may be an excellent place in which to study the natural course of institutionalized demented persons. These units can also serve as sites for controlled trials of interventions, such as a restraint-free environment, the effectiveness of exercise in improving sleep patterns, reality orientation and feeding programs, and the effects of certain drugs on behaviors and cognition. Observation of noncommunicative residents during interactions with staff or in response to environmental stimuli such as music, light/darkness, and food may provide insight into the complex issue of quality of life in the demented elderly, so that better units can be designed in the future.

SUGGESTED READINGS

American Psychiatric Association: *Diagnostic and Statistical Manual of Mental Disorders* (3d ed, revised). Washington DC, American Psychiatric Association, 1987.

Calkins MP: *Design for Dementia: Planning Environments for the Elderly and the Confused.* Baltimore, National Health Publishing, 1988.

Cummings JL, Miller BL (eds): *Alzheimer's Disease: Treatment and Long Term Management.* New York, Marcel Dekker, Inc, 1990.

Holmes D, et al: Impact associated with special care units in long term care facilities. *Gerontologist* 30(2):178–183, 1990.

Lipkowski ZJ: Delirium (acute confusional states). *JAMA* 258:1789–1792, 1987.

Mace NL (ed): *Dementia Care: Patient, Family, and Community.* Baltimore, Johns Hopkins University Press, 1990.

Moletta G (ed): Treatment considerations for Alzheimer's disease and related dementing illnesses. *Clinics in Geriatric Medicine,* vol 4. Philadelphia, WB Saunders Co, 1988.

NIH Consensus Conference: Differential diagnosis of dementing diseases. *JAMA* 258:3411–3416, 1987.

Ramsdell JW, Rothrock JF, Werd HW, Volk DM: Evaluation of cognitive impairment in the elderly. *J Gen Intern Med* 5:55–66, 1990.

Winograd CH, Jarvik LF: Physician management of the dementia patient. *J Am Geriatr Soc* 34:285–308, 1986.

PSYCHIATRIC AND BEHAVIORAL DISORDERS

A hallmark of a good nursing home (NH) is adequate attention to the identication and appropriate management of psychiatric and behavioral disorders. The prevalence of psychiatric and behavioral disorders among NH residents has been estimated to be between 68 and 94 percent. Psychological problems in the NH include depression, cognitive disorders, late-life paranoia, anxiety and panic disorders, and behavioral disorders. In addition, NH personnel need to be aware of psychopathology among relatives of residents; they must also be able to deal with psychological reactions among staff caregivers. This chapter reviews the diagnosis and management of common psychiatric and behavioral disorders seen in the NH. The diagnosis and management of dementia and delirium are discussed in Chap. 9.

DEPRESSION

The prevalence of major depression among NH residents has been reported to range from 9 to 38 percent. In addition, dysphoria, particularly at the time of admission to the NH, is common. The diagnosis of depression in older individuals involves the same diagnostic criteria as those utilized in younger persons (Table 10–1). To be considered depressed, the resident must have had at least a 2-week period of dysphoria or loss of interest or enjoyment in activities. In addition, at least two of the following symptoms must be present: appetite disturbance or weight loss, fatigue or decreased energy, psychomotor agitation or retardation, guilt, sleep disturbance, altered cognition

Table 10-1 Diagnostic criteria for depression

A. At least five of the following symptoms have been present during the same 2-week period and represent a change from previous functioning; at least one of the symptoms is either (1) depressed mood or (2) loss of interest or pleasure. (Do not include symptoms that are clearly due to a physical condition, mood-incongruent delusions or hallucinations, incoherence, or marked loosening of associations.)

  1. Depressed mood most of the day, nearly every day, as indicated either by subjective account or observation by others
  2. Markedly diminished interest or pleasure in all or almost all activities most of the day, nearly every day (as indicated either by subjective account or observation by others of apathy most of the time)
  3. Significant weight loss or weight gain when not dieting (e.g., more than 5 percent of body weight in a month) or decrease or increase in appetite nearly every day
  4. Insomnia or hypersomnia nearly every day
  5. Psychomotor agitation or retardation nearly every day (observable by others, not merely subjective feelings of restlessness or being slowed down)
  6. Fatigue or loss of energy nearly every day
  7. Feelings of worthlessness or excessive or inappropriate guilt (which may be delusional) nearly every day (not merely self-reproach or guilt about being sick)
  8. Diminished ability to think or concentrate, or indecisiveness, nearly every day (either by subjective account or as observed by others)
  9. Recurrent thoughts of death (not just fear of dying), recurrent suicidal ideation without a specific plan, a suicide attempt, or a specific plan for committing suicide

B. 1. It cannot be established that an organic factor initiated and maintained the disturbance
   2. Disturbance is not a normal reaction to the death of a loved one (uncomplicated bereavement)

C. At no time during the disturbance have there been delusions or hallucinations for as long as 2 weeks in the absence of prominent mood symptoms (i.e., before the mood symptoms developed or after they have remitted)

D. Not superimposed on schizophrenia, schizophreniform disorder, delusional disorder, or psychotic disorder

Source: American Psychiatric Association, *DSM III Revised,* 1987.

or concentration, and suicidal ideas. Older persons with depression are more likely to have weight loss and less likely to express suicidal ideation. Nursing home residents with depression often have atypical presentations (Table 10–2).

Delusions and agitated behavior may be particularly common presentations of depression in the NH. Pain syndromes such as jaw, abdominal or musculoskeletal pains for which there is no obvious explanation may also constitute the presentation of depression. Malnutrition is another very common presentation of depression in NH residents.

On admission to the NH, all residents should be screened with an objective test such as the Yesavage Geriatric Depression Scale (YGDS) (Table 10–3). Residents with a score of 15 or greater should be considered for treat-

Table 10-2   Atypical presentation of depression in the nursing home

Anxiety/agitation
Delusions
Depressive dementia ("pseudodementia")
Malnutrition
Atypical pain syndromes
Passive suicide

Table 10-3   Yesavage Geriatric Depression Scale (YGDS)

Choose the best answer for how you felt the past week:		
1. Are you basically satisfied with your life?	Yes	No[a]
2. Have you dropped many of your activities and interests?	Yes	No
3. Do you feel that your life is empty?	Yes	No
4. Do you often get bored?	Yes	No
5. Are you hopeful about the future?	Yes	No[a]
6. Are you bothered by thoughts you can't get out of your head?	Yes	No
7. Are you in good spirits most of the time?	Yes	No[a]
8. Are you afraid that something bad is going to happen to you?	Yes	No
9. Do you feel happy most of the time?	Yes	No[a]
10. Do you often feel helpless?	Yes	No
11. Do you often get restless and fidgety?	Yes	No
12. Do you prefer to stay at home, rather than going out and doing new things?	Yes	No
13. Do you frequently worry about the future?	Yes	No
14. Do you feel you have more problems with memory than most?	Yes	No
15. Do you think it is wonderful to be alive now?	Yes	No[a]
16. Do you often feel downhearted and blue?	Yes	No
17. Do you feel pretty worthless the way you are now?	Yes	No
18. Do you worry a lot about the past?	Yes	No
19. Do you find life very exciting?	Yes	No[a]
20. Is it hard for you to get started on new projects?	Yes	No
21. Do you feel full of energy?	Yes	No[a]
22. Do you feel that your situation is hopeless?	Yes	No
23. Do you think that most people are better off than you are?	Yes	No
24. Do you frequently get upset over little things?	Yes	No
25. Do you frequently feel like crying?	Yes	No
26. Do you have trouble concentrating?	Yes	No
27. Do you enjoy getting up in the morning?	Yes	No[a]
28. Do you prefer to avoid social gatherings?	Yes	No
29. Is it easy for you to make decisions?	Yes	No[a]
30. Is your mind as clear as it used to be?	Yes	No[a]

[a] These questions are scored 1 point for a "no" answer; other questions are scored 1 point for a "yes" answer. Mean scores are as follows: normal (not depressed), 5; mildly depressed, 15; very depressed, 23. Scores of 15 and above generally indicate depression (see text and Fig. 10-1).

ment of depression. Residents with scores between 10 and 14 often revert to nondepressed levels within 4 to 6 weeks without pharmacological therapy. For this reason, we recommend repeating the YGDS 6 weeks after admission for residents with scores in this range. The utility of the YGDS is limited among residents with moderate to marked dementia.

When the diagnosis of depression is made, it is important to exclude any treatable medical causes (Table 10–4). In addition, physicians need to be aware that following a stroke, 1 in 3 NH residents will develop depression within the next 2 years. Thus, these NH residents should be screened for depression every 3 months for 2 years following a stroke. A careful review of all medications must be conducted for any depressed resident, because many medications may contribute to depression (Table 10–4).

An approach to the treatment of depression among NH residents is illustrated in Fig. 10–1. When the diagnosis of depression is made and the resident is not agitated and has no major sleep disturbance, treatment is initi-

Table 10-4   Treatable medical causes of depression

Endocrine
    Thyroid disease
    Hyperparathyroidism

Chronic infections

Malnutrition

Tumors
    Central nervous system
    Pancreatic carcinoma
    Other

Electrolyte imbalances and dehydration

Medications
    Antihypertensives
        Propranolol
        Reserpine

    Psychotropics
        Neuroleptics
        Benzodiazepines

    Hormones
        Corticosteroids

    Analgesics
        Indomethacin

    Other
        Narcotics
        Digoxin
        Amantadine

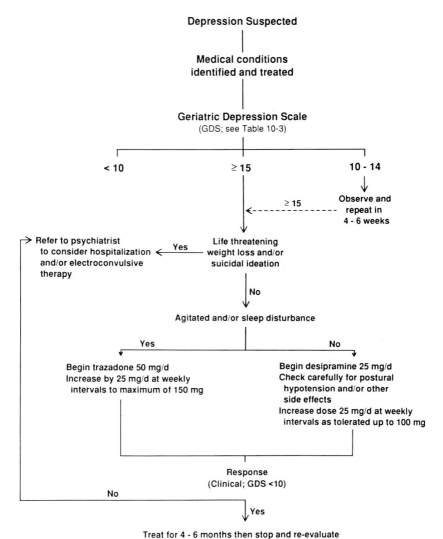

Figure 10-1. Approach to depression in the nursing home

ated with desipramine 25 mg in the evening for 3 days. It is then increased to 50 mg. Postural vital signs should be monitored at least once or twice per week during this time, and other potentially bothersome side effects should be identified (see below). Residents with prolonged PR intervals or QRS durations on electrocardiogram should have a repeat electrocardiogram to identify any progression of heart block. After 2 weeks, the YGDS is repeated. If the score is still greater than 15, the dose of desipramine is increased to 75 mg daily for 1 week and then to 100 mg daily. The depression scale is repeated 3 weeks later. If the resident is still depressed, she/he is referred to a psychiatrist. At the start of therapy, nursing staff are informed that the resident is depressed. They are asked to increase positive verbal interactions with the resident and to consistently encourage her/him to become involved in group activities.

If the resident is agitated or has severe sleep disturbances, then trazodone (which has mild to moderate sedative effects) is used instead of desipramine, starting at a dose of 50 mg in the evening for 1 week and increasing the dose by 25 mg every week to a maximum dose of 150 mg a day. If this fails to normalize the YGDS, referral to a psychiatrist is appropriate.

Desipramine is preferred to nortriptyline because it has slightly less anticholinergic side effects. The major anticholinergic side effects of these secondary amines are urinary retention in residents with prostatic enlargement, decreased visual acuity, constipation, and dry mouth. A major potential side effect is orthostatic hypotension, which can result in falls. Orthostatic blood pressure measurements should be done at regular intervals (at least twice per week) while a NH resident is being stabilized on an appropriate dose of desipramine. Trazodone produces a greater degree of sedation and less anticholinergic side effects than desipramine. Occasional residents may benefit from the addition of small doses of lithium to the antidepressant. If lithium is prescribed, blood levels should be monitored carefully. The use of methylphenidate (Ritalin) is sometimes effective, but it should be limited to prescription and oversight by psychiatrists. Fluoxetine should generally not be used in NH residents, because it can precipitate agitated behavior and also cause life-threatening weight loss. Side effects of monoamine oxidase inhibitors usually limit their use in the NH population, but they may occasionally stimulate appetite in malnourished residents.

In severely depressed residents with significant weight loss, malnutrition, or high suicide potential, electroconvulsive therapy (ECT) is the treatment of choice. It should also be considered for residents who fail an adequate trial of antidepressant therapy. Serum levels of antidepressants should be obtained to demonstrate that a sufficiently high dosage was given before treatment was considered unsuccessful.

Severely depressed residents should be given a room near the nursing station to permit regular observation. These residents should be carefully monitored to identify any suicidal ideation. As a first step, residents should be asked directly if they have any suicidal thoughts or wish to die. If they respond positively, they should be asked if they have made any specific plans. Residents who have specific plans (e.g., hoarding pills, suffocation) should be taken seriously and hospitalized for more intensive management. In most NHs, staffing is inadequate to monitor these residents for suicide attempts. Severely depressed residents should be checked regularly, especially after being outside the NH or in the hospital, to ensure that they are not hiding medications that could be used to commit suicide. The early phase of recovery from depression is also a time of higher risk for suicide.

LATE-LIFE PARANOIA

Isolated late-life paranoia is a relatively unusual condition, but residents who develop it can be very disruptive. They may become suspicious and develop delusions that caregivers or other residents are trying to poison them or steal from them. The affected resident may focus on a single fellow resident or staff member and attempt to enlist the help of other staff and residents to prove the guilt of the person who has been singled out. As stealing and other unacceptable behaviors can occur among staff, the resident's paranoid complaints should be evaluated carefully. When paranoid delusions are present and disruptive, the resident may respond well to low doses of haloperidol (see Chap. 21).

ANXIETY AND PANIC DISORDERS

Anxiety is a common problem in NH residents. Approximately 20 percent of NH residents exhibit some degree of anxiety. Common signs and symptoms of anxiety include palpitations, tremors, hyperventilation, insomnia, confusion, hypochondriasis, generalized fears, and feelings of hopelessness and helplessness. When a NH resident develops these symptoms, a careful assessment should be undertaken to exclude treatable medical conditions that might underlie the symptoms. Anxiety may also be based on a legitimate concern, such as the fear of falling, that is then blown out of proportion.

Whenever possible, anxiety should be treated nonpharmacologically. Acute adjustment reactions to NH admission are best treated by supportive psychotherapy. Biofeedback and relaxation techniques and participation in activity programs may be useful for some residents with anxiety. Buspirone or short-acting benzodiazepines without active metabolites may be useful (see Chap. 21). Once symptoms are under control, an attempt should be made to wean anxious residents from drug therapy, and nonpharmacologic interventions should be provided.

Late-life onset of panic disorders is being more commonly recognized. Buspirone, a nonbenzodiazepine anxiolytic, may be particularly useful in treating NH residents with panic disorders. Late-life onset of mania must also be recognized, as the treatment of choice for this disorder is lithium. When supportive measures and drug treatment fail, residents with severe anxiety or panic disorders should be evaluated by a psychiatrist.

SLEEP DISTURBANCES

With advancing age there is a tendency for older individuals to spend more time in bed, sleep less, take longer to fall asleep, have decreased sleep efficiency, and have increased episodes of wakefulness after falling asleep. For this reason, complaints about sleep tend to increase with advancing age, and it is important to distinguish pathological sleep disturbances from the normal age-related changes.

Insomnia can be transient, such as the sleeplessness that may occur on first being admitted to a NH or when a resident's room is changed. Reassurance that normal sleep patterns will return is usually sufficient in these cases. Insomnia lasting for more than 3 weeks requires a careful diagnostic workup. The major causes of chronic insomnia are listed in Table 10–5.

The treatment of insomnia involves explaining to the resident the normal, age-related changes in sleep patterns as well as the appropriate management of the treatable causes, listed in Table 10–5. A list of simple techniques for promoting improved sleep for residents with insomnia is given in Table 10–6. Some residents may benefit from administration of a bright

Table 10-5   Causes of chronic insomnia in the nursing home

Excessive daytime naps

Resident being awakened after falling asleep at night (e.g., for medication dosage)

Psychological disturbances
  Depression
  Dementia
  Anxiety
  Late-life panic disorder
  Mania

Medical conditions
  Heart failure (orthopnea, nocturia)
  Esophageal reflux
  Hyperthyroidism
  Head injury
  Venous insufficiency (nocturia)

Insufficient light during day (midwinter insomnia/indoor insomnia)

Chronic pain

Sleep apnea

Nightmares/night fears

Nocturnal myoclonus

Drugs
  Withdrawal from alcohol or sedative/hypnotics
  Caffeine
  Theophylline

Table 10-6   Sleep improvement program in the nursing home

Avoid daytime naps
Do not awaken resident after he/she has fallen asleep
Implement consistent times for sleep and awakening
Do not allow resident to rest frequently in bed or to be on the bed to watch television or read
See that resident exercises in the afternoon
Reduce resident's caffeine intake
Do not allow resident to fall asleep immediately after evening meal
Provide hot milk and a snack at bedtime (tryptophan loading)
Do not restrain resident in bed, so that normal sleep movements can occur
If the resident is not asleep within 30 min, have him or her get up for at least 30 min before
  making another attempt to go to sleep
Use muted night light if resident has anxiety or night fears
Keep disturbing noises and lights to a minimum
Restrict fluids for 3 h before bedtime in order to decrease nocturia when necessary

light (2500 lux) for an hour in the morning. Nocturnal myoclonus may respond to treatment with a muscle relaxant (e.g., baclofen or a short-acting benzodiazepine). Daytime exercises and the planning of meals and social activities so as to keep the resident awake later at night may also be useful. Use of hot milk before sleep remains an excellent placebo. When the contaminant which caused muscle disease is removed, L-tryptophan may again be a good choice for insomnia, though it may be nothing more than a placebo. Sedatives and hypnotics are discussed in Chap. 21. The long-term use of hypnotics should be avoided whenever possible. At the St. Louis V.A. Nursing Home Care Unit, a majority of residents have been successfully weaned from sleeping medications without any appreciable difference in complaints concerning sleep.

Hypersomnolence during the daytime hours is also not a rare phenomenon in the NH. The most common causes are obstructive sleep apnea and nocturnal myoclonus. Narcolepsy is a rare condition. Fatigue following infection and other acute illnesses and day-night reversal among residents with dementia may both result in excessive sleep during the day. Drugs are probably the major cause of excessive sleepiness during the day. Carryover sleepiness from benzodiazepines given the previous evening is very common. Antihistamines, trazodone and other antidepressants, methyldopa, and antipsychotic drugs can all cause hypersomnolence and should be discontinued if this becomes a problem.

BEHAVIORAL DISORDERS—GENERAL

Behavioral disorders are common among NH residents. They may be expressed as overtly aggressive antisocial behaviors or as passive aggression. In some cases, the behavioral disorder is a symptom of an underlying psychiatric disorder. When this is the case, therapy should be directed toward the underlying disorder. In other cases, behavioral disorders represent the expression of a lifelong personality disorder. Inappropriate methods that the resident may have used to cope with stressors in the past may become accentuated in his or her later years. These individuals often show marked dependency and require constant reassurance and direction. Other individuals may have outbursts of anger when frustrated. Phobias concerning potential injury may discourage the resident from leaving his or her chair or cause inappropriate screams for help.

A major reason for the onset of new behavioral disturbances is related to the loss of locus of control that many residents experience on entry to the NH. These residents may respond by attempting to regain their locus of control by using manipulative behaviors. Refusal to eat is one such behavior. Others will constantly demand attention. In some cases, residents will be verbally abusive toward staff in an attempt to prove that they can still be in charge. This can lead to a vicious cycle in which the abused staff member retaliates, potentially creating a situation of resident abuse. Early recognition of this problem and the provision of support groups for staff are important steps in preventing resident abuse.

An outline of behavioral disorders commonly observed in the NH is given in Table 10–7. Management of these disorders begins by recognizing

Table 10-7 Behavioral problems commonly seen among nursing home residents

Disruptive
  Shouting
  Breaching privacy of others
  Deliberately attempting to interfere with staff when they are busy

Demanding
  Attention seeking
  Food refusal
  Continuous seeking of reassurance
  Inappropriately summoning staff
  Dependency behaviors

Distressful
  Hitting
  Biting
  Crying
  Other forms of agitation (see Table 10-9)
  Paranoia
  Emotional lability

Offensive
  Verbal abuse
  Sexually inappropriate behavior
  Undressing in public
  Abnormal feeding behaviors (e.g., sloppiness, pica)

their existence. The first approach should be to provide residents with reassurance that their needs will be met. An approach of rewarding appropriate behaviors and not rewarding inappropriate behaviors is often successful. When behaviorally difficult residents are recognized, the staff should receive support and recognition of the difficulties involved in handling such residents. Staff should be encouraged to express their anger to other staff and should be made aware of the fact that anger and dislike resulting from problematic resident behaviors are appropriate feelings. However, the staff must be aware that it is inappropriate to express such feelings to the resident or to allow them to interfere with the care plan. Recognition and elimination of environmental and staff problems that trigger behavioral disorders represent an important part of the management. Short-acting benzodiazepine anxiolytics or buspirone may be useful in allowing the resident to adapt to the environment and benefit from appropriate attempts by staff at behavior modification. All residents who are excessively demanding should have a contract drawn up with the staff, setting forth clearly defined limits. It is important that all staff work together in this regard, not allowing the resident to manipulate one staff member against another. The establishment of a monthly support group for staff, where they can discuss their problems with behaviorally disruptive residents in a supportive environment, often dissipates latent anxiety among the staff and may decrease unplanned leave.

BEHAVIORAL DISORDERS ASSOCIATED WITH DEMENTIA

In the NH, the major need in the management of residents with dementia is to control the secondary symptoms (Table 10–8). Table 10–9 illustrates an agitation inventory developed by Dr. Jiska Cohen-Mansfield that may be helpful to NH staff in identifying the nature and frequency of specific behaviors, and for monitoring the response of these behaviors to the various management approaches. Agitated behavior may be worse at night ("sundown-

Table 10-8   Examples of behavioral disturbances seen in residents with dementia

---

Agitated behaviors (see Table 10-9)
Aggressive behavior (verbal, physical)
Wandering
Repetitive questions
Inappropriate sexual behavior
Screaming
"Sundowning"
Overreliance on staff for self-care skills
Social isolation/withdrawal
Depression

Table 10-9 The Cohen-Mansfield Agitation Inventory[a]

Frequency of the following behaviors are rated by nursing staff for the previous 2 weeks on a 7-point scale:

1 = Never
2 = Less than once/week
3 = Once or twice/week
4 = Several times/week
5 = Once or twice/day
6 = Several times/day
7 = Several times/h

Pacing, aimless wandering
Inappropriate dress or disrobing
Spitting (include at meals)
Cursing or verbal aggression
Constant unwarranted requests for attention or help
Repetitive sentences or questions
Hitting (including self)
Kicking
Grabbing onto people
Pushing
Throwing things
Strange noises (weird laughter or crying)
Screaming
Biting
Scratching
Trying to get to a different place (e.g., out of the building)
Intentional falling
Complaining
Negativism
Eating/drinking inappropriate substances
Hurting self or other (cigarette, hot water, etc.)
Handling things inappropriately
Hiding things
Hoarding things
Tearing things or destroying property
Performing repetitive mannerisms
Making verbal sexual advances
Making physical sexual advances
General restlessness

[a]Copyright Cohen-Mansfield, 1986. Reprinted with permission.
Source: Cohen-Mansfield J, Marx MS, Rostenthal AS: A description of agitation in a nursing home. *J Gerontol* 44(3):M77–M84, 1989.

ing"). Sundowning that occurs after the evening meal may be due to glucose fluctuations and may be improved by the use of frequent small snacks. Sometimes residents with dementia who become agitated at night respond to frequent reorientation. Night lights should be kept on in the rooms of residents with sundowning. Residents who frequently pace at night should be placed in exercise programs. Residents who are agitated at night should be carefully observed for precipitating causes of their agitation; where possible, these causes should be removed. Only when behavior modification fails should the use of low-dose neuroleptics (such as haloperidol) or short-acting benzodiazepines be tried. In some cases trazodone (50 to 100 mg) at night will prove to be useful. High doses of a beta blocker may decrease agitation in some residents for whom there are no contraindications to these agents.

Aggressive behavior can be either physical or verbal. Verbally aggressive behavior may sometimes be controlled by ignoring the resident during the outbursts and increasing attention at other times. Verbal aggression may be precipitated by the inability of the resident to hear or understand complex instructions or answers to questions. Thus, simplification of dialogue with the resident may result in improved behavior. Verbal aggression should never be treated with psychotropic drugs. Physical aggression is best treated by giving residents sufficient space of their own. Many staff wittingly or unwittingly taunt residents and precipitate physical outbursts. Residents with Alzheimer's disease have visual defects which cause them to startle easily when rapidly approached, especially from behind. This can give the appearance of violent behavior. If physical aggression is unresponsive to behavior modification, isolation of the resident in his or her own room may be appropriate. Low doses of an antipsychotic may also be necessary in some cases and would be acceptable under OBRA regulations provided that the need is documented (see Chap. 21 and the Appendix).

Approximately 10 percent of NH residents are wanderers. Positive effects of wandering include exercise and decreased tension. Negative effects of wandering include the risk of being lost or sustaining injury, the problem of invading the privacy of others, and the creation of staff stress and an increase in time necessary to observe the resident. The wanderer costs a NH approximately $2500 per year extra in staff time in order to monitor the wandering behavior.

The management of wandering requires both staff and environmental modifications (Table 10–10). Restraints (physical or chemical) should *never* be used to manage the wandering resident. Exercise programs and other organized group activities represent a cost-effective response to monitoring groups of wanderers. Elimination of stressors that may trigger wandering is an important part of the overall approach. A lounge or garden specifically designed for wandering can be particularly useful. Adequate signposting to help residents to find their own rooms, the bathroom, and the dining room is very important. The placement of a picture of the resident at the entrance to his or her room may be most useful in this regard. A strip of masking tape on the floor may be a sufficient barrier for some residents. For others, the use of "Dutch doors" (half doors) or door-locking devices that work on a code known only to the staff may be appropriate.

Table 10-10   Approaches to managing wandering behavior

Staff intervention
   Adequate and repeated resident orientation
   Exercise
   Planned group activities
   Distraction techniques
   Elimination of stressors that trigger wandering
   Placing pictures and items from home in resident's room
   Behavior modification
   Placing picture of resident outside room
   Using bracelets to identify residents

Environmental modifications
   Clear sign posting
   Dutch doors
   Wandering garden/lounge
   Door-monitoring systems
   Perimeter monitoring systems
   Door-locking devices
   Electronic locator systems

Administrative modifications
   Environmental design and space allocation
   Staff training
   Staff support

The advent of high technology in the NH has led to the development of a number of sophisticated systems to monitor wandering residents. Door monitoring systems can be activated to sound an alarm when residents wearing bracelet activators pass though them. Other units allow the wanderer to wear a transmitter which activates an alarm in a receiver when a preselected perimeter distance is exceeded. One company has developed a locator system that displays the locations of individuals on a microcomputer screen.

Inappropriate sexual behavior is most often represented by public masturbation and verbal and sexual overtures to staff and other residents. Residents who masturbate should be encouraged to do this in private, and staff should be counseled that this is a normal behavior. Residents who make verbal or physical sexual overtures should be counseled and firmly told that such behavior is unacceptable. The need of some residents to touch and hug other people should be distinguished from true sexual overtures. When two demented or demented and nondemented residents form romantic attachments, a number of ethical questions arise. Overall, the major criteria for allowing such relationships should be the ability of both residents to understand the implications of their behavior. It should not be automatically assumed that mildly demented residents cannot carry on normal relationships. Finally, all NHs should provide a quiet room where residents can be assured privacy to entertain a spouse or partner when so desired. In-service programs for staff should include discussions of normal and acceptable sexual behavior in the NH. Staff should also be encouraged to express their feelings about these matters.

Screaming is a particularly disturbing problem in some residents. Frequent orientation and keeping the resident near the nurses' station may decrease the frequency of screaming. High-dose beta blockers and/or trazodone may also be useful for some of these residents. Good results may be obtained with some chronic screamers through the use of electroconvulsive therapy.

Social isolation and withdrawal are common problems in demented residents. This behavior may lead to depression and deterioration in self-care skills. Care must be taken to see that attempts to increase socialization result in meaningful experiences for the residents. Social interaction can be increased by, for example, arranging chairs in small groupings and having refreshment areas throughout the NH. Spirituality groups which emphasize touching and overt religious expression may be especially useful for some residents. Tai chi (Chinese exercise) done to music may also increase participation in social activities. Television and radio may play a role in keeping residents in touch with society. However, some demented residents may incorporate events seen on television or heard on the radio into their versions of reality. Hallucinations or delusions may, in fact, be the reality of a television program.

Self-care skills can sometimes be improved by retraining, even among residents with dementia. Rewarding the performance of self-care tasks by tokens redeemable for small luxuries or treats has been reported to increase some NH residents' self-care skills. Such a reward system may slow the development of disability.

Many demented residents respond to reality orientation. This involves constant reminders about real events that are going on in the NH and the community. Correction of mistaken ideas is undertaken. Residents are continuously reminded of where they are and oriented to time and place. Staff are instructed to work with the residents to establish positive attitudes. Such approaches can greatly improve both resident and staff morale. Finally, reminiscing may be very helpful for some residents and can be carried out in a group setting.

PHYSICAL RESTRAINTS

A common response to agitated behaviors, wandering, or a fear of falling has been to restrain NH residents physically. Restraint usage has been increasing in the United States. Up to 50 percent of NH residents are in some type of physical restraint for some portion of the day. This is in stark contrast to the extremely rare use of restraints in Europe. The most common types of restraints are wrist, chest, and jacket restraints. Sheet restraints confining agitated residents to their beds are not rare. Bed rails are virtually universal. The OBRA regulations should decrease the use of restraints in the United States (see Appendix).

The major reasons for the use of restraints are listed in Table 10–11. However, a majority of these have no scientific basis. In one Canadian nursing home, reduction in the use of physical restraints resulted in no significant increase in falls. At the St. Louis Veterans Administration Medical Center's 150-bed Nursing Home Care Unit, reduction of physical restraints from 38 to 9 percent resulted in a significant decrease in falls. Other studies have suggested that the application of restraints increases agitated behavior. Recent court cases in the United States have found liability for the NH when residents injure themselves while they are being restrained. The rationale in these cases has been that the application of physical restraints to an individual implies that the resident is in danger and requires 24-hour-a-day observation. On the other hand, courts have failed to assign culpability to the institution in most cases when a nonrestrained resident falls.

The application of physical restraints has been associated with a number of adverse effects (Table 10–12). Table 10–13 lists examples of management decisions that result in restraint reduction. The single most impor-

Table 10-11   Rationale given for the application of physical restraints in nursing homes

Rationale	Evidence that restraints are useful for this purpose
To prevent falls	No
To prevent wandering	Yes, but at expense of resident freedom
To reduce agitated behavior	No, actually increases such behavior
To avoid litigation	No
For posture improvement	In some cases
To substitute for insufficient staffing	May utilize more staff time if properly monitored
To satisfy staff and administration	Yes
As a punitive measure in cognitively impaired residents for "misbehaving"	Certainly punitive but no evidence that it produces appropriate behavior modification
Protection of staff and residents from violent behavior	In most cases confinement to a room is better
To allow medical treatment, such as feeding tubes and intravenous lines, to be administered without interference	In some cases necessary, but alternatives should be tried first

Table 10-12 Potential adverse effects of physical restraints

Deconditioning
Falls and injuries
Death
   Strangulation
   Overall increased mortality
Abrasions, sheet burns
Incontinence
Contractures
Increased agitation
Depression
Anxiety (e.g., inability to get out in case of fire)
Anorexia and protein-energy malnutrition
Dehydration
Decreased functional status
Loss of locus of control
Osteopenia
Regressive behavior
Pressure sores

---

tant decision is for managers not to demand restraints to prevent injury. Restraint programs work better when the nurses' aides and licensed nurses are asked to come up with strategies allowing the removal of restraints. Monthly feedback on number of restraints in the facility and number of falls also reinforces a restraint-reduction program and is an excellent proactive quality-assurance measure. In some cases, the use of seat belts like those

Table 10-13 Approaches to restraint reduction

Administration should mandate restraint reduction and remove pressures from staff when residents wander or fall
Staff education concerning problems associated with restraints
Emotional appeal to staff: "How would you like to be tied down?"
Licensed nurses and nurses' aides should be asked for their suggestions for restraint reduction and rewarded for good suggestions
Measure restraints and falls on a monthly basis, graph results, and share with staff
Consider use of seat belts like those on airplanes (Posey)
Identify high-risk fallers and place them near nursing station
Document resident feelings about restraints and their comments after removal
Institute conditioning program for deconditioned residents
Increase awareness that many falls occur in bathrooms
Develop contractual arrangements with residents not to leave chairs without help
Continual reinforcement and praise

Table 10-14 Sample care plan for complex, behaviorally disturbed residents

Behaviors

 Yelling and screaming on frequent basis

 Insomnia

 Uncooperativeness

 Demandingness

 Attention seeking

 Restlessness

 Abusive language

 Potential assaultiveness to staff

 Disruption of unit and staff with noise (i.e., crying out and shouting at mealtime—demanding immediate service)

 Unsteady gait with need at present for restraints

 Request for bathroom after every few minutes

Goals

 To resolve pain sustained from fall

 To decrease agitation precipitated by fall and the use of restraints

 To achieve safe ambulation as soon as possible

 Reevaluation of behavioral changes and mobility every 2 weeks

Interventions

 Follow-up psychiatric consultation

 Toilet resident every hour *only* at appointed hour and explain procedure to resident. With each toileting, have resident ambulate as much as possible. At night, toilet when resident awakes and asks to be toileted.

 May use geri-chair *only* for mealtime. If resident becomes disruptive to the rest of the residents, move resident out of the dining hall to finish meal.

 If resident is agitated, try

  Walking with resident in the halls

  Moving resident to another area

  Sitting and talking calmly with resident. Find a topic of interest (e.g., resident's relatives, past life experiences)

  Sitting quietly with resident, holding his/her hand and offering reassurance

 If behavior becomes disruptive, noisy, and out of control, use unit manager's office as a quiet room until resident calms down. Do not leave resident alone.

 Under *no* circumstances allow a resident who is shouting and asking for assistance to be ignored

 When resident is quiet and cooperative, give praise and reward resident's good/appropriate behavior. Rewards are

  Praise

  Attention

  Sweets (candy bars)

  Popcorn

 Medicate freely as needed for hip and thigh pain

 Give resident sleep medication at night as needed

 Give haloperidol prn as ordered for agitation that is not resolved by other measures

 Protect resident from injury; use Posey seat belt if necessary for safety

 Set limits firmly but with kindness and tell resident when behavior is *not* appropriate

 Do *not* reward resident for inappropriate behavior

 Rotate staff to work with resident throughout the shift to prevent exhaustion and burnout

on airplanes (manufactured by J. T. Posey Co., Arcadia, California 91006) will remind the resident not to rise from the chair while still allowing her/him freedom to remove the belt.

SUMMARY

The management of psychiatric and behavioral disorders among NH residents is a difficult and challenging task. The precise nature and frequency of these disorders must be carefully defined, and treatable medical conditions that can cause or exacerbate these disorders should be identified and treated. Optimal management requires an interdisciplinary team approach. Psychiatrists and psychologists as well as clinical social workers should work together with medical and nursing staff to identify and treat these disorders. An example of an interdisciplinary care plan for a complex resident with severe behavioral disturbances is outlined in Table 10–14. Physical restraints and psychotropic medications should be avoided in the management of behavioral disturbances. When they are used, the reasons should be clearly documented and the behavioral responses closely monitored. Attempts should be made to reduce or eliminate the use of these interventions as soon as feasible.

SUGGESTED READINGS

Cohen-Mansfield J, Marx MS, Rosenthal AS: A description of agitation in a nursing home. *J Gerontol* 44(3):M77–M84, 1989.

Cohen-Mansfield J, Werner P, Marx MS: Screaming in nursing home residents. *J Am Geriatr Soc* 38:785–792, 1990.

Evan LK, Stumpf NE: Tying down the elderly: A review of the literature on physical restraints. *J Am Geriatr Soc* 37:65–74, 1989.

Fitten LJ, Morley JE, Gross PL, et al: Depression. *J Am Geriatr Soc* 37:459–472, 1989.

Gillin JC, Byerly WF: The diagnosis and management of insomnia. *N Engl J Med* 322:239–247, 1990.

Grossberg G, Massan R, Szwabo P, et al: Psychiatric problems in the nursing home. *J Am Geriatr Soc* 38:907–917, 1990.

Powell C, Mitchell-Pedersen L, Fingerote E, Edmund L: Freedom from restraint: Consequences of reducing physical restraints in the management of the elderly. *Can Med Assoc J* 141:561–564, 1989.

Werner P, Cohen-Mansfield J, Braun J, Marx MS: Physical restraints and agitation in nursing home residents. *J Am Geriatr Soc* 37:1122–1126, 1989.

Winograd CH, Jarvik LF: Physician management of the demented patient. *J Am Geriatr Soc* 34:295–308, 1986.

ELEVEN

NUTRITION

Malnutrition is very common in the nursing home (NH). The prevalence varies based on the case mix and socioeconomic status of the resident population in different institutions. The most common form of malnutrition among NH residents is protein-energy malnutrition, which occurs in up to 66 percent. Insufficient caloric intake has been documented in 5 percent to 18 percent of NH residents. Along with malnutrition, vitamin and trace mineral deficiencies occur in a substantial proportion of NH residents. This chapter highlights the specific nutritional problems often seen in NH residents and gives a practical approach to their management.

PROTEIN-ENERGY MALNUTRITION

Diagnosis

Protein-energy malnutrition can present either with weight loss alone with maintenance of serum albumin levels (marasmus) or with low serum albumin levels (kwashiorkor). A marasmuslike picture is a more common presentation, as most older individuals in institutions are ingesting at least 800 to 1000 calories, which is sufficient to maintain serum albumin at the expense of muscle protein. In patients with marasmus, the onset of infection leads to release of interleukins and tumor necrosis factor, which results in a decrease in serum albumin levels.

The best indicators of protein-energy malnutrition in a NH resident are weight loss, low body weight, low mid-arm muscle circumference, low cholesterol levels and low albumin levels (Table 11-1). The single best predictor of death in a malnourished NH resident is a cholesterol below 150 mg/dl. Other predictors of death are recent weight loss, low mid-arm muscle circumference, albumin below 4 g/dl, and hematocrit below 41 percent. The use of regular monthly weights is recommended for monitoring NH residents. It is essential that the scales be checked regularly, and standard procedures for weighing should be used (e.g., no shoes, no jackets, no sweaters, and empty pockets). There must be regular in-service training on procedures for weighing, and a random sample (e.g., 5 percent) of residents should have their weights checked by a registered nurse (RN) supervisor on a monthly basis. In residents who have fluid shifts—such as those with congestive heart failure, renal failure, or dehydration—measurement of mid-arm circumference should replace weighing. However, use of skin-fold thickness generally shows too high an interindividual variation to be useful as a routine method of assessing nutritional status. Table 11-2 lists average body weights and normal mid-arm circumference values.

Causes

The major causes of protein-energy malnutrition are outlined in Table 11-3. Every effort should be made to separate the less impaired from the more impaired residents at mealtimes. This allows residents to enjoy their meals and, where possible, promotes social interaction. Room dividers can be very useful in this regard. Eating habits of different residents need to be carefully observed and table pairings made on this basis. Ethnic food preferences also need to be determined.

Restrictive diets in NHs are more likely to cause protein-energy malnutrition than they are likely to improve the status of other diseases. For example, the prescription of severely sodium-restricted diets in NHs has been questioned. In one study, switching NH residents from a 3 g to a 4 g sodium diet resulted in no significant changes in control of heart failure. Similarly,

Table 11-1 Indicators of protein-energy malnutrition

Indicator	Critical level
Weight loss	5 lb in 6 months or less
Low body weight	Less than 10% of average weight
Mid-arm circumference	Less than 10.4 in.
Albumin	Less than 4.0 g/dl in ambulatory and less than 3.5 g/dl in recumbent
Cholesterol	Less than 150 mg/dl

Table 11-2   Limits for standard body weight per inch of height (± 10 percent)

Height, inches	Age, year					
	65–69	70–74	75–79	80–84	85–89	90–94
Men						
61	156–128	153–125	151–123			
62	158–130	155–127	153–125	148–122		
63	161–131	157–129	155–127	150–122	146–120	
64	164–134	161–131	157–129	152–124	148–122	
65	166–136	164–134	160–130	155–127	153–126	143–117
66	169–139	167–137	163–133	158–130	156–128	146–120
67	172–140	170–140	166–136	162–132	160–130	150–122
68	175–143	174–142	169–139	165–135	163–133	154–126
69	179–147	178–146	174–142	169–139	167–137	158–130
70	184–150	182–148	178–146	175–143	172–140	164–134
71	189–155	186–152	183–149	180–148	176–144	169–139
72	195–159	190–156	188–154	187–153	182–148	
73	200–164	196–160	192–158			
Women						
58	146–120	138–112	135–111			
59	147–121	140–114	136–112	122–100	121–99	
60	148–122	142–116	139–113	130–106	124–102	
61	151–123	144–118	141–115	133–109	128–104	
62	153–125	147–121	144–118	136–112	132–108	131–107
63	155–127	151–123	147–121	141–115	136–112	131–107
64	158–130	154–126	151–123	145–119	141–115	132–108
65	162–132	158–130	154–126	150–122	146–120	136–112
66	166–136	162–132	157–128	154–126	152–124	142–116
67	170–140	166–136	161–131	158–130	156–128	
68	175–143	170–140				
69	180–148	176–144				

Source: After Master A, Lasser R. *JAMA* 172:658, 1960.

there is little evidence that ADA diabetic diets have a major role in NH residents. A "no free sugar" diet may be equally effective and allow residents more variety. There is also no evidence that low-cholesterol diets benefit NH residents. An optimal cholesterol level for a NH resident is 240 to 280 mg/dl. In addition to a routine diet order, bedtime nourishment should be offered to all NH residents.

Depression is a common, treatable cause of weight loss. All NH residents with weight loss should be screened for depression. The multiple other causes of weight loss in NH residents with dementia are outlined in Table 11-4. One study demonstrated that 18 minutes per day was spent feeding demented NH residents, compared with 99 minutes per day when the same

Table 11-3   Causes of protein-energy malnutrition in the nursing home

Social
   Monotonous institutional meals
   "Disgust" with surroundings and/or behaviorally disturbed residents
   Lack of ethnic foods
   Unnecessary dietary restrictions (e.g., low salt, low cholesterol, ADA diabetic)

Psychological
   Depression
   Dementia
   Anorexia nervosa
   Anorexia (tardive)
   Sociopathy—loss of locus of control
   Late-life paranoia
   Mania
   Overwhelming burden of life (passive suicide)

Medical
   Increased metabolism
      Hyperthyroidism
      Pheochromocytoma
   Anorexia
      Drugs
         Digoxin
         Psychotrophics
         Fluoxetine
      Esophageal candidiasis
      Hyperparathyroidism
      Intestinal ischemia
      Zinc deficiency
      Altered taste and smell
   Malabsorption
   Cancer
   Chronic obstructive pulmonary disease (increased metabolism and anorexia)
   Dysphagia

Table 11-4   Causes of weight loss in nursing home residents with dementia

Inadequate time spent feeding
Apraxia of swallowing
Lack of recognition of need to eat
Coexistent depression
Pacing (increased exercise)
Behavioral disorders (e.g., pica)

individuals were managed at home. The use of a semicircular table where one aide can feed four or five residents at a time is one innovative solution to this problem. To overcome the apraxia of swallowing, nurse's aides need to be taught to instruct the residents to swallow. Residents with loss of locus of control often attempt to use food to regain this control. Thus, food refusal may represent a manipulative behavior. Other residents notice that residents who are not eating get extra attention; thus they may also refuse to eat to obtain more interactive time with staff.

Anorexia nervosa can recur in older women who had an episode of this condition as teenagers. Older men and women may develop extremely abnormal attitudes toward eating and an abnormal body image. In some cases, this is related to a desire for immortality and to the belief that calorie restriction or low cholesterol levels will extend life. This disorder has been called *anorexia tardive*. Recognition of these abnormal attitudes about eating is essential for appropriate management. In addition to depression, other psychiatric disorders may also be related to poor nutritional intake. Late-life paranoia can present with refusal to eat because of the belief that the food is poisoned. Mania can result in weight loss due to increased energy utilization.

In some NH residents, failure to eat is related to a perception of life as an overwhelming burden and as such represents a form of passive suicide. In these residents, treatable depression must be excluded. At present, there is no single clear ethical principle that determines whether a NH resident who can make decisions for herself or himself should be allowed to starve to death. In the case of the severely demented individual, a written advance directive authorizing withholding or withdrawal of feeding appears legally necessary. Passive suicide should be distinguished from the normal failure to eat that is often noted in the last few weeks of life in very old individuals. Ethical issues surrounding artificial feeding and hydration are discussed further in Chap. 25.

Several medical disorders and medications can contribute to weight loss (Table 11-3). Among the medical causes of weight loss, apathetic hyperthyroidism should not be missed. Among NH residents with severe weight loss in whom hypertension is difficult to control, the presence of pheochromocytoma should be considered. Malnutrition occurs in 25 percent of residents on digoxin, and anorexia improves when this drug is discontinued. High doses of psychotropics often result in malnutrition. Severe wasting may occur when residents are treated with fluoxetine for depression. Early satiety may represent a presentation of intestinal ischemia. This condition may respond to nitrates or calcium channel antagonists. Residents with chronic obstructive pulmonary disease often become dyspneic when eating. These residents should have several (at least six) small meals a day.

Difficulties with swallowing are a major problem in NH residents.

Table 11-5 Techniques for oral feeding

Proper positioning to maximize ability to swallow
Nondistracting environment
Food preparation
    Palatably warm—not hot
    Gelatinous consistency
    Avoid rice and applesauce
    Try macaroni and cheese, meatloaf and gravy
    If there is excessive mucus, exclude milk products and chocolate

Besides leading to aspiration pneumonia, swallowing disorders can also result in a conditioned aversion to feeding. The single most important management strategy for dysphagic individuals is an upright posture, allowing maximum use of gravity. Feeding in a nondistracting environment is another important feature of the management of swallowing disorders such as dysphagia. Other techniques for feeding residents with dysphagia are outlined in Table 11-5. All dysphagic NH residents should have a modified barium swallow and evaluation by a speech therapist.

Management

The management of protein-energy malnutrition involves the early and aggressive use of supplements. Before the institution of tube feeding, documentation that both hand feedings and swallowing therapy have been attempted must appear in the resident's record. Most studies suggest that enteral feedings usually produce only weight maintenance, not weight gain. These data suggest the need for early introduction of enteral feeding to prevent malnutrition. Alternatively, the calories administered need to be increased to more than 2000 per day until weight gain occurs. For reimbursement, this requires documentation that lower levels of calories failed to produce weight gain. The indications for tube feeding are outlined in Table 11-6, and the major complications of enteral feeding are outlined in Table 11-7. Before switching from elemental to blenderized formulas, the presence of diarrhea should be documented. Table 11-8 lists other potential

Table 11-6 Indications for enteral nutrition in long-term-care setting

Protein-energy malnutrition with inadequate oral intake for 5 days
Less than 50% of required nutrient intake for 7 to 10 days
Severe dysphagia
Radiation or chemotherapy with anorexia
Organ failure with anorexia

Table 11-7   Potential complications of enteral feeding

Problems with tube placement
Intolerance of tube
Aspiration
Gastric erosions
Diarrhea
Selenium deficiency
Fluid intolerance
Hypotension (with bolus feeding)
Glucose intolerance
Electrolyte imbalance (low blood levels of potassium, phosphorus, calcium, sodium, magnesium)

approaches to diarrhea associated with tube feeding. Table 11-9 gives the composition of some of the commonly used enteral products.

The feeding tube may be placed through the nose or through the skin, or it can be implanted surgically. It appears that overall there is little difference in complications regardless of the method of placement. Thus the choice should be dictated by resident and/or staff preference. There is no clear advantage to percutaneous gastrostomy tube placement over jejunostomy tube placement. Tubes placed in the stomach pose a greater risk of aspiration than tubes placed in the small intestine. They have the advantage, however, of allowing bolus feedings. Aspiration from endogenous secretions continues to occur after tube placement, no matter what type of tube is placed. Placing a soft small-bore tube in ice before insertion may facilitate placement by the nasogastric route. Alternatively, a small-bore tube may be attached to a larger nasogastric tube, either by holding the two together with a gelatin capsule or placing the small-bore tube inside the larger tube after it has been split open lengthwise. Both these techniques are associated with a greater rate of mechanical complication during insertion.

Table 11-8   Management of diarrhea among tube-fed residents

Rule out treatable causes of diarrhea
    Medication side effects
    Antibiotic-associated enterocolitis
    Fecal impaction
    Other
Dilution of formula may work, but results in decreased intake of calories
Switch to a lactose-free feeding
Switch to blenderized formula
Give banana chips orally
Try a high-fiber diet among those who take food orally

Table 11-9 Composition of some commonly used enteral feeding products

	Calories (per ml)	Protein (g/liter)	Sodium (meq/liter)
Ensure (Ross)	1.1	37	37
Isocal (Mead-Johnson)	1.1	34	23
Osmolite (Ross)	1.1	37	28
Replete (Clinitec Nutrition)	1.0	62	22
Sustacal (Mead-Johnson)	1.5	49	36
Resource (Sandoz)	1.1	37	37
Jevity (Ross)[a]	1.1	45	40
Sustacal with fiber[a] (Mead-Johnson)	1.1	46	31
Compleat (Sandoz)[b]	1.1	43	57
Mentene Liquid (Sandoz)[b]	1.0	69	48
Ensure Plus (Ross)	1.5	55	50
Isocal MN (Mead-Johnson)	2.0	75	35
Nutren 2.0 (Clinitec Nutrition)	2.0	80	43
Two Cal MN (Ross)	2.0	84	46
Sustagen (Mead-Johnson)[b]	1.7	112	55

[a] Contains fiber.
[b] Contains lactose.

Among the methods of tube feeding, bolus feedings are the most poorly tolerated, are most likely to result in missed feedings, and involve the most staff time. Cyclical feeding at night frees the resident from being attached to a pump during the day and allows him or her optimal opportunity to eat. Cyclical feeding is often better tolerated psychologically as well. Continuous feedings have better gastrointestinal tolerance and more easily achieve adequate calorie delivery than do cyclical feedings. They also smooth metabolic control. Their major disadvantage is that the resident is "tube tied" throughout the day and night.

Elemental formulas containing 1.0 to 1.5 calories/ml should be sufficient for most NH residents (see Table 11-9). Residents who develop infections should be switched to high-protein formulas. Low-protein formulas are used for residents with renal failure. High-fat formulas can be used for residents with chronic obstructive pulmonary disease, because they decrease the amount of oxygen needed for the metabolism of the food and may smooth the control of patients with diabetes mellitus. High-fiber formulas should be given only to residents who are ambulatory, because they can produce constipation in immobile residents. All residents receiving tube feeding should be supplemented with 100 μg of sodium selenite daily unless the formula contains selenium.

VITAMIN DEFICIENCY

Vitamin deficiency is not rare in the NH population. The presence of vitamin deficiency closely parallels that of protein-energy malnutrition. Individuals with cheilosis, angular stomatitis, and a magenta tongue have vitamin B_2 (riboflavin) deficiency. Pyridoxine (B_6) deficiency may present similarly but without the magenta tongue. Individuals with vitamin B_{12} (cobalamin) deficiency often have a beefy red, large tongue. Dermatological findings suggestive of these vitamin deficiencies that can be seen in NH residents include cheilosis and dermatoses. It therefore appears prudent to give a B-complex vitamin to any NH resident with a low caloric (less than 1200 calories per day) intake.

Pernicious anemia occurs in 1 percent to 2.5 percent of persons over 60 years of age. Vitamin B_{12} deficiency is classically associated with megaloblastic anemia, subacute combined degeneration of the spinal cord, and/or dementia. It is now recognized that in individuals with both iron and vitamin B_{12} deficiencies, the anemia may be either normo- or microcytic. Dementia can occur in the face of vitamin B_{12} deficiency without the development of anemia. NH residents with dementia may also develop a secondary vitamin B_{12} deficiency associated with malnutrition. In these cases, some cognitive improvement may be obtained by treatment with vitamin B_{12}. If this approach is taken, a vitamin B_{12} level below the normal range should be documented. The resident's cognitive status should also be documented, and this should be repeated every 3 months, using a standard scale to measure improvement.

Vitamin C (500 mg per day) may be useful for NH residents with pressure sores or other poorly healing skin lesions. Higher doses of vitamin C appear to offer no benefit. Vitamin C must be withdrawn at least 72 h before testing for blood in the stool, as it can cause false-negative occult blood tests.

MINERAL DEFICIENCY

NH residents often have a borderline zinc status. This is especially true among those receiving thiazide diuretics and those with diabetes mellitus or liver disease. The putative effects of zinc deficiency are outlined in Table 11-10. The major indications for zinc supplementation in a NH resident are poorly healing skin ulcers and anorexia without an obvious cause. Age-related macular degeneration may also be slowed by administration of zinc. The preferred dosage is zinc sulfate 220 mg three times a day with meals. The sulfate may cause gastrointestinal distress. Breaking the zinc capsule

Table 11-10   Putative effects of zinc deficiency

Anorexia
Hypogeusia
Poor wound healing
Immune dysfunction
Age-related macular degeneration

and mixing the contents with water may alleviate the gastrointestinal distress.

Selenium deficiency may occur in tube-fed NH residents and can be associated with muscle weakness and/or pain and nail changes (i.e., thickened and fragile, with rough, ridged surfaces). Residents with selenium deficiency can also have humoral and cellular immune dysfunction and may have a greater propensity to develop candidiasis. Treatment consists of supplementation with 100 μg of sodium selenite daily.

WATER

Water is the single most abundant part of the body's composition yet it is most likely to be forgotten. Screening for dehydration can be carried out by identifying all residents with a blood urea nitrogen to creatinine ratio of greater than 20:1. Further diagnosis then depends on demonstrating a postural blood pressure drop or an increasing pulse rate in response to standing for 2 min.

Several factors make NH residents susceptible to dehydration. Older individuals do not recognize thirst as readily as younger ones do. In addition, older individuals may have impaired access to fluids because of physical restraints or because of inherent impaired mobility. Incontinent residents sometimes self-limit fluid intake in an attempt to decrease urinary frequency. Increased fluid loss occurs with fever; special attention must be paid to the fluid needs of such residents. For these reasons, it is essential that NH residents be offered fluids at regular intervals.

SUGGESTED READINGS

Morley JE: Nutritional status of the elderly. *Am J Med* 81:679–695, 1986.
Morley JE, Glick Z, Rubenstein LZ: *Geriatric Nutrition: A Comprehensive Review.* New York, Raven Press, 1990.
Morley JE, Mooradian AD, Silver AJ, et al: Nutrition in the elderly. *Ann Intern Med* 109:890–904, 1988.

TWELVE

PRESSURE SORES AND OTHER SKIN DISORDERS

PRESSURE SORES

Pressure sores and other skin disorders are prevalent among nursing home (NH) residents and present a challenge for both prevention and management. Pressure sores are commonly used as indicators of poor quality of care. Most studies have been conducted among older hospitalized patients in acute care hospitals and report prevalence rates of between 20 and 30 percent. The true incidence of pressure sores in NHs is not known. It is estimated that 60,000 people die per year from complications of pressure sores. In addition to the human toll, the financial aspects are significant. Nursing time per NH resident doubles for the resident with a pressure sore. Cost estimates to heal each pressure sore range from $5000 to $40,000. The annual national cost of care for pressure sores is estimated at $3.5 to $7 billion. In addition, medical outcomes associated with pressure sores can be devastating. For example, a fourfold risk of death has been reported for institutionalized patients who develop pressure sores.

Etiology and Pathogenesis

Table 12-1 describes primary and secondary factors associated with the development and healing of pressure sores. As their name implies, pressure is the causative factor leading to these lesions. Normal capillary pressure in humans is about 35 mmHg. Pressure between a bony prominence and a hard resting surface can exceed 300 mmHg. The concentration of pressure

145

Table 12-1   Factors associated with the
development of pressure sores

Primary factors	Secondary factors
Pressure over bony prominences	Malnutrition
Shearing forces	Immobility
Tissue tolerance	Moisture
	Friction
	Anemia
	Vascular insufficiency
	Diabetes mellitus
	Sensory impairments

over a limited area reduces capillary blood flow to near zero at the point of pressure. High pressure can be tolerated, but only if it is relieved intermittently. Mobile people with intact sensation can sense the ischemia as discomfort and shift their position periodically. Thus, NH residents with impaired mobility are at increased risk for developing pressures that produce pressure sores. Pressure as low as 70 mmHg can produce irreversible tissue damage if it is applied for more than 2 h. Microscopic examination of damaged tissue shows characteristic ischemic changes of cellular infiltration, extravasation, and hyaline degeneration. A cone-shaped area of ischemia develops from the point of pressure to a wider area in the deeper tissues. The skin itself may be the last tissue layer to demonstrate ischemic changes. Ischemia and subsequent inflammatory changes therefore show a predilection for sites overlying bony prominences, particularly below the belt line. Most pressure sores develop on the sacrum, ischial tuberosities, greater trochanters, heels, and lateral malleoli (Fig. 12-1).

Another primary factor implicated in the development of pressure sores is the shearing forces caused by sliding adjacent surfaces. These forces are encountered clinically when the head of a bed is raised, causing the patient's torso to slide down while the sacral skin remains fixed. This can cause stretching and agitation of small blood vessels, with subsequent thrombosis. Friction also contributes to the development of pressure sores by removing the skin's outer protective layer. Moisture, regardless of the source, also promotes maceration and skin breakdown.

With continued pressure on skin that has become ischemic, a dermatitis-like picture develops. Edema and softening of the skin allow further damage due to friction. Bacterial invasion of damaged tissue can take place when the epithelium is disrupted. Infection can cause major delay in healing because of tissue damage and bacterial competition for oxygen.

Other secondary factors contributing to the development and healing of pressure sores are listed in Table 12-1. There remains some disagreement

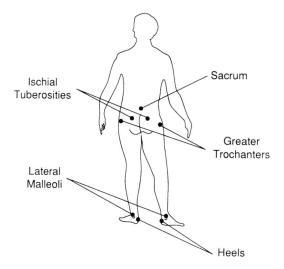

Ischial
Tuberosities

Sacrum

Greater
Trochanters

Lateral
Malleoli

Heels

Figure 12-1 Most common sites of development of pressure sores in NH residents.

regarding risk factors and their role in the development of pressure sores. One study identified hypoalbuminemia, fecal incontinence, and hip fracture as independent risk factors for developing pressure sores. Other reported risk factors include immobility, weight loss, and hypotension. All these factors are common among NH residents, making them especially vulnerable to pressure sores.

Assessment

Proper assessment of pressure sores requires careful examination of the sore. Most sores cannot be accurately assessed until all eschar and purulent material has been removed. Several descriptive assessment tools can be found in the literature. All use depth of the lesion as a grading criterion. The classification of Shea, which describes four stages, is used most often and helped form the basis of the National Pressure Ulcer Advisory Panel's Consensus Conference Statement in 1989 (Table 12-2).

Determining the stage of the pressure sore is only one aspect of assessment. The wound should also be assessed for location, size (length and width in centimeters), depth, undermining or tunneling, exudate (type, amount), odor, color of wound bed, surrounding tissue status, necrotic tissue (type, color, and amount), and granulation tissue. It is important to review previous treatment strategies and to identify contributing factors that may also affect the progress of healing.

Closed pressure sores, usually covered by eschar, may involve large areas of destruction under the skin, with only a small area of overlying skin

Table 12-2   The staging of pressure sores

Stage I	Nonblanchable erythema on intact skin; the heralding lesions of skin ulceration
Stage II	Partial-thickness skin loss involving epidermis and/or dermis. The ulcer is superficial and present clinically as an abrasion, blister, or shallow crater
Stage III	Full-thickness skin loss involving damage or necrosis of subcutaneous tissue; this may extend down to but not through underlying fascia. The ulcer presents clinically as a deep crater with or without undermining of adjacent tissue
Stage IV	Full-thickness skin loss with extensive destruction, tissue necrosis, or damage to muscle, bone, or supporting structures (e.g., tendon, joint capsule, etc)

Source: National Pressure Sore Advisory Panel Consensus Conference Statement (1989).

appearing to be involved. These sores can be deceptive and may require debridement or radiological evaluation (CT, MRI, or sinography) for accurate assessment.

Management of Pressure Sores

Prevention. The best strategy for preventing the development of pressure sores is to avoid immobility and pressure. High-quality nursing care is critical. A reliable risk-assessment or screening tool to identify high-risk NH residents has yet to be perfected. The often used Norton scale has been criticized for its lack of overall predictive value and validity. Other scales are in use but suffer from similar limitations. Familiarity with the known risk factors (Table 12-1) leads to the development of a preventive strategy, such as the one described in Table 12-3. The development of specific protocols for the prevention and treatment of pressure sores can be useful to nursing staff in order to standardize their approach to the problem. Standards of care for pressure sores are available from the International Association of Enterostomal Therapists (IAET, Irvine, California), and they may help form the basis of such protocols.

Staff education and appropriate nursing management techniques are especially important to assure compliance and accountability for proper body positioning and the prevention of immobility (i.e., walking the resident, changing positions), which are critical elements in the prevention of pressure sores. Figure 12-2 illustrates various body positions relative to pressure sore development.

Primary physicians should work with nursing staff to carefully and systematically observe NH residents at high risk for pressure sores and to identify and treat early sores before they become deeper. The use of enteros-

Table 12-3   Guidelines for the prevention of pressure sores

A. Reduce and/or relieve pressure

   Rationale: In providing effective pressure relief, both pressure and time must be considered.

   1. Pressure relieving devices

   Rationale: Capillary closing pressure is 25 to 32 mmHg. *Pressure relieving* devices are those which *consistently* reduce pressure below this level and can be used to prevent pressure breakdown.

   Candidates

   Residents who cannot tolerate turning.

   Residents who have skin breakdown or who are at risk for skin breakdown involving multiple surfaces.

   Examples

   Low airloss bed therapy.

   Air fluidized bed therapy.

   2. Pressure reducing devices

   Rationale: Pressure reducing devices lower pressure, as compared to standard hospital mattresses or chair surfaces. They *do not* reduce pressure below capillary closing levels on a consistent basis and must be used in conjunction with a turning or position change schedule.

   Candidates

   Residents who *can* be turned.

   Residents with skin breakdown or at risk for skin breakdown involving only one surface.

   Examples

   Dynamic—pressure reducing devices, which *move* (eg, alternating air mattress), reduce pressure locally.

   Static—pressure reducing devices, which are stationary (such as foam mattresses, gel cushions, water beds, and air mattresses), also reduce pressure locally.

   3. Establish schedule for major position changes and weight shifts. Generally turning every 2 h is sufficient, but some individuals may require more frequent turning.

B. Reduce and/or relieve shearing

   Rationale: Shearing is caused when tissue layers slide against each other and results in angulation or disruption of blood vessels, usually at the fascial level.

   1. When not contraindicated, keep head of bed at or below 30° angle and flat.

   2. If not contraindicated, use knee gatch when head of bed is elevated.

   3. Use padded foot board.

C. Reduce and/or relieve friction

   Rationale: Friction—caused when the skin rubs against another surface—can cause superficial skin damage.

   1. Use assistive devices and/or techniques—such as turning sheets, trapeze bar, lifts, transfer boards—to facilitate movement.

   2. Use powder or cornstarch on surfaces contacting skin to reduce surface friction and absorb moisture.

D. Reduce excessive moisture

   Rationale: Excessive moisture and/or contact with urine or stool causes maceration and/or chemical erosion of the skin.

   1. Institute measures to contain fecal and/or urinary incontinence and to protect the skin.

E. Evaluate nutritional and hydration status

   Rationale: Tissue hydration and positive nitrogen balance are critical elements in wound healing.

   1. Consult dietician and provide nutrition and hydration support as required.

Site of
Pressure Sore   Allowed Positions   Positions to Avoid

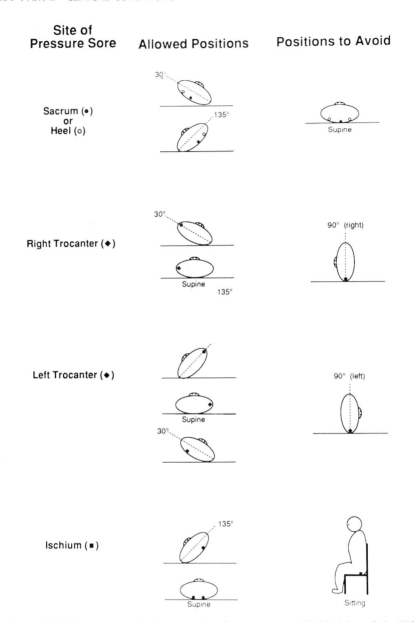

Figure 12-2 Body position and the prevention of pressure sores. Modified from Sieler WO, Stahelin HS: *Geriatrics* 40(7):53–60, 1985.

tomal therapy (ET) nurses, who have special education in pressure sore management, or other nurse consultants in NHs can enhance pressure sore care and staff education. The management of medical conditions that place residents at high risk for pressure sores should be optimized (e.g., anemia, vascular disease, diabetes). It is important to note that many pressure sores develop during an acute hospital stay; it is the NH staff that then has to deal with them. It has unfortunately been the practice of long-term care regulatory agencies to penalize NHs for the presence or aggravation of pressure sores. Effective prevention and management of pressure sores must therefore involve a cooperative effort between acute hospital and NH staffs. Regulatory agencies should focus on assisting such cooperative efforts rather than trying to find someone to blame for the development of individual pressure sores.

Treatment. Pressure sores differ little from other skin wounds, and general principles of wound care are applicable to their management. Although not specifically discussed in this chapter, the general principles of managing lower extremity venous and arterial ulcers are similar to those of managing pressure sores. General medical care should focus on nutritional repletion to reverse protein catabolism and promote wound healing. Table 12-4 reviews the functions of nutritional elements in wound healing. (For more detailed information on wound healing, see Suggested Readings.) Correction of anemia, control of underlying medical conditions such as diabetes, and improvement in oxygenation and tissue perfusion may also enhance wound healing.

The objectives of managing pressure sores include the relief of pressure, prevention of further tissue damage, wound debridement and the elimination of local infection, and the promotion of a healing environment. In severe cases, excision and closure of defects may be necessary. Some 70 to 90 percent of pressure sores are superficial (stage II or less) and may be managed with conservative therapy.

Relief of pressure can be accomplished in a variety of ways, including frequent turning in order to prevent prolonged exposure to one area (see Fig. 12-1) and the use of local padding or pressure-reducing beds. It is important to note that use of local skin padding such as "donuts" should be avoided because of their propensity to impede circulation, and worsen the already present ischemia. Heel protectors are useful in preventing friction and shearing, but they require monitoring to ensure that they do not cause undue pressure. Several types of pressure-reducing devices and beds are available. Egg-crate foam mattresses are probably the least expensive and most convenient. Their advantages are offset by the fact that they offer the least pressure reduction and are generally considered devices that serve only to enhance comfort if the foam-rubber projections are less than 4 in.

Table 12-4   Function of various nutritional elements in wound healing

Element	Function	Effect of deficiency
Protein	Cell proliferation, collagen metabolism	Delayed healing
Carbohydrate	Energy source	Altered leukocyte function
Fats	Membrane function	Not known
Vitamin C	Enzyme cofactor in collagen metabolism	Rickets, altered collagen formation, delayed healing
Vitamin A	Antagonizing effect of steroids	Not well known
Thiamine	Energy metabolism	Decreased cell proliferation and collagen metabolism
Vitamin E	Membrane stabilization	None known
Vitamin K	Coagulation cofactor	Excessive bleeding, hematoma, wound disruption
Water and salts (sodium, potassium, chlorine)	Membrane function, hydration	Volume depletion, decreased tissue profusion
Phosphorus	ATP metabolism	Altered cell replication and protein metabolism
Calcium, magnesium, manganese	Enzyme cofactors in collagen metabolism	Altered collagen formation, delayed healing
Zinc	RNA metabolism	Altered cell replication, delayed healing
Iron, copper	Enzyme cofactors in collagen metabolism	Delayed healing, anemia

high (including bases and peaks). Water beds provide modest pressure reduction, but their inflation pressure is critical. Over- or underinflation results in less than optimal pressure reduction. The materials used for these mattresses is usually plastic or rubber, and moisture may become a problem. Air mattresses provide better pressure reduction, and aerated models also help to decrease moisture. Air fluidized and low airloss beds provide a levitation medium (air or fiberglass spheres). These units provide adequate pressure dispersion, pressure relief, and labor conservation (requiring less turning and changes of linen). They provide a dry environment, decreasing the effect of perspiration and incontinence, and a freely movable surface that may decrease the forces of friction and shear. Recent reports suggest these beds—as opposed to foam mattresses—may have a significant positive effect on large pressure sores during the first week of wound care. Because air fluidized beds are costly, their use should be considered only for residents with large stage III and stage IV wounds for whom positioning is difficult. The average NH cannot afford the cost of these beds unless supplemental coverage by insurance is available. With proper staff and physician documentation, the NH can fill out a treatment authorization report (TAR) and be reimbursed for the use of the bed by some Medicaid programs. Medicare Part A recognizes the selective need for this modality and frequently authorizes its use, reimbursing the cost through the NH's cost reporting mechanism.

Table 12-5 provides examples of protocols for the management of various types of pressure sores. Many NH nurses have their own favorite protocols. Many of these protocols do work, but none have been adequately tested in randomized controlled trials. The effective management of stage I and stage II pressure sores involves pressure relief, the optimization of nutrition, treatment of underlying medical conditions, and excellent local care. Superficial cultures have *no* role in the management of stage I and stage II sores and should not be ordered routinely (see Chap. 17). Debridement must be added to management protocols for stage III and stage IV sores, for which removal of necrotic tissue is essential. Debridement is done by surgically removing eschar and necrotic debris, followed by coverage with saline-soaked mesh gauze. This is allowed to dry for 4 to 8 h ("wet to dry"). Then the gauze is removed and replaced by newly soaked gauze. This removes loose necrotic debris and effectively lowers the bacterial count. Alternatively, one may use "slow" chemical debridement using proteolytic enzymes to help liquify the necrotic tissue. Collagenase is capable of digesting undenatured collagen, which is found in most eschar. Semiocclusive dressings (e.g., hydrocolloid) may be applied after a wound is cleaned and debrided. This provides an environment conducive to healing. Topical antibiotics or oxidizing agents offer no advantage and may actually retard healing by being toxic to new cells or by encouraging the growth of resistant bacteria. The reduction of moisture and fecal contamination is also essential. Absorptive pads are preferable to indwelling catheters to manage incontinence because of the risk of sepsis, although the temporary use of an indwelling catheter may be necessary to help heal some pressure sores. Adequate staffing and intensive nursing care are necessary to provide the frequent cleaning that may be required for incontinent residents with pressure sores.

Control of infection is achieved mostly by debridement and removal of

Table 12-5 Examples of protocols for the management of various stages of pressure sores[a]

A. Pressure sore classification: stage I, epidermis intact
  1. Wound cleansing
    a. No special cleansing necessary
  2. Topical treatment: goal—protect and maintain intact epidermis
    a. Transparent semipermeable membrane
      Rationale: Protects intact epidermis yet allows visualization of area.
      Procedure: Apply to clean, dry skin. Change every 7 days in p.m.
    b. Skin barrier film
      Rationale: Protects intact epidermis yet allows visualization of area.
      Procedure: Available as wipes or spray. Apply to clean, dry area once a day.

B. Pressure sore classification: stage II, partial-thickness wounds and/or stage III, shallow, full-thickness wounds with little exudate
  1. Wound cleansing
    a. Normal saline
      Rationale: Normal saline is physiologic and has no deleterious effects on the wound-healing process. Wound cleansing promotes removal of wound debris and bacteria from wound surface.
  2. Topical treatment: goal—keep wound surface clean, moist, and free of secondary infection.
    a. Transparent semipermeable membrane
      Rationale: Provides a moist wound-healing environment by trapping wound exudate under dressing; allows visualization of wound.
      Procedure: Apply to clean wound with at least 2 cm of dressing extending beyond wound. Dressing should be changed every 7 days and/or whenever wound fluid leaks from underneath dressing.
    b. Hydrocolloid dressing
      Rationale: Provides a moist wound-healing environment by trapping wound exudate under dressing. Many encourage angiogenesis as most are occlusive dressings.
      Procedure: Apply to clean wound with at least 2 cm of dressing extending beyond wound. Dressing should be changed every 7 days and/or whenever wound fluid leaks from underneath dressing. If more frequent dressing changes are needed, use smaller dressing with less extending around wound.
    c. Gel dressing
      Rationale: Provides a moist wound-healing environment. May absorb some wound exudate. Used with other dressings (transparent semipermeable membrane, hydrocolloid, or gauze).
      Procedure: Apply gel to clean wound and cover with secondary dressing of choice (transparent semipermeable membrane, hydrocolloid, gauze). Change according to secondary dressing used (usually every 3 to 4 days). If gauze is used, change every day or every other day.
    d. Calcium alginate dressing
      Rationale: Provides a moist wound-healing environment. Absorbs wound exudate.
      Procedure: Apply enough to cover wound bed on clean wound. If wound is fairly dry, moisten dressing with small amount of normal saline. After application, cover with gauze dressing and change when drainage strikes through cover dressing, generally every 3 to 5 days. Alternatively, cover with transparent semipermeable membrane and change every 7 days and/or when there is leakage of exudate from underneath dressing.
    e. Moist gauze dressing
      Rationale: If applied correctly, will provide a moist wound-healing environment. Absorbs small amount of wound exudate.

Procedure: Use gauze instead of cover sponges. Moisten gauze with normal saline, fluff, and apply to clean wound. Cover with dry cover sponge. Change every 4 h. Gauze should not be allowed to dry out, as this will retard wound healing.

f. Lubricating spray

Rationale: Provides a moist wound-healing environment.

Procedure: Spray in clean wound bed and cover with gauze dressing. Change dressing every day to every shift, depending on amount of wound exudate.

C. Pressure sore classification: stage III and/or stage IV; full-thickness wounds, deep craters, or wounds with excessive or pooled exudate

1. Culture and sensitivity, after cleansing of the wound base, in the following circumstances: symptoms or signs of clinical infection (e.g., cellulitis) bone/joint involvement; sepsis when the etiology is unknown

   Rationale: All dermal wounds are contaminated; culture is indicated *only* for evidence of clinical infection or potential for osteomyelitis. Surface swab cultures are of *no* value; culture should be taken from deep necrotic tissue or bone.

2. Wound cleansing

   Rationale: Thorough cleansing at each dressing change promotes removal of wound debris and bacteria from wound surface. Many commonly used solutions have deleterious effects on the wound healing process and should be used with caution if used at all. For example:

   Povidone-iodine—inhibits and/or destroys macrophages and fibroblasts

   Hydrogen peroxide—provides mechanical cleansing through effervescence but also destroys fibroblasts even when diluted

   Dakin's solution (potassium hypochlorite)—controls odor, is effective for staphylococcal and streptococcal infections, helps liquify necrotic tissue, but also destroys fibroblasts.

   Acetic acid—appropriate for *pseudomonas* infections, but also destroys fibroblasts even when diluted.

   a. Normal saline

      Rationale: Normal saline is physiologic and has no deleterious effects on the wound healing process. It is appropriate for all wounds.

      Procedure: May be used as a solution for irrigation or for less aggressive cleansing.

3. Topical treatments: Goal—keep wound surface clean, moist, and free of secondary infection; pack wound to obliterate dead space without damaging tissue.

   a. Absorption dressing—copolymer starches and dextranomers

      Rationale: Absorption dressings absorb excess exudate, obliterate dead space, and provide a moist wound-healing environment.

      Procedure: Mix or prepare dressing according to manufacturer's guidelines and apply to clean wound bed, taking care to pack dead space. Cover with gauze dressing and change once a day or more frequently depending on wound exudate.

   b. Absorption dressing—calcium alginates

      Rationale: Absorbs excess exudate, obliterates dead space, and provides a moist wound-healing environment.

      Procedure: Gently pack dead space and apply to clean wound bed. Cover with gauze dressing and change when drainage strikes through dressing. (In heavily exudating wounds, this may be once or twice a day; less frequently for wounds with less exudate.)

   c. Absorption dressing—moist gauze

      Rationale: Absorbs excess exudate, obliterates dead space, and provides a moist wound-healing environment.

Procedure:	Use gauze instead of cover sponges. When packing wounds with large amounts of dead space, it is best to use rolled gauze for easy removal. Moisten gauze with desired solution; normal saline is appropriate for all wounds (see notes on wound cleansing solutions under C2, above.) Gently pack dead space and fluff to apply to clean wound bed.

D. Pressure sore classification: stage III and/or stage IV, with necrotic tissue present
   1. Topical treatments: Goal—debridement of necrotic tissue

     Rationale: Necrotic tissue is an impediment to wound healing and must be removed

     a. Conservative instrumental debridement

Rationale:	Conservative debridement can be used in conjunction with other topical therapy to enhance the process without the risks involved in surgical debridement.
Procedure:	May be done by enterostomal therapy (ET) nurses and/or other nurse specialists depending on state nurse practice acts and education. Removal of tissue is done by scalpel or sharp scissors and is limited to clearly identified necrotic tissue.

     b. Enzymatic debriding ointments

Rationale:	Enzymatic agents chemically break down necrotic tissue; effectiveness is dependent on appropriate use.
Procedure:	Many wound cleaning solutions interfere with the action of enzymatic debriding ointments; if used, they must be thoroughly rinsed from wound bed with normal saline. Apply ointment to necrotic tissue only and cover with gauze dressing. Some ointments work better with a moist gauze dressing. Most should be changed every 8 h (check manufacturer's guidelines for duration of action). If the necrotic tissue is hard or eschar is present, scoring or cross-hatching of the hard eschar may be required prior to use of enzymatic ointment.

     c. Physiologic debridement using transparent semipermeable membrane dressings

Rationale:	Transparent semipermeable membrane dressing enhance leukocyte migration and resultant autolysis of necrotic tissue.
Procedure:	Especially effective on hard eschar necrotic tissue. Apply to clean wound with at least 2 cm of dressing extending beyond wound. Change every 7 days or whenever wound fluid leaks from underneath dressing.

     d. Mechanical debridement using wet-to-dry dressings and/or water propulsion therapy

Rationale:	Wet-to-dry dressings are a nonselective debriding approach; granulation tissue may be removed in addition to necrotic tissue. Water propulsion provides mechanical removal of *loose* necrotic tissue.
Rationale:	Moisten gauze (not cover sponges), fluff; apply to wound bed and cover with cover sponge: allow gauze to dry prior to next dressing change (usually 4 h) and pull dry gauze out of wound bed. Gauze should not be moistened to ease removal, as this contradicts the purpose of the dressing. This debridement method can be painful, and pain medication may be needed prior to dressing changes. Water propulsion can be performed by needle and syringe, Water Pik, or whirlpool therapy. Water propulsion will remove only necrotic tissue that is already loose.

     e. Once debridement of necrotic tissue is accomplished, topical treatments include those identified in C, above.

---

[a] All protocols should be accompanied by prevention strategies (see Table 12-3) and optimization of nutrition and management of other medical conditions.

Source: International Association for Enterostomal Therapy: *Standards of Care Dermal Wounds: Pressure Sores*. Irvine, California, 1987.

necrotic material. Use of systemic antibiotics should be limited to lesions complicated by cellulitis, osteomyelitis, bacteremia, or sepsis. The management of infected pressure sores is discussed in detail in Chap. 17.

OTHER SKIN DISORDERS

Dry Skin (Xerosis)

Dry skin is one of the most common dermatologic problems affecting the elderly. It usually occurs on exposed surfaces, including the hands, feet, and face. The sides of the torso are also frequently involved. The clinical signs of xerosis include scaling, flaking, cracks, and fissures. Symptomatically, xerosis manifests itself by pruritus, which may be intense and can cause excoriations complicated by superinfection. Since many other skin disorders (e.g., contact dermatitis, seborrheic dermatitis, allergic reactions, psoriasis) as well as some medical conditions (e.g., renal failure, hyperbilirubinemia) can cause pruritus, a careful assessment should be done before pruritus is ascribed simply to dry skin.

Prevention of xerosis is largely dependent upon retarding the loss of moisture from the surface of the stratum corneum. Table 12-6 lists some general guidelines for the prevention of dry skin. Many NH residents develop dry skin in winter because indoor heated air is very low in humidity, and forced-air heating systems keep air currents moving past exposed skin. Use of a humidifier to maintain adequate humidity (i.e., above 40 percent) may be important in preventing xerosis, pruritus, and other complications. Sebum from sebaceous glands helps preserve epithelial hydration. When combined with sweat, sebum forms an emulsion that coats the skin, forming a barrier against transdermal water loss. Commercial moisturizing creams, lotions, and oils act by producing an occlusive or semiocclusive film that coats the surface and helps the sebaceous glands to reduce evaporation. These products also lubricate the skin, making rough, dry, scaly skin smoother and less irritated. Any treatment for dry skin should be supplemented by an effort to replace the moisture lost through perspiration and evaporation. Nursing home residents should be encouraged to drink several

Table 12-6   Strategies to prevent dry skin and pruritus

1. Encourage adequate fluid intake.
2. Use tepid baths and bath oils to preserve skin moisture.
3. Apply moisturizing creams or lotions after baths and two to three times per day.
4. Use soft, absorbent clothing.
5. Prescribe topical steroid creams sparingly to avoid skin atrophy.
6. Whenever possible, avoid antihistamines unless severe pruritus is causing excoriations or disrupting sleep.

glasses of water per day. This will help to prevent not only dry skin but also dehydration and its complications.

Dermatitis and Eczema

The terms *dermatitis* and *eczema* are often used interchangeably or in combination. Both imply superficial inflammation of the skin due to irritant exposure, allergic sensitization, and/or other factors that contribute to skin irritation. Pruritus can result in erythema and edema of the skin, which may progress to vesicle formation, oozing, crusting, and scaling. Table 12-7 describes several types of dermatitis that are seen in the NH population.

Table 12-7   Types of dermatitis seen in the nursing home population

Condition	Description/characteristics	Management
Idiopathic eczema of the hand	Persistent erythema and scaling of the palms or lateral digits without an obvious precipitating cause.	Emollients, topical steroids; overnight occlusion to intensify steroid absorption.
Contact dermatitis	Skin inflammation caused by contact with irritant or allergic substance.	Avoid contact with irritant such as soaps, detergents, solvents. Acute eczema with blister formation should be referred to a dermatologist.
Stasis dermatitis	Inflammation occurring as a result of venous hypertension in the lower leg.	Well-fitting support stockings to control edema; keep limb elevated as much as possible.
Drug-caused eruptions	Eruption of the skin that occurs after administration of a drug. Starts 1 to 10 days after the resident first takes the drug and may last for 14 days after it is discontinued.	Drug should be removed; symptomatic treatment of lesions; severe reactions may require the use of systemic corticosteroids.
Toxic epidermal necrolysis	Severe eruption that begins with general malaise, skin tenderness, and erythema; rapidly progresses to blistering.	Remove drug (NSAID, sulfa, penicillin); systemic steroids; diphenylhydantoin; severe reactions may require care in a burn unit.
Psoriasis	Well-defined erythematous plaques covered with a silver scale. Affects especially knees, elbows, scalp, and buttocks.	Coal tar or cream or paste (0.1% to 0.4%); topical corticosteroids; phototherapy; methotrexate.
Seborrheic dermatitis	Scaly erythematous eruption affecting face, eyebrows, eyelids, scalp, nasolabial folds, and body flexures. May cause blepharitis and conjunctivitis.	Topical hydrocortisone creams or ointments; tar-containing shampoos for scalp involvement.

Many NH residents develop a dermatitis of unknown etiology. Treatment consists of avoiding the excessive use of products that might irritate the skin, such as drying soaps and detergents. Clothing made of nonirritant materials such as cotton should be worn next to the skin. Emollients should be used liberally, especially after bathing. Corticosteroid creams or ointments should be applied three times daily to affected areas. Once symptoms are alleviated, use of the topical corticosteroid can be reduced and often discontinued in favor of emollients alone. Antihistamines may be necessary to reduce severe pruritus and help the resident sleep. However, these agents must be used with caution in elderly NH residents, since they have anticholinergic effects and may produce paradoxical agitation.

Herpes Zoster ("Shingles")

Herpes zoster is a cutaneous eruption caused by the reactivation of a varicella zoster viral infection. The lesions begin as pustules and then rupture, with resultant crusting in a unilateral dermatomal distribution. Occasionally secondary bacterial infection becomes a serious problem. After 2 to 4 weeks, the skin lesions resolve, sometimes leaving some scarring. Pain in the dermatome may precede the onset of the lesions and persist for weeks or months after the skin lesions heal (postherpetic neuralgia). The management of herpes zoster is discussed in Chap. 17.

Scabies

Scabies is an eruption caused by the mite *Sarcoptes scabiei*. The female mite burrows into the skin and deposits eggs, which hatch into larvae in a few days. Scabies is transmitted by skin-to-skin contact and can rapidly spread throughout a NH. Scabies may present less typically and may mimic eczema or exfoliative dermatitis, with thick crusted lesions. Erythroderma and generalized lymphadenopathy may be present. The mite must be excavated with a needle or a scalpel blade in order to make the diagnosis. In long-standing cases with widespread excoriation, a mite may be impossible to find. In these cases, treatment based on a presumptive diagnosis may be the best option. This consists of applying a lotion or cream containing lindane 1 percent (i.e., Kwell) to the entire body, from the neck down. After 24 h, the resident should be bathed and all clothing and bed linens should be machine-laundered in hot water or dry-cleaned. Any close personal contacts such as other residents, nurses' aides, or other clinical staff and their household contacts should be treated to avoid spreading scabies to individuals as yet asymptomatic. A second application of the cream or lotion, also left on the body for 24 h, is indicated 7 days later to ensure that any newly hatched larvae are killed. The itching may not subside for 1 to 2 weeks after the resident has been treated. Persistent itching can be treated effectively with topical corticosteroids or, in very severe cases, with a tapering course of an oral corticosteroid.

Pediculosis (Lice)

Lice may infest the head (pediculosis capitis) and/or the body (pediculosis corporis). NH residents are at risk for head and body lice. Pediculosis capitis is transmitted through personal contact or through hairbrushes and head wear. Infected individuals develop severe itching of the scalp, often with secondary eczematous changes and impetiginization. Cervical lymphadenopathy may also be present. On examination, small gray or white mites (ova) are seen on the hair shafts. Unlike scales, they cannot easily be removed. Pediculosis corporis produces intense generalized itching that, in turn, can lead to the development of eczematous changes, excoriations, and secondary bacterial infections. Lice or mites may be found in the seams of clothing.

For head lice, shampoo containing 1 percent lindane is applied to the scalp and left in place for 4 to 6 min. After rinsing, the hair should be combed with a fine tooth comb. The procedure should be repeated in 10 days to destroy any remaining mites. Combs and brushes should be soaked in the shampoo for 1 h. For body lice, the resident's clothing should be dry-cleaned or washed in a machine (hot cycle). The seams of the clothing should be pressed with a hot iron. Alternatively, the clothing can be disinfected with an insecticidal powder such as DDT 10 percent or malathion 1 percent. Eczema and/or infection that develops as a result of the infestation should be treated appropriately.

Bullous Pemphigoid

Bullous pemphigoid is an autoimmune disorder of the skin that occurs most commonly in the elderly. Pathologically, immunoglobulin (IgG) is deposited along the basement membrane of the skin. Sometimes the mucosa is also involved. Clinically, bullous pemphigoid presents as intact tense blisters that occur on normal or erythematous skin. Crusting occurs after the bullae rupture. This disorder is usually well controlled by systemic corticosteroid therapy. Other immunosuppressive drugs such as azathioprine and methotrexate are also used in some cases. Some reports have linked bullous pemphigoid with malignant neoplasms, but there is no evidence that individuals with bullous pemphigoid have a higher rate of cancer than the general elderly population.

Skin Tumors

Skin malignancies are strongly related to aging and are therefore common in the NH population. Virtually all skin cancers can be recognized early. Most can be cured with appropriate medical or surgical therapy. Table 12-8 describes several malignant skin tumors. It is important for primary care physicians to recognize these lesions and refer residents for dermatologic

Table 12-8   Examples of malignant skin tumors seen in the geriatric nursing home population

	Description	Treatment
Basal cell carcinoma	Lesion on sun-exposed areas of fair-skinned individuals. Slow-growing, superficial, reddened or pearly with irregular border. Metastases are rare.	Superficial lesions: topical 5-fluorouracil. Small tumors: curettage and cauterization cryotherapy. Larger tumors: excision with closure or split-thickness skin graft; radiotherapy.
Squamous cell carcinoma	Arise in sun-damaged skin in fair-skinned people. Commonly a shallow ulcer surrounded by a wide, elevated, indurated border. Ulcer may be covered by crust, which conceals the red base. May present as a persistent nonhealing ulcer. Lesions on lips or genitals are likely to metastasize.	Well differentiated: surgical treatment. Poorly differentiated: radiotherapy. Cryotherapy used for multiple lesions.
Malignant melanoma	Pigmented macular lesion with irregular border on sun-exposed areas.	Wide local excision. Close follow-up for irregular pigmentation, nodularity, or bleeding.
Superficial spreading melanoma	Accounts for about 60% of all melanomas. Can occur on any part of the body. Irregular border with pigmentation.	Wide local excision. Close follow-up for irregular pigmentation, nodularity, or bleeding.
Kaposi's sarcoma	An indolent tumor in elderly men of central European origin. One or more purple or dark blue macules on legs; these slowly enlarge to nodules and ulcers.	Simple excision or radiotherapy.

evaluation when a malignant lesion is suspected. In addition to malignant skin tumors, benign and premalignant lesions are also commonly seen in the geriatric population. The most common benign lesions are seborrheic keratoses. These are brown, sharply demarcated, slightly raised lesions that are found in areas where sebaceous glands are plentiful, such as the trunk, face, and extremities. They do not need treatment unless they become irritated and are bothersome. The rapid appearance or increase in size of seborrheic keratoses in a previously blemish-free area (sign of Heser-Trelat) is associated with internal malignancy. Actinic keratoses are well demarcated, scaly, rough papules on sun exposed areas. These are premalignant lesions and can be managed by a number of different techniques [e.g., cryotherapy, curettage, topical 5-fluorouracil (5FU), excisional surgery]. Bowen's disease is a form of squamous cell carcinoma in situ. Lesions are often multiple and appear as slowly enlarging erythematous patches with sharp but irregular borders and crusting. These lesions are treated in a manner similar to squamous cell carcinoma (see Table 12-8).

SUGGESTED READINGS

Allman RM: Pressure ulcers among the elderly. *N Engl J Med* 320:850, 1989.

Allman RM, Laparda CA, Noel LB, et al: Pressure sores among the elderly. *Ann Intern Med* 105:377, 1986.

Balin AK: Aging of the human skin, in Hazzard WR, Andres R, Bierman EL, Blass JP (eds): *Principles of Geriatric Medicine and Gerontology.* New York, McGraw-Hill 1990, pp 383–412.

Ferrell BA, Osterweil D: Pressure sores and nutrition, in Morley J, Glick Z, Rubenstein LZ (eds): *Geriatric Nutrition.* New York, Raven Press, 1990, pp 363–379.

Phillips TJ, Gilchrest BA: Skin changes and disorders, in Abrams WB, Berkow R (eds): *The Merck Manual of Geriatrics.* Rahway, New Jersey, Merck Sharp & Dohme Research Laboratories, 1990, pp 1025–1053.

Reuler JB, Cooney TG: The pressure sore: Pathophysiology and principles of management. *Ann Intern Med* 94:661, 1981.

THIRTEEN

INCONTINENCE

PREVALENCE AND MORBIDITY

Urinary incontinence (UI) affects approximately half of nursing home (NH) residents. The prevalence varies among individual facilities depending upon case mix; rates may be as low as 40 percent to as high as 70 percent or even higher in facilities with a very functionally impaired resident population. In contrast to UI among ambulatory community-dwelling geriatric patients, UI among NH residents is more severe and more commonly associated with stool incontinence. Incontinent NH residents generally have multiple episodes of UI throughout the day and night, and approximately half also have stool incontinence more than once per week.

UI in the NH is associated with substantial morbidity and cost. Although data demonstrating a cause-and-effect relationship are lacking, UI has been shown to be associated with several physical conditions including skin irritations, urinary tract infections (UTI), and falls. For those afflicted, UI is uncomfortable; it can lead to skin irritation and make pressure ulcers difficult to heal, it can result in UTI when urinary retention with overflow UI remains undiagnosed or when UI is inappropriately managed by a chronic indwelling catheter, and it may lead to falls among residents with urge UI and impaired balance or gait. The adverse psychological effects of UI have been difficult to document systematically, but incontinent residents who are not severely demented are often embarrassed and frustrated by their condition. The NH staff generally consider UI to be one of the most onerous and difficult conditions for which they care and perceive that they spend a disproportionate amount of time on incontinent residents.

163

The economic costs of UI in the NH are less difficult to document. Conservative estimates of the costs of managing UI range from $0.5 to $2 billion annually, including staff time, laundry, and supplies.

Although it is unrealistic to expect to cure UI or dramatically reduce the costs of its management in the NH, it is realistic and, in fact, appropriate to attempt to identify selected residents who may benefit from specific therapeutic approaches, to implement reasonable policies and procedures for bladder and bowel management programs and catheter care, and to utilize containment devices such as padding and incontinence undergarments in a cost-effective manner.

BASIC PRINCIPLES OF MANAGING INCONTINENCE IN THE NURSING HOME

As is emphasized throughout this text, NH residents are heterogeneous. A realistic and appropriate goal for one type of resident may be totally unrealistic and inappropriate for another. The approach to UI brings this concept into sharp focus. A resident undergoing active rehabilitation after a hip fracture or a stroke may, after a thorough incontinence assessment, benefit from a specific bladder retraining protocol and/or pharmacologic therapy for detrusor hyperactivity. Incontinence undergarments and indwelling catheters are unlikely to be appropriate for this type of resident. On the other hand, a resident with end-stage dementia and severe agitation may be most appropriately managed by a containment device without any specific evaluation for UI.

Thus, an extremely important aspect of incontinence care is to determine, through the interdisciplinary care-planning process, if a particular resident has the potential to respond to specific interventions for UI. Because even severely impaired residents may respond very well to a prompted voiding program (see the discussion under "Assessment" and "Behavioral Interventions," below), a bias in favor of assessment and a therapeutic trial is appropriate.

Several other basic principles of incontinence management for the NH are outlined in Table 13-1. Each of these principles will be discussed in more detail in subsequent sections of this chapter. First, however, a brief review of the basic types and causes of UI will be presented in order to put the specific recommendations into context.

BASIC TYPES AND CAUSES OF URINARY INCONTINENCE

The pathogenesis of UI among NH residents is often multifactorial, involving urological/gynecological conditions, neurological disorders, behavioral and

**Table 13-1   Basic principles of managing incontinence
in the nursing home**

1. Identify a physician and nurse who will oversee an incontinence management program
2. Develop written policies and procedures where applicable
3. Provide in-service education on incontinence to medical and nursing staffs
4. Assess the continence status of all new residents at admission and periodically thereafter
   a. A legible bladder record should be used (Fig. 13-1)
   b. Recent onset of incontinence should prompt a search for reversible causes (Table 13-2)
5. Make an interdisciplinary decision about the resident's potential
   a. Do not automatically attribute incontinence to functional disability and manage palliatively
   b. Develop realistic goals: e.g., reduction of frequency of UI (versus cure), elimination of daytime UI with palliative management at night
6. Perform a basic diagnostic evaluation focusing on the identification of reversible factors (Table 13-2)
7. Use specific criteria to refer selected residents for further evaluation (Table 13-4)
8. Develop standardized bladder retraining and prompted voiding protocols (Tables 13-8 and 13-9)
9. Systematically monitor the response to specific therapeutic interventions using a bladder record (Fig. 13-1) and modify the approach if necessary
10. Do not overuse padding, incontinence undergarments, and indwelling catheters
    a. Specific indications for indwelling catheters should be documented (Table 13-10)
    b. Implement a catheter-care protocol for residents who are managed by chronic indwelling catheterization (Table 13-11)

psychological factors, and functional impairments. Thus, the approach to assessment and treatment must be comprehensive and should include all of these potential factors.

The most important factors to consider are those that are *reversible.* While identification and management of these reversible factors may not cure the UI, it may reduce its frequency and make it more manageable by other interventions (e.g., prompted voiding). Reversible factors are more commonly found among residents with recent-onset incontinence, which may be the situation for many newly admitted NH residents. It is essential to recognize, however, that reversible factors may also be contributing to persistent forms of UI that have been present for months or even years. As outlined in Table 13-2, reversible factors can be remembered by using the acronym DRIP.

Table 13-3 illustrates a basic classification of the types of persistent UI. Three important features of this classification should be noted. First, from a neurourological perspective, this classification is greatly simplified and does not include all the pathophysiological types of UI. Nonetheless, it is helpful in attempting to develop a basic approach to the assessment and treatment of UI in the geriatric population. Second, many incontinent NH residents have mixtures of these types of UI. The predominant abnormality

Table 13-2   Reversible (DRIP) factors that may contribute to urinary incontinence

D	Delirium	New-onset UI may be associated with delirium due to acute underlying conditions requiring diagnosis and treatment
R	Restricted mobility	Acute conditions causing immobility may precipitate UI; environmental manipulation and scheduled toileting are appropriate until condition resolves
	Retention	Urinary retention may be precipitated by many drugs (see below) or may occur acutely due to anatomic obstruction; immobility and large fecal impactions may also contribute
I	Infection	Acute cystitis may precipitate urge UI Otherwise asymptomatic bacteriuria may contribute to urinary frequency and should be eradicated before any urodynamic evaluations are carried out
	Inflammation	Atrophic vaginitis and urethritis can cause irritative voiding symptoms, including UI
	Impaction	Fecal impaction may be associated with UI (as well as fecal incontinence)
P	Polyuria	Poorly controlled diabetes with glucosuria can contribute to urinary frequency and UI Edema due to congestive heart failure and/or venous insufficiency can cause nocturia and exacerbate nocturnal UI
	Pharmaceuticals	These include rapid-acting diuretics (urge UI), psychotropics (sedation, immobility), anticholinergics, alpha agonists, beta agonists, calcium channel blockers, narcotics (urinary retention), alpha antagonists (stress UI), and alcohol (sedation, immobility, polyuria)

of lower urinary tract functioning found among NH residents is *detrusor hyperactivity* (involuntary bladder contractions found on cystometry; also termed *detrusor instability, unstable bladder,* and *detrusor hyperreflexia*—the latter in the presence of a neurological disorder). Although most often associated with urge-type UI, detrusor hyperactivity is commonly seen in conjunction with sphincter weakness and stress UI among women, obstruction in men with benign or malignant prostatic enlargement, and with impaired bladder contractility resulting in incomplete bladder emptying (termed *detrusor hyperactivity with impaired contractility,* or DHIC). Thus, depending on the type of therapeutic approach being considered, it may be very important to identify these mixed types of UI (see "Assessment," below). Third, and most important, functional-type UI should be a diagnosis of exclusion, because most NH residents have impairments of cognitive and/or physical functioning that may interfere with toileting skills. These residents may also have other potentially treatable conditions contributing to their UI. Thus, a search for reversible factors and other types of UI should be completed before labeling a NH resident's UI as functional.

Table 13-3   Basic types and causes of persistent urinary incontinence

Type	Definition	Common causes
Stress	Involuntary loss of urine (usually small amounts) with increases in intra-abdominal pressure (e.g., cough, laugh, or exercise)	Weakness and laxity of pelvic floor musculature Bladder outlet or urethral sphincter weakness
Urge	Leakage of urine (usually larger volumes) because of inability to delay voiding after sensation of bladder fullness is perceived	Detrusor hyperactivity isolated or associated with one or more of the following: Local genitourinary condition such as cystitis, urethritis, tumors, stones, diverticula, outflow obstruction; impaired bladder contractility (DHIC) Central nervous system disorders such as stroke, dementia, parkinsonism, suprasacral spinal cord injury or disease
Overflow	Leakage of urine (usually small amounts) resulting from mechanical forces on an overdistended bladder or from other effects of urinary retention on bladder and sphincter function	Anatomic obstruction by prostate, stricture, cystocele Acontractile bladder associated with diabetes mellitus or spinal cord injury Neurogenic (detrusor-sphincter dyssynergy) causes associated with multiple sclerosis and other suprasacral spinal cord lesions
Functional	Urinary leakage associated with inability to toilet because of impairment of cognitive and/or physical functioning, psychological unwillingness, or environmental barriers	Severe dementia and other neurological disorders Psychological factors such as depression, regression, anger, and hostility

ASSESSMENT

An assessment of bladder and bowel function is a requirement for all newly admitted NH residents. A bladder and bowel record is helpful in document-ing the continence status of new residents and can also be used as a com-ponent of periodic reassessments. A 3- to 5-day monitoring period is enough to document the timing, amount, and situations associated with any incon-tinence. A legible record, such as the one shown in Fig. 13-1 should be employed. The specific symbols used are not important, but there should be a simple way of documenting wetness, dryness, appropriate toileting, bowel status, and comments. Records such as the one shown in Fig. 13-1 can be reduced photographically so that several records can fit on one page.

INCONTINENCE MONITORING RECORD

INSTRUCTIONS: EACH TIME THE PATIENT IS CHECKED:
1) Mark *one* of the circles in the BLADDER section at the hour closest to the time the patient is checked.
2) Make an X in the BOWEL section if the patient has had an incontinent or normal bowel movement.

🖉 = Incontinent, small amount	⊘ = Dry	X = Incontinent BOWEL
🔴 = Incontinent, large amount	⧄ = Voided correctly	X = Normal BOWEL

PATIENT NAME _____ ROOM # _____ DATE _____

	BLADDER				BOWEL			
	INCONTINENT OF URINE		DRY	VOIDED CORRECTLY	INCONTINENT X	NORMAL X	INITIALS	**COMMENTS**
12 am	●	●	O	△ cc ____				
1	●	●	O	△ cc ____				
2	●	●	O	△ cc ____				
3	●	●	O	△ cc ____				
4	●	●	O	△ cc ____				
5	●	●	O	△ cc ____				
6	●	●	O	△ cc ____				
7	●	●	O	△ cc ____				
8	●	●	O	△ cc ____				
9	●	●	O	△ cc ____				
10	●	●	O	△ cc ____				
11	●	●	O	△ cc ____				
12 pm	●	●	O	△ cc ____				
1	●	●	O	△ cc ____				
2	●	●	O	△ cc ____				
3	●	●	O	△ cc ____				
4	●	●	O	△ cc ____				
5	●	●	O	△ cc ____				
6	●	●	O	△ cc ____				
7	●	●	O	△ cc ____				
8	●	●	O	△ cc ____				
9	●	●	O	△ cc ____				
10	●	●	O	△ cc ____				
11	●	●	O	△ cc ____				
TOTALS								

Figure 13-1 Example of a NH bladder and bowel record for assessing and following response to therapy. (Copyright, Regents of University of California, 1984; reprinted with permission.)

This type of record is also helpful in monitoring responses to therapeutic interventions.

Because many newly admitted residents come from acute-care hospitals, they frequently arrive at the NH with an indwelling bladder catheter. In this situation it is essential to determine why the catheter was placed (i.e., to monitor urinary output versus urinary retention versus management of UI) and to consider the resident for a bladder retraining program, as described under "Behavioral Interventions," below. The catheter should be removed unless there is an appropriate indication for keeping it in place (see "Catheters and Catheter Care," below).

After this initial assessment and documentation, an interdisciplinary decision should be made about whether the resident should undergo further assessment or be managed palliatively with containment devices. It is important to reemphasize in this regard that UI should not automatically be attributed to functional disability for at least two reasons: (1) although functional disability may be contributing to the UI, specifically treatable conditions can also be detected; and (2) many very functionally impaired NH residents respond well to a simple prompted voiding program. Specific predictors of responsiveness to prompted voiding are outlined later in this chapter.

Table 13-4 outlines key aspects of the clinical assessment. The objectives of this assessment include the following:

1. Identification of potentially reversible factors (Table 13-2).
2. Identification of conditions that may require further urological, gynecological, and/or complex urodynamic evaluation (see below and Table 13-5).
3. Determination of the type of UI (i.e., urge, stress, overflow, functional, mixed)

Figure 13-2 depicts the basic diagnostic assessment strategy. It can be argued that once objectives 1 and 2 are met, it may not be critical to determine the exact type of UI *if* the initial approach will be to treat all residents with a behavioral intervention such as prompted voiding. This may, in fact, be a reasonable initial approach, because some studies of prompted voiding suggest that it reduces the frequency of different types of UI. If, however, drug therapy is being contemplated or if the resident does not respond well to prompted voiding, further assessment by some type of urodynamic evaluation will be necessary in order to guide further therapy.

Table 13-6 and Fig. 13-4 detail procedures for a simplified urodynamic evaluation. The simplified urodynamic evaluation can be carried out even among residents with moderate to severe dementia. Several caveats should, however, be briefly mentioned. First, the resident must be communicative enough to understand the instructions and cooperate with the testing. Second, misleading results can be obtained if the tests are not performed prop-

**Table 13-4   Key aspects of the clinical assessment
of incontinence in the nursing home**

History
   Often difficult to obtain from resident
   Important symptoms:[a]
      Irritative (suggestive of urge UI and detrusor hyperactivity): frequency, urgency,
      nocturia, bed-wetting, leakage without warning

      Voiding difficulty (suggestive of obstruction and/or bladder contractility problem):
      hesitancy, poor or intermittent stream, straining to finish voiding

      Stress incontinence: leaks with straining, coughing, changing position, or leaks
      continuously

   Nursing observations can be helpful, such as signs of urgency, stress incontinence, or
   voiding difficulty
Physical examination
   Mental status among residents with dementia
      Ability to accurately perceive wetness versus dryness

      Ability to locate toilet and initiate voiding appropriately

      Ability to respond appropriately to a prompt to void
   Mobility
      Ability to use a toilet or toilet substitute, manage cleaning and clothing
   Lumbosacral innervation
      Detection of focal finding or neuropathy
   Abdominal
      Suprapubic palpation after voiding (may not be sensitive in detecting significant urinary
      retention)
   Rectal for fecal impaction and prostate exam
   Pelvic
      Significant prolapse (see Fig. 13-3)

      Atrophic vaginitis (patchy erythema, telangiectasias, friability, bleeding)
Urinalysis and urine culture
   May be difficult to obtain a clean specimen

   For men, clean penis with antiseptic solution, apply a clean condom catheter, and collect
   specimen from first void

   For women, very small catheters available

   Should be done in conjunction with postvoid residual determination
Postvoid residual determination
   Can be done by portable ultrasound device if available

   [a] These symptoms are not specific and may, in fact, be deceiving.

erly. This is especially true if the stress test, observation of voiding, and
residual volume determination are done when the resident's bladder is not
very full (i.e., <150–200 ml). Third, the individual performing the tests must
have a sound understanding of lower urinary tract functioning and what
they are looking for. Fourth, involuntary bladder contractions are very common in this population, but because they can occur with conditions other

than pure urge UI (e.g., sphincter weakness, outlet obstruction), their presence must be interpreted cautiously and in the context of other findings. Finally, like any other diagnostic tests, these tests should only be performed if the results will make a difference in the resident's care.

APPROACHES TO THERAPY

Reversible Factors

The first step in treating incontinence is to reverse the reversible (Table 13-2). Bacteriuria should be eradicated, not because this will cure the UI but because it may reduce its frequency in some residents and make them more responsive to other therapeutic interventions. Although published data do not support treating "asymptomatic" bacteriuria among NH residents because such treatment does not appear to alter morbidity or mortality, data are not yet available on the effects of eradicating bacteriuria on the frequency of UI. Thus, until adequate studies are available, we recommend eradicating bacteriuria (once) when assessing and treating UI in the NH.

Atrophic vaginitis should be treated by either vaginal estrogen cream (1–2 g to be applied 3 to 5 nights per week) or oral conjugated estrogen at a dose of 0.3–0.625 mg/day. There is no standard treatment protocol, but we recommend a 1- to 2-month trial. Like eradicating bacteriuria, the goal is not necessarily to cure the UI but to reduce its frequency and possibly make the resident more responsive to other forms of treatment. If there is a clear response, estrogen therapy can either be continued or alternatively withdrawn and reinstituted if symptoms and signs recur. Estrogen is contraindicated in women with a history of breast cancer, and women given estrogen for long periods of time should have mammography if they have not already had routine mammography in the past year.

Fecal impaction is often a recurrent problem. The management of constipation is discussed in Chap. 19.

Factors contributing to polyuria and/or nocturia should be addressed. Although it may be difficult to control diabetes tightly in some NH residents (see Chap. 16), the osmotic diuresis induced by glucosuria can certainly exacerbate UI and an attempt should be made at achieving better glucose control. Edema due to congestive heart failure and/or venous insufficiency may be mobilized in the evening and night hours and cause bothersome nocturia. This may even be hazardous in some residents who are prone to falls. It is therefore reasonable, in some situations, to initially manage the UI by adding (or increasing the dose of) a rapid-acting diuretic in the morning to reduce the edema and to make the resident urinate more often when there is better access to a commode.

Drugs which may be contributing to the UI should be removed whenever possible, especially if urinary retention is present. If it is not possible to discontinue them, reducing the dose may help manage the UI.

Table 13-5 Criteria for referral of incontinent nursing home residents for urological, gynecological, and/or complex urodynamic evaluation

Criteria	Definition	Rationale
History		
Recent history of lower urinary tract or pelvic surgery or irradiation	Surgery or irradiation involving the pelvic area or lower urinary tract within the past 6 to 12 months	A structural abnormality relating to the recent procedure should be sought
Relapse or rapid recurrence of a symptomatic urinary tract infection	Onset of dysuria, new or worsened irritative voiding symptoms, fever, suprapubic or flank pain associated with significant growth of a urinary pathogen; symptoms and bacteriuria return within 4 weeks of treatment	A structural abnormality or pathologic condition in the urinary tract predisposing to infection should be excluded
Physical examination		
Marked pelvic prolapse (see Fig. 13-3)	Pronounced uterine descensus to or through the introitus or a prominent cystocele that descends the entire height of the vaginal vault with coughing during speculum examination	Anatomic abnormality may underlie the pathophysiology of the incontinence and may require surgical repair
Stress incontinence that has failed or cannot be managed by nonsurgical therapy or stress incontinence in a man	Stress incontinence demonstrated standing or supine; urine, generally drops or small volumes, leaks coincident with increasing abdominal pressure	Surgical procedures are generally well tolerated and successful in properly selected women who have stress incontinence that responds poorly to more conservative measures; stress incontinence in a man suggests sphincter damage

Marked prostatic enlargement and/or suspicion of cancer	Gross enlargement of the prostate on digital exam; prominent induration or asymmetry of the lobes	An evaluation to exclude prostate cancer that requires curative or palliative therapy should be undertaken
Severe hesitancy, straining and/or interrupted urinary stream	Straining to begin voiding and a dribbling or intermittent stream at a time the patient's bladder feels full	Signs suggestive of obstruction or poor bladder contractility are present
Postvoid residual		
Difficulty passing a 12- or 14-French straight catheter	Catheter passage is impossible or requires considerable force or a larger, more rigid catheter is required	Anatomic blockage of the urethra or bladder neck may be present
Postvoid residual volume >200 ml	Volume of urine remaining in the bladder within 5 to 10 min after the patient voids spontaneously in as normal a fashion as possible	Anatomic or neurogenic obstruction or poor bladder contractility may be present
Urinalysis		
Hematuria (sterile)	Greater than 5 red blood cells per high power field on microscopic exam in the absence of infection	A pathologic condition in the urinary tract should be excluded
Uncertain diagnosis	After the history, physical exam, simple tests of lower urinary tract function, and urinalysis, none of the other referral criteria are met and an appropriate treatment plan cannot be developed based on the findings	A complex urodynamic evaluation may help better define and reproduce the symptoms associated with the incontinence and target treatment

Continence assessment on admission using bladder/bowel record

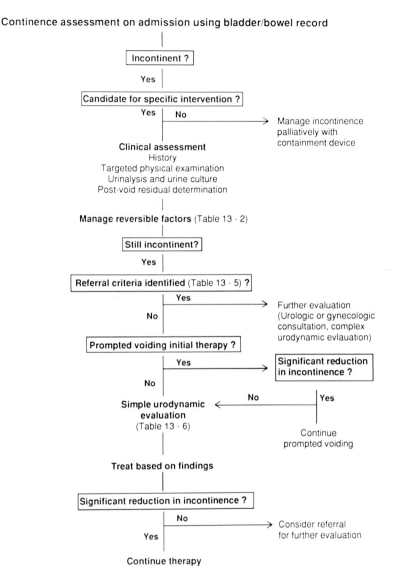

Figure 13-2 General strategy for diagnostic assessment and management of incontinence among NH residents.

Behavioral Interventions

Most NHs have "bladder training" protocols which consist of simple scheduled toileting on an every-2-h basis. While this is practical for staff and may help some residents, it is probably not the most efficient procedure and should be combined with other techniques whenever feasible.

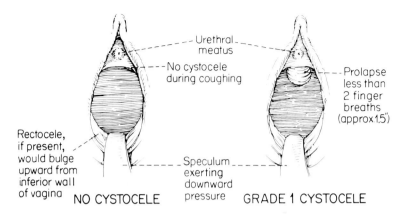

Urethral meatus

No cystocele during coughing

Prolapse less than 2 finger breaths (approx 1.5")

Rectocele, if present, would bulge upward from inferior wall of vagina

NO CYSTOCELE

Speculum exerting downward pressure

GRADE 1 CYSTOCELE

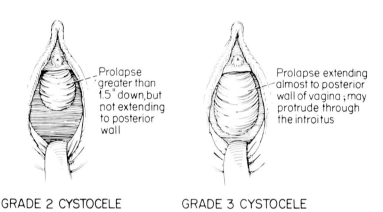

Prolapse greater than 1.5" down, but not extending to posterior wall

Prolapse extending almost to posterior wall of vagina ; may protrude through the introitus

GRADE 2 CYSTOCELE   GRADE 3 CYSTOCELE

Figure 13-3 Example of a grading system for cystoceles. A grade 3 cystocele would be a criterion for further evaluation. See Table 13-5. (Reprinted with permission, *J Am Geriatr Soc* 37:715–724, 1989.)

Behavioral interventions can be divided into two basic types, "patient-dependent" and "caregiver-dependent" (Table 13-7). Patient-dependent procedures such as bladder retraining require highly functional and motivated individuals and are most relevant for residents with recent-onset UI, especially those who are admitted to the NH with an indwelling catheter. An example of a bladder retraining protocol is depicted in Table 13-8. The precise protocol will depend on the resident's bladder function. If the catheter was placed to measure urine output or to manage UI during a hospitalization, the bladder is likely to be irritable and of small capacity; in this instance an attempt can be made to progressively increase the intervoiding interval. In highly functional residents, pelvic muscle exercises and other behavioral

Table 13-6 Procedures for simple tests of lower urinary tract function[a]

Procedure	Observations	Interpretation
Stress maneuvers		
If possible start the tests when the resident feels fullness in the bladder; ask the resident to relax and cough forcefully three times in the standing position with a small pad under the urethral area	Timing (coincident or after stress) and amount (drops or larger volumes) of any leakage	Leakage of urine coincident with stress maneuver confirms presence of stress incontinence
Normal voiding		
Ask the resident to void privately in that resident's normal fashion into a commode containing a measuring "hat" after a standard prep for clean urine specimen collection	Signs of voiding difficulty (hesitancy, straining, intermittent stream)	Signs of voiding difficulty may indicate obstruction or bladder contractility problem
	Voided volume	
Postvoid residual determination		
A 12- or 14-French straight catheter is inserted into the bladder using sterile technique within a few minutes after the resident voids	Ease of catheter passage	If there is great difficulty passing the catheter, obstruction may be present (easy passage does not exclude obstruction)
	Postvoid residual volume	If the residual volume is elevated (e.g., over 100 ml) after a normal void, obstruction or a bladder contractility problem may be present
Bladder filling (see Fig. 13-4)		
For females, position a fracture pan under the buttocks; for males, have a urinal available to measure any leakage during filling.	First urge to void ("I'm starting to feel a little full")	Involuntary contractions or severe urgency at relatively low bladder volume (e.g., <250–300 ml) suggest urge incontinence, especially if consistent with presenting symptoms

A 50-ml catheter-tip syringe without piston is attached to the catheter and used as a funnel to fill the bladder. The bladder is filled with room-temperature sterile water, 50 ml at a time, by holding the syringe so that it is approximately 15 cm above the pubic symphysis (bladder pressure should not normally exceed 15 cm of water during filling) until the resident feels the urge to void; this is continued in 25-ml increments until bladder capacity is reached (an involuntary contraction or "I would rush to the toilet now, I can't hold anymore")

The catheter is then removed

Repeat stress maneuvers

The resident is asked to relax and cough forcefully three times in the supine and standing positions

Bladder emptying

The resident is asked to empty his/her bladder again privately into the commode with the measuring "hat"

Presence or absence of involuntary bladder contractions—detected by continuous upward movement of the column of fluid (sometimes accompanied by leaking around or expulsion of the catheter) in the absence of abdominal straining, which the resident cannot inhibit.

Amount lost with involuntary contraction and subsequent bladder emptying.

Bladder capacity—amount instilled before either an involuntary contraction or the strong urge to void is perceived

Timing (coincident or after stress) and amount (drops or larger volumes) of any leakage

Signs of voiding difficulty (see above)

Voided volume

Calculated postvoid residual (amount instilled minus amount voided)

Involuntary contractions may occur in association with conditions other than pure urge incontinence. Thus, the results of this test must be interpreted carefully in the context of other findings (see text)

See above

Stress maneuvers with a full bladder are more sensitive for detecting stress incontinence

See above

Calculated postvoid residual may be more valid than postvoid residual obtained by catheter if resident did not feel full at beginning of tests

---

[a] See text for caveats about these tests.

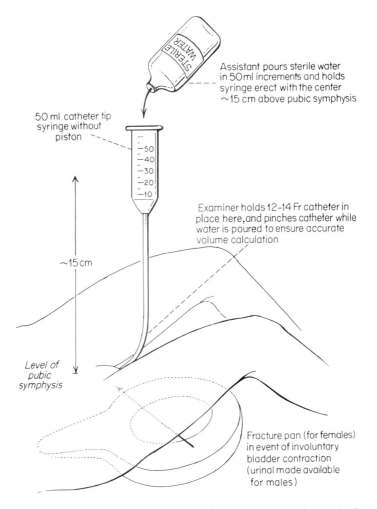

Assistant pours sterile water
in 50 ml increments and holds
syringe erect with the center
~15 cm above pubic symphysis

50 ml catheter tip
syringe without
piston

—50
—40
—30
—20
—10

Examiner holds 12-14 Fr catheter in
place here, and pinches catheter while
water is poured to ensure accurate
volume calculation

~15 cm

Level of
pubic
symphysis

Fracture pan (for females)
in event of involuntary
bladder contraction
(urinal made available
for males)

Figure 13-4 Illustration of simple cystometry procedure. See Table 13-6 for details. (Reprinted with permission, *J Am Geriatr Soc* 37:706–714, 1989.)

techniques may be helpful. If the catheter was placed for urinary retention, the bladder muscle may be decompensated; in this situation regular attempts to void should be combined with routine postvoid or intermittent catheterizations. It may take weeks for the bladder to begin refunctioning. If postvoid residuals remain elevated and the resident remains incontinent, a urological evaluation should be considered. Note that in either situation clamping the catheter before removal is not necessary; it has never been shown to be beneficial and may be harmful to residents who already have

Table 13-7 Examples of behavioral interventions for urinary incontinence

Procedure	Definition	Types of incontinence	Comments
PATIENT-DEPENDENT			
Pelvic muscle (Kegel) exercises	Repetitive contraction of pelvic floor muscles	Stress and urge	Requires adequate functioning and motivation May be done in conjunction with biofeedback
Biofeedback	Use of bladder, rectal, or vaginal pressure recordings to train residents to contract pelvic floor muscles and relax bladder	Stress and urge	Requires equipment and trained personnel Relatively invasive Requires adequate cognitive and physical functioning and motivation
Behavioral training	Use of educational components of biofeedback, bladder records, pelvic floor and other behavioral exercises	Stress and urge	Requires trained therapist, adequate cognitive and physical functioning, and motivation
Bladder retraining[a]	Progressive lengthening or shortening of intervoiding interval, with adjunctive techniques[b] such as intermittent catheterization in residents recovering from bladder overdistension with persistent retention	Acute (e.g., postcatheterization with urge or overflow, poststroke)	Goal is to restore normal pattern of voiding and continence Requires adequate cognitive and physical functioning and motivation
CAREGIVER-DEPENDENT			
Scheduling toileting	Fixed toileting schedule	Urge and functional	Goal is to prevent wetting episodes Can be used in patients with impaired cognitive or physical functioning Requires staff/caregiver availability and motivation

Table 13-7 *(Continued)* Examples of behavioral interventions for urinary incontinence

Procedure	Definition	Types of incontinence	Comments
Habit training	Variable toileting schedule based on pattern of voiding with positive reinforcement	As above	As above
Prompted voiding[c]	Regular (every 1–2 h) prompts to void with positive reinforcement	As above	As above

[a] See Table 13-8.
[b] Techniques to trigger voiding (running water, stroking thigh, suprapubic tapping), empty bladder completely (bending forward, suprapubic pressure), and alteration of fluid or diuretic intake patterns.
[c] See Table 13-9.

a decompensated bladder after urinary retention. Other patient-dependent procedures, such as pelvic muscle exercises and biofeedback, are relevant only to a small number of NH residents. Electrical stimulation, which can be used as an adjunct to these techniques, appears promising, but it has not been adequately tested in the NH population.

Although all the caregiver-dependent techniques have been shown to be effective, we recommend prompted voiding because it is the most practical, efficient, and well-studied technique.

An example of a prompted voiding protocol is depicted in Table 13-9. As opposed to bladder retraining (Table 13-8), the goal here is *not* necessarily to restore a normal pattern of voiding and continence; it is, rather, to prevent wetness. When motivated staff implement it properly, prompted voiding has been shown to be highly effective in reducing incontinence frequency during the day and evening hours. Because it appears to be effective in NH residents with different types of lower urinary tract dysfunction and is virtually free of side effects, it is a reasonable initial approach to managing most incontinent NH residents (Fig. 13-2). Note that the best results from prompted voiding have been documented when the protocol is implemented from 7 a.m. to 7 p.m. It is not clear whether the potential benefits of regular toileting throughout the nighttime hours are outweighed by disruption of the resident's sleep. In addition, staffing patterns at night may preclude an effective prompted voiding program, even in targeted residents. Thus, until further data are available, NHs should modify the protocol for nighttime hours and/or use incontinence undergarments.

Table 13-8   Example of a bladder retraining protocol

Goal: To restore a normal pattern of voiding and continence after the removal of an indwelling catheter[a]

1. Remove the indwelling catheter (clamping the catheter before removal is not necessary)[b]
2. Treat urinary tract infection if present[c]
3. Initiate a toileting schedule
   a. Begin by toileting the resident:
      (1) Upon awakening
      (2) Every 2 h during the day and evening
      (3) Before getting into bed
      (4) Every 4 h at night
4. Monitor the resident's voiding and continence pattern with a record[d] that allows for the recording of
   a. Frequency, timing, and amount of continent voids
   b. Frequency, timing, and amount of incontinence episodes
   c. Fluid intake pattern
   d. Postvoid or intermittent catheter volume
5. If the resident is having difficulty voiding (complete urinary retention or very low urine outputs, e.g., <240 ml in an 8-h period while fluid intake is adequate):
   a. Perform in and out catheterization, recording volume obtained, every 6 to 8 h until residual values are <100 ml[e]
   b. Instruct the resident on techniques to trigger voiding (e.g., running water, stroking inner thigh, suprapubic tapping) and to help completely empty bladder (e.g., bending forward, suprapubic pressure, double voiding)
6. If the resident is voiding frequently (i.e., more often than every 2 h):
   a. Perform postvoid residual determination to ensure that resident is emptying the bladder completely
   b. Encourage the resident to delay voiding as long as possible and instruct him/her to use techniques to help empty bladder completely (above)
7. If the resident continues to have frequency and nocturia with or without urgency and incontinence and there is no infection:
   a. Rule out other reversible causes (e.g., medication effects, hyperglycemia, congestive heart failure)
   b. Consider urodynamic evaluation to rule out detrusor hyperactivity

---

[a] Indwelling catheters should be removed from all residents who do not have an indication for their acute or chronic use (see text and Table 13-10).

[b] Clamping routines have never been shown to be helpful and are not appropriate for residents who have had overdistended bladders.

[c] Significant bacteriuria with pyuria (>10 white blood cells per high power field on a spun specimen).

[d] See Fig. 13-1.

[e] In residents who have been in urinary retention, it may take days or weeks for the bladder to regain normal function. If residuals remain high, urological consultation should be considered before the resident is committed to a chronic indwelling catheter.

Table 13-9 Example of a prompted voiding protocol

Goal: To reduce the frequency of wetness in selected residents from 7 a.m. to 7 p.m.

Assessment period (4–6 days)
1. Contact the resident every hour from 7 a.m. to 7 p.m. for 2–3 days, then every 2 h for 2–3 days
2. Focus resident's attention on voiding by asking whether he/she is wet or dry.
3. Check for wetness, record on bladder record, and give feedback on whether resident was correct or incorrect.
4. Whether wet or dry, ask resident if he/she would like to use the toilet (or urinal).
   a. If resident says yes:
      (1) Offer assistance
      (2) Record the results on the bladder record
      (3) Give positive reinforcement by spending an extra minute or two talking with resident.
   b. If resident says no:
      (1) Repeat the question once or twice
      (2) Inform him/her that you will be back in an hour and request that resident try to delay voiding until then
      (3) In the event that resident has not attempted to void in the last 2 to 3 h, repeat the request to use the toilet once or twice more before leaving
5. Measure voided volumes as often as possible by
   a. Placing a measuring "hat" in commode
   b. Preweighing and then reweighing incontinence pads or garments

Targeting
1. Prompted voiding is more effective in some residents than others
2. The best candidates for continuing on an effective prompted voiding program are residents who show the following characteristics during the assessment period[a]:
   a. Are correct more often than not about their wet/dry status
   b. Void in the toilet, commode, or urinal (as opposed to being incontinent in a pad or garment) more than half the time
   c. Have a maximum voided volume of 200 ml or more
   d. Show substantial reduction in incontinence frequency on the every 2-h prompt
3. Residents who do not show any of these characteristics may be candidates for either:
   a. Further evaluation to determine the specific type of incontinence
   b. Palliative management by containment devices and a checking-and-changing protocol

Prompted voiding (ongoing protocol)
1. Contact the resident every 2 h from 7 a.m. to 7 p.m.
2. Use same procedures as for the assessment period (items A2 through A4 above)
3. For nighttime management, use either a modified prompted voiding schedule or a containment device
4. If a resident who has been responding well has an increase in incontinence frequency despite adequate staff implementation of the protocol, he/she should be evaluated for reversible factors (Table 13-2)

[a] These criteria are based on limited data but appear to be highly accurate in identifying good responders to this protocol.

Though preliminary, there are some data to suggest that residents who will respond very well to prompted voiding can be identified during an initial assessment period (see Table 13-9). Residents who are better able to correctly identify themselves as wet or dry, who more frequently void in a toilet or toilet substitute during the assessment period, and who have a maximum voided volume of 200 ml or greater appear to be highly responsive. These criteria may be helpful in targeting a prompted voiding program and making it more efficient for staff.

Drug Therapy

Because of the close association between functional disability and UI among NH residents, drug therapy for UI is generally an adjunct to some form of toileting program.

Drug therapy for UI in the NH is directed at one of two abnormalities of lower urinary tract functioning or a combination of both. *Detrusor hyperactivity* (involuntary bladder contractions on urodynamic testing) is the most common urodynamic abnormality found in incontinent NH residents and is generally associated with urge-type UI. Drug treatment for detrusor hyperactivity involves an anticholinergic agent. Although several are available, none have been adequately studied in the NH setting. New types of drugs and long-acting preparations (e.g., slow-release capsules, skin patches) are under investigation but are not currently available. Until better data are available, we recommend that detrusor hyperactivity in the NH residents with urge-type UI be treated with oxybutynin. The starting dose should be 2.5 mg two or three times per day (and/or at bedtime for nocturnal UI); this can be increased to 5 mg three to four times per day. Two to four weeks is an adequate therapeutic trial. Careful observation for anticholinergic side effects (dry mouth, constipation or fecal impaction, blurry vision, worsening cognitive function, urinary retention) should be undertaken.

For *sphincter weakness* with stress-type UI in women, drug treatment involves a combination of estrogen and an alpha agonist. Estrogen can be given in the form of vaginal cream (1–2 g at bedtime) or as an oral tablet (0.3–0.625 mg conjugated estrogen daily). Either pseudoephedrine (30 to 60 mg three times per day) or phenylpropanolamine (75 mg twice daily) can be used as the alpha agonist. Drug treatment for stress UI should be combined with a toileting program (to keep the bladder volume as low as possible) and pelvic muscle exercises (for residents who can cooperate). Women who have prominent pelvic prolapse or who fail a 3- to 6-month trial of drug and/or behavioral therapy should be considered for surgical intervention (see Table 13-5 and under "Surgery," below).

For women with mixed urge and stress UI, a combination of the above approaches can be used. Imipramine (10 to 25 mg three times per day) may be used as a combination anticholinergic-alpha agonist. This drug is, however, contraindicated in the presence of cardiac conduction abnormalities and can, in addition to its anticholinergic side effects, cause significant postural hypotension in NH residents who are ambulatory.

Drug treatment for overflow UI is usually not effective on a chronic basis. Cholinergic agonists (e.g., bethanechol) have been used in patients with poor bladder contractility, and alpha antagonists (e.g., prazosin) have been used for increased sphincter tone. Neither of these pharmacologic approaches is, however, generally recommended for the chronic therapy of overflow UI in the NH setting.

Surgery

Surgical intervention for UI is a consideration for a small but important subgroup of incontinent NH residents. Since UI is not a life-threatening problem, it must be bothersome enough to the resident to justify the pursuit of elective surgical treatment.

Surgery for UI is basically of two types. First, women with stress UI associated with significant pelvic prolapse (Fig. 13-3) and/or intrinsic sphincter weakness ("type 3" stress incontinence) may benefit from bladder neck suspension and repair of the pelvic prolapse if indicated. In properly selected cases, the short-term (1 to 5 years) success of this type of surgery by an experienced surgeon is high (probably in the range of 75 percent for significant reduction or elimination of wetness). Thus, NH residents who have bothersome stress UI and who fail to respond adequately to nonsurgical approaches might be referred for further evaluation if an experienced surgeon is available.

The other type of surgical intervention for UI is the removal of anatomic obstruction, most commonly an enlarged prostate in males or a urethral stricture or bladder neck contracture. Detailed discussion of the evaluation and surgical treatment of lower urinary tract obstruction is beyond the scope of this chapter. Suffice it to say that NH residents who meet the criteria outlined in Table 13-5 with regard to possible obstruction should be referred to a urologist who is experienced with complex urodynamic evaluation.

Although artificial urinary sphincters are available for the management of UI, they are only rarely a consideration for NH residents. New surgical techniques, such as periurethral injection of Teflon or collagen, are being tested, but they have not been studied in the NH population.

Pads and Undergarments

Highly absorbent launderable or disposable pads and incontinence undergarments are the most common method of managing UI in the NH. This method of management is certainly appropriate for the subgroup of incontinent NH residents who are identified for palliative incontinence care. Pads and garments may also be very helpful at night for residents who are managed by prompted voiding and/or other interventions during the day and evening.

These containment devices should not, however, be used as the sole solution to UI in the NH or in a manner that fosters further dependency. When pads or garments are used, residents should still be regularly checked, toileted, and/or changed if necessary in order to avoid skin irritation and breakdown.

Catheters and Catheter Care

Three basic types of catheters and catheterization procedures are used for the management of urinary incontinence in NHs: external catheters, intermittent straight catheterization, and chronic indwelling catheterization. External catheters consist of some type of condom connected to a drainage system. Improvements in design and observance of proper procedure and skin care when applying the catheter will decrease the risk of skin irritation as well as the frequency with which the catheter falls off. Studies of complications associated with the use of these devices have been limited, but existing data suggest that male NH residents with external catheters are at increased risk of developing symptomatic UTIs. External catheters should therefore be used only to manage intractable incontinence in male residents who do not have urinary retention and who are extremely physically dependent. As with incontinence undergarments and padding, these devices should not be used as a matter of convenience, since they may foster dependency. Contrary to popular belief, by simply cleaning the penis with betadine, applying a new catheter, and collecting the first voided urine, one can use the external catheter to collect urine specimens that accurately reflect bladder urine. Use of this simple technique will avoid false-positive cultures and the discomfort of straight catheterization in residents suspected of having an infection. An external catheter for use in females is now commercially available, but its safety and effectiveness have not been well documented in the NH setting.

Intermittent catheterization is used in the management of urinary retention and overflow incontinence. The procedure involves straight catheterization two to four times daily, depending on residual urine volumes. Studies conducted largely among younger paraplegics have shown that this technique is practical and, as compared with chronic catheterization, reduces the risk of symptomatic infection. Intermittent self-catheterization has also been shown to be feasible for elderly female outpatients who are functional and both willing and able to catheterize themselves. However, studies carried out in young paraplegics and elderly female outpatients cannot automatically be extrapolated to the NH population. The technique may be useful for certain NH residents, such as women who have undergone bladder neck suspension or following removal of an indwelling catheter in a bladder retraining protocol (Table 13-8). However, the practicality and safety of this procedure in the NH setting have never been documented. Elderly NH residents, especially men, may be difficult to catheterize, and the anatomic abnormalities commonly found in the lower urinary tract of NH residents may increase the risk of infection due to repeated straight catheterizations. In addition, using this technique in an institutional setting (which may have an abundance of organisms relatively resistant to many commonly used antimicrobial agents) may pose an unacceptable risk of nosocomial infections. Using sterile catheter trays for these procedures would be very expensive. Thus, it may be extremely difficult to implement such a program in a typical NH setting.

Chronic indwelling catheterization is probably overused in the NH and has been shown to increase the incidence of a number of complications, including chronic bacteriuria, symptomatic UTI, bladder stones, periurethral abscesses, and even bladder cancer. Elderly NH residents, especially men, managed by this technique are at relatively high risk of developing symptomatic UTI. Given these risks, it seems appropriate to recommend that the use of chronic indwelling catheters be limited to specific situations (Table 13-10). When indwelling catheterization is used, sound principles of catheter care should be observed in order to minimize complications (Table 13-11).

Fecal Incontinence

Fecal incontinence is less common than urinary incontinence, but a large proportion (about 50 percent) of residents with frequent urinary incontinence also have episodes of fecal incontinence. Defecation, like urination, is a physiological process that involves smooth and striated muscles, central and peripheral innervation, coordination of reflex responses, mental awareness, and physical ability to get to a toilet. Disruption of any of these factors can lead to fecal incontinence.

The most common causes of fecal incontinence are problems with constipation and laxative use, hyperosmotic enteral feedings, neurological dis-

Table 13-10   Indications for use of a chronic indwelling catheter

1. Urinary retention that
   a. Is causing persistent overflow incontinence, symptomatic infections, or renal dysfunction
   b. Cannot be corrected surgically or medically
   c. Cannot be managed practically with intermittent catheterization
2. Skin wounds, pressure sores, or irritations that are being contaminated by incontinent urine
3. Care of the terminally ill or severely impaired for whom bed and clothing changes are uncomfortable or disruptive
4. Preference of resident when he/she has failed to respond to more specific treatments

Table 13-11   Key principles of chronic indwelling catheter care

Maintain sterile, closed gravity drainage system

Avoid breaking the closed system

Use clean techniques in emptying and changing the drainage system; wash hands between residents

Secure the catheter to the upper thigh or lower abdomen to avoid perineal contamination and urethral irritation due to movement of the catheter

Avoid frequent and vigorous cleaning of the catheter entry site; washing with soapy water or antibacterial solution once per day is sufficient

Do not routinely irrigate; change the catheter every 4 to 8 weeks or if symptomatic infection occurs

If bypassing occurs in the absence of obstruction, consider the possibility of a bladder spasm, which can be treated with a bladder relaxant

If catheter obstruction occurs frequently, increase the resident's fluid intake and acidify the urine if possible (dilute acidic irrigations may be useful)

Do not routinely use prophylactic or suppressive urinary antiseptics or antimicrobials

Do not do routine surveillance cultures to guide management of individual patients, because all chronically catheterized individuals have bacteriuria (which is often polymicrobial) and the organisms change frequently

Do not treat infection unless the patient develops symptoms; symptoms may be nonspecific and other possible sources of infection should be carefully excluded before attributing symptoms to the urinary tract

If a symptomatic infection does occur, change the catheter before obtaining a specimen for culture (cultures obtained through the old catheter may be misleading)

If a resident develops frequent symptomatic UTI, a genitourinary evaluation should be considered to rule out pathology such as stones, periurethral or prostatic abscesses, and chronic pyelonephritis

orders, and colorectal disorders (Table 13-12). Constipation is extremely common in the elderly and when chronic can lead to fecal impaction and incontinence. The hard stool (or scybalum) of fecal impaction irritates the rectum and results in the production of mucus and fluid. This fluid leaks around the mass of impacted stool and precipitates incontinence.

Table 13-12.   Causes of fecal incontinence

Fecal impaction	Colorectal disorders
Laxative overuse/abuse	Diarrheal illnesses (see Chap. 17)
Hyperosmotic enteral feedings	Diabetic autonomic neuropathy
Neurological disorders	Rectal sphincter damage
Dementia	
Stroke	
Spinal cord disease	

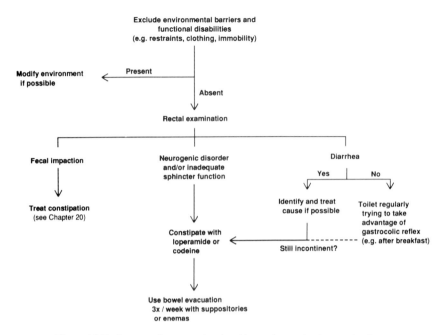

Figure 13-5 Strategy for managing fecal incontinence in the nursing home.

Appropriate management of constipation will prevent fecal impaction and resultant fecal incontinence. The management of constipation is discussed in Chap. 20.

Fecal incontinence due to neurological disorders is sometimes amenable to biofeedback therapy, although most elderly residents with dementia are unable to cooperate. For those residents with end-stage dementia, a program of alternating constipating agents (if necessary) and laxatives on a routine schedule (such as giving laxatives and enemas three times a week) is effective in controlling defecation and preventing fecal incontinence. Figure 13-5 depicts an approach to managing fecal incontinence in the NH setting.

SUGGESTED READINGS

Prevalence, Associated Factors, Morbidity

Ouslander JG and Fowler E: Incontinence in VA nursing home care units. *J Am Geriatr Soc* 33:33–40, 1985.

Ouslander JG and Kane RL: The costs of urinary incontinence in nursing homes. *Med Care* 22:69–79, 1984.

Ouslander JG, Kane RL, and Abrass IB: Urinary incontinence in elderly nursing home patients. *JAMA* 248:1194–1198, 1982.

Starer P and Libow LS: Obscuring urinary incontinence: Diapering the elderly. *J Am Geriatr Soc* 12:842–846, 1985.

Types and Causes of Incontinence

Pannill FC III, Williams TF, and Davis R: Evaluation and treatment of urinary incontinence in long term care. *J Am Geriatr Soc* 36:902–910, 1988.

Resnick NM, Yalla SV, and Laurino E: The pathophysiology of urinary incontinence among institutionalized elderly persons. *N Engl J Med* 320:1–7, 1989.

Diagnostic Evaluation

Ouslander JG, Leach G, and Staskin D: Simplified tests of lower urinary tract function in the evaluation of geriatric urinary incontinence. *J Am Geriatr Soc* 37:706–714, 1989.

Ouslander JG, Uman GC, and Urman HN: Development and testing of an incontinence monitoring record. *J Am Geriatr Soc* 34:83–90, 1986.

Treatment

Burgio KL and Burgio LD: Behavior therapies for urinary incontinence in older people. *JAMA* 256:372–379, 1986.

Colling J: Educating nurses to care for the incontinent patient. *Nurs Clin North Am* 23:279–289, 1988.

Hadley E: Bladder training and related therapies for urinary incontinence in older people. *JAMA* 256:372–379, 1986.

Hu T-W, Igou JF, Kaltreider DL, et al: A clinical trial of a behavioral therapy to reduce urinary incontinence in nursing homes. *JAMA* 261:2656–2662, 1989.

McCormick K, Scheve A, and Leahy E: Nursing management of urinary incontinence in geriatric inpatients. *Nurs Clin North Am* 23:231–264, 1988.

Ouslander JG, Greengold BA, and Chen S: Complications of chronic indwelling urinary catheters among male nursing home patients: A prospective study. *J Urol* 138:1191–1195, 1987.

Schnelle JF, Newman DR, and Fogarty T: Management of patient continence in long term care nursing facilities. *Gerontologist* 30:373–376, 1990.

Schnelle JF, Sowell VA, Hu T-W, and Traughber B: Reduction of urinary incontinence in nursing homes: Does it reduce or increase costs? *J Am Geriatr Soc* 36:34–39, 1988.

Warren JW, Damron D, Tenney JH, et al: Fever, bacteremia and death as complications of bacteriuria in women with long-term urethral catheters. *J Infect Dis* 155:1151–1158, 1987.

Wendland CJ and Ouslander JG: *A Rehabilitative Approach to Urinary Incontinence in Long-Term Care: Monograph for Nurses.* Pasadena, California, The Beverly Foundation, 1986.

General

Resnick NM and Ouslander JG (eds): NIH Conference on Urinary Incontinence. *J Am Geriatr Soc* 38:263–386, 1990.

FOURTEEN

GAIT DISORDERS AND FALLS

Falls among nursing home (NH) residents are a monumental problem, accounting for substantial morbidity, mortality, and cost. Falls, which inhibit residents' courage and threaten their independence, are one of the primary justifications for the widespread use of restraints. Falls may also be a marker for preexisting morbidity that requires assessment and management. In this chapter we review the epidemiology of gait instability and falls in the NH, their causes, and approaches to their evaluation and prevention.

PREVALENCE, INCIDENCE, AND MORBIDITY

Forty to 50 percent of residents in NHs have difficulty with walking. Falls are common, even among nonambulatory residents. The estimated annual incidence ranges from 0.6 to 3.6 falls per NH resident or 1600 falls per 1000 beds per year. Approximately 10 to 20 percent of falls result in serious injury; 2 to 6 percent result in fractures; and 5 to 10 percent cause serious injuries other than fractures—such as hematomas, lacerations, and dislocations—which require medical care or result in restricted activity for more than a few days. Subdural hematomas or cervical fractures, the most devastating injuries, are rare. The frequency, costs, and lasting morbidity of injuries other than hip fractures have not been studied thoroughly enough to provide accurate estimates in the NH population.

There are approximately 200,000 hip fractures annually in the United

States, most due to falls by older persons. Although many hip fractures occur among elderly NH residents, most occur in the community-dwelling geriatric population. A majority of these fractures require at least a brief stay in a NH for rehabilitation.

One-year mortality from hip fractures is estimated to be 25 percent in the United States (12 to 67 percent elsewhere). In some proportion of hip fractures, the victim falls and fractures his or her hip (traumatic fracture), while in others, the order of events is reversed due to osteoporotic bone (pathologic fracture). The relative proportion of these two types of hip fractures is not known. It is noteworthy that osteoporosis, falling, and hip fractures are more common in elderly women and that somewhat more trauma is generally required for a male to fracture his hip. However, mortality after hip fracture is higher at all ages for males than for females.

NORMAL GAIT

Multiple factors interact to produce a fall. Abnormalities of gait and balance are the leading factors, followed closely by environmental factors. It is important to understand some of the basic biomedical and physiological factors relating to normal gait in the aged in order to understand the pathophysiology of falls.

Figure 14–1 illustrates the normal gait cycle. It begins when the right heel strikes the floor, an event that initiates the "stance phase" for the right leg. The "swing phase" begins when the right toe leaves the floor. The stance phase for the legs overlaps, so that 20 to 25 percent of the time both feet are on the ground (double limb support). Flexor muscles are active in the swing phase and extensor muscles during the stance phase. Modern gait laboratories have helped to assess the elements of this gait cycle. The most important elements appear to be gait velocity, gait cadence, and stride length. The coordination of the complex task of ambulation is mediated by the spinal cord and integrated in the brain. Balance is maintained by keeping the center of gravity over the base of support, an area bounded by foot contact. Adjustments of the trunk and leg muscles occur during stance, beginning roughly 100 ms after a shift in the support surface. The automatic responses in maintaining dynamic equilibrium during walking require reliable afferent information from the visual system, the vestibular system, and the proprioceptors in the lower limbs.

Aging has several potential effects on balance and gait. During normal aging, body sway while standing increases, postural support responses are slowed, and there is a change in the capacity to integrate sensory information, with greater reliance on proprioception. While the elderly are more dependent on afferent information to maintain balance, these sensory systems are vulnerable to age-related changes and disease. Because so much of the nervous system is called on to support ambulation, changes in gait

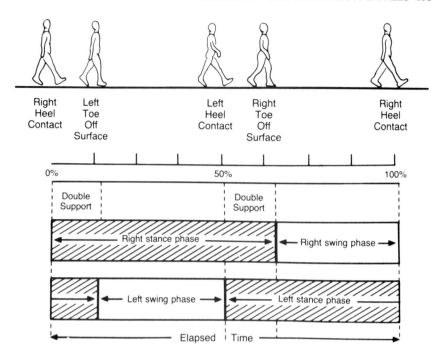

| Right Heel Contact | Left Toe Off Surface | | Left Heel Contact | Right Toe Off Surface | Right Heel Contact |

Figure 14-1 The normal gait cycle. (Reprinted from Sudarsky L: Gait disorders in the elderly. *N Engl J Med* 322:1441–1445, 1990.)

are often associated with neurological diseases which are common in the elderly. Elderly individuals demonstrate a shorter, broader-based stride, reduced pelvic rotation and joint excursions, and increased reliance on double-limb support. Normal velocity for a fit person at the age of 80 is 1.0 to 1.2 m/s, which represents a 10 to 20 percent decline from the value for younger persons. When the decrease in gait velocity with age is compounded by profound slowness or an abnormal pattern of ambulation, a gait disorder is present.

CAUSES OF INSTABILITY AND FALLING

Intrinsic Factors

Commonly described causes of gait instability and falling are either related to the individual (intrinsic) or are environmental (extrinsic). Instability and falling may result from a single intrinsic or extrinsic cause or, very often among NH residents, from the combined effects of multiple intrinsic and extrinsic factors. Table 14–1 lists the most common intrinsic risk factors for falling.

Table 14-1 Intrinsic factors that contribute to falls

Factor	History	Potential etiologies
Sensory		
Vision; near, distant, perception, dark adaptation		Age-related, cataract, glaucoma, macular degeneration
Vestibular	Vertigo; past use of aminoglycosides, furosemide, aspirin; ENT surgery, ear or mastoid infections	Age-related, drugs, tumors, previous surgery, infections, benign positional vertigo
Proprioceptive		
Peripheral nerves, spinal cord	Balance worse in dark, on uneven ground or thick rugs	Age-related, diabetes, vitamin B_{12} deficiency, tabes dorsalis
Cervical	Same as above, worse with head turning, vertigo, history of whiplash injury	Spondylosis, degenerative disease, Paget's disease, rheumatoid arthritis
Central neurological		
Any central nervous system lesion impairing problem solving and judgment	Variable, depends on disease	Variable
Musculoskeletal		
Arthritides, especially of the lower extremities	"Knee gave out," pain, stiffness	Degenerative, inflammatory
Muscle weakness, contractures	Variable	Many
Foot disorders		
Systemic diseases		
Postural hypotension	Light-headedness, worse with position change or walking, complaints consistent with predisposing disease (e.g., Parkinson's disease, diabetes)	Age-related, Parkinson's disease, diabetes, autonomic dysfunction, deconditioning, medications
Cardiac, respiratory, metabolic disease	Variable	Any systemic disease
Depression	Vegetative complaints, poor concentration, apathy	Reactive or endogenous
Medications		
All	Confusion, light-headedness, vertigo, fatigue, weakness	Any medication

Source: Tinetti ME: Instability and falling in elderly patients, in Jenkyn L (ed): *Seminars in Neurology*. Volume 9, Number 1, New York, Thieme Medical Publishers, Inc, 1989.

Physical changes in the lower extremities and spine have a direct effect on the gait. Osteoarthritic changes in the weight-bearing joints are seen radiographically in 85 percent of the population of age 75 or above. These changes may cause pain, which in turn may result in an antalgic and unsteady gait.

Cervical spondylosis is usually generalized to include any degenerative lesion of the cervical spine. Symptoms include numbness and tingling of the fingers and clumsiness with fine motor tasks such as buttoning shirts. Later there may be mild spastic quadriparesis and impaired perception of vibration because of compression of the posterior columns. The gait abnormalities and postural instability result from a combination of motor dysfunction and impaired proprioception. Computed tomography, magnetic resonance imaging, or myelography may be used to establish the diagnosis. Lumbar stenosis may coexist with cervical spondylosis or occur independently as a cause of gait abnormalities and instability. The most common presenting symptom is pseudoclaudication, defined as pain, numbness, or weakness in the buttocks, thighs, or legs on standing, walking, or exercise associated with extension. Symptoms are generally relieved when the resident is sitting or lying. Physical findings include mild muscle weakness (S1 distribution) and decreased ankle and knee reflexes. Normal-pressure hydrocephalus (NPH) is a syndrome consisting of "slowness and paucity of thought and action, unsteadiness of gait, and unwitting incontinence," with hydrocephalus and a cerebrospinal fluid pressure below 180 mmHg. The gait is characterized by reduced cadence ("stuck to the floor") and poor balance; it is similar to the frontal lobe gait. Many elderly persons with gait impairment have enlarged ventricles, so the diagnosis of NPH depends on the demonstration of a dynamic abnormality of cerebrospinal fluid circulation by radioactive scanning techniques. The diagnostic evaluation is aimed at identifying the subgroup of patients with the best chance of responding to a shunt procedure. The clinical response to the removal of 40 to 50 ml of cerebrospinal fluid may be an acceptable screening test among those with a high suspicion for this syndrome.

Some investigators have postulated that specific patterns of central nervous system pathology are associated with gait and balance disorders. Increased ventricular size and white matter loss have been noted with unexplained balance and gait problems. Magnetic resonance imaging has in some cases shown an association between multiple infarcts with gait and balance disorders even among those without a known history of strokes. Gait disorders in hypertensive residents are frequently associated with white matter lesions from small vessel disease (Binswanger's disease). The gait is characterized by hesitation in starting, shuffling, difficulty in picking the feet up off the floor ("magnetic foot response"), difficulty with turns, and poor standing balance. This pattern of abnormality is also termed frontal gait disorder or gait apraxia. The radiologic abnormality is frequently asymptomatic, and the pathological correlate has not been well characterized. White matter lesions have, however, been associated with recurrent falls in the elderly.

In Parkinson's disease, the gait is characterized by flexed posture, a diminished arm swing, a tendency to festination (starting slowly and gradually becoming more rapid), and difficulty with the initiation of motion and turns. Disturbance of balance occurs later, when postural support responses are compromised. Gait can be improved by drug therapy, but balance is not always restored.

Cerebellar disorders of balance and motor control can present with unsteady gait and a tendency to fall. Gait is characterized by a lateral instability of the trunk, erratic foot placement, and a widened stance. Many balance and gait disorders are related to the afferent systems. Sensory ataxia of tabetic neurosyphilis is a classic but rare example. Neuropathy affecting large-fiber afferents is a "modern" equivalent. The stance in such individuals is destabilized by eye closure (Romberg test). Selective loss of muscle spindle afferents has been proposed as a mechanism for some "senile" gait disorders. Multiple sensory deficits is a syndrome of imbalance resulting from deficits in proprioception, vision, and vestibular sense that impair postural support mechanisms. Age-related changes, such as impaired dark adaptation and lens accommodation, in combination with diseases such as macular degeneration are common and can contribute to the risk of falling. Visual perception (i.e., visual orientation in space) may be more relevant to falling than visual acuity. In view of decreased proprioception and vision, there is a tendency to rely on vestibular senses. Vestibular dysfunction, manifesting as true vertigo or dizziness with specific head movements and worsening instability in the dark, is common among older persons.

A recent prospective study found three significant and independent risk factors for falls among NH residents: hip weakness, low balance score, and the number of prescription medication taken. Sedating medications, particularly neuroleptic agents and long-acting benzodiazepines, affect postural reflexes and increase the risk of falls. The same applies to vasodilators. Since disorders due to drugs are reversible, their identification should have a high priority. Postural hypotension can be caused by many different drugs and may precipitate falls, but it was not found to independently contribute to the risk of falling in this study. It should be recognized that, even after extensive evaluation, no cause for gait disturbances can be found in 10 to 20 percent of the elderly.

Extrinsic Factors

Environmental or extrinsic causes are implicated in approximately 30 percent of falls in the NH. In a randomized prospective study conducted at the Jewish Homes for the Aging of Greater Los Angeles, most falls occurred in the resident's room. Almost half occurred between the hours of 6 p.m. and 6 a.m., and about 12 percent occurred while the resident was exiting the bed or in the bathroom. Table 14–2 lists some of the environmental factors that are important in the cause and prevention of falls in the NH. The floor surface is among the environmental hazards most frequently mentioned. Very shiny and smooth floors—as well as a transition from a high-friction surface such as a carpet to a low friction surface such as tile or polished linoleum—may precipitate falls in frail elderly. Spotlights or skylights on these surfaces can cause startle responses and falling in NH residents with Parkinsonism and other gait and balance abnormalities. Lighting plays an important role in providing a safe environment. Very bright and direct sources of light, such as fluorescent bulbs reflected against a highly polished linoleum floor, may be as big a hazard as poorly illuminated areas, since the glare so produced may have a blinding effect on elderly persons with cataracts and poor lens accommodation.

Bedroom falls occur most often at the bedside while the resident is getting in or out of bed. Falls are frequently associated with the use of bed rails. Contrary to common belief and practice, bed rails may increase the seriousness of falls. The same applies to other types of bed or wheelchair restraints. A recent report describes strangulation resulting in death with the use of "soft restraints." Therefore, bed rails or any other form of physical restraint should not substitute for a more practical and less restrictive approach to safety. New federal regulations (OBRA 1987) require very strict restrictions on the use of restraints (see Appendix). The use of physical

Table 14-2   Important environmental safety features in the NH

Interior
Non-slip surfaces
Securely fastened handrails
Sufficient light
Glare-free lights
Low lying objects avoided so as to minimize tripping hazard
Telephone and call button accessible
Chairs of the proper height and equipped with armrests to assist in transferring
Time-delayed automatic doors to allow for slow-moving residents

Bathroom
Door wide enough to provide unobstructed entering with or without a device
Skidproof strips or mats in the tub or shower
Toilet and tub/shower grab bars
Elevated toilet seat to assist in transfers

Bedroom
Bedside or night lights for nighttime ambulation
Unobstructed pathway from the bed to the bathroom
Height-adjustable beds to allow safe transfers
Completely recessible bed rails
Sag-resistant mattress edges to provide good sitting support
Closet shelves reachable without standing on tiptoe or chair
Fall-management sensors where applicable

restraints in the NH is discussed in more detail in Chap. 10. The features of a safe bedroom include a bed that can be lowered so that its height is approximately 19 in. (62 cm) or less from the top of the mattress to the floor. This will allow for safer transfers. Institutions purchasing beds should seek height-adjustable high-low beds with a frame that is approximately 14 in. (30 cm) in height when the bed is at its lowest position. Other safety features for the bedroom are outlined in Table 14–2.

The bathroom is another common site of falls in the NH. Most falls are the result of transferring on or off the toilet, or they occur while the resident is hurrying to urinate or defecate. In addition to appropriate toileting assistance, several environmental designs can improve safety around the bathroom. These include doors that are wide enough to provide entrance for wheelchairs and walkers, toilet and shower grab bars, and elevated toilet seats which assist with transfers.

An adjunct to bedroom/bathroom safety is an institutional fall prevention program involving all levels of staff. Administrative aspects of such programs are discussed at the end of this chapter. Specially designed sensors may be a useful addition to fall-prevention programs. Figure 14–2 illus-

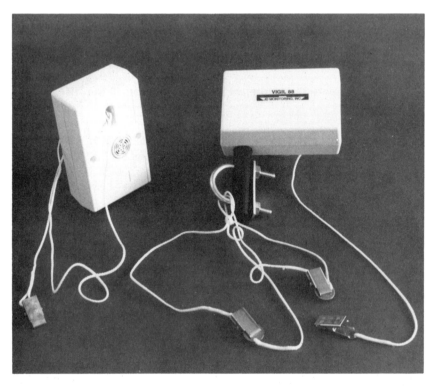

Figure 14-2 Examples of sensor devices that detect movement from a bed or a wheelchair. These devices can be linked with a call system to alert nursing staff when a high-risk resident is in danger of falling.

trates one example of such a sensor. These sensors are designed to alert caregivers when resident's motion exceeds a predetermined safety zone, indicating that the resident is in danger of falling. The sensor can be used with the nurse-call system or with a separate wireless system, providing local (resident's room) as well as remote (hallway, nurse's station) alarms. One manufacturer provides a sensor that mounts on a wheelchair, which is a common site associated with falls of unattended NH residents. The sensor allows staff to go about their activities while monitoring the resident at risk for falling. Preliminary studies have shown that environmental fall prevention programs geared to residents at risk result in a 25 percent annual decrease in falls. While there are no randomized prospective published studies to document the effectiveness of these approaches, we believe that combining comprehensive fall-prevention and safety programs with the use of "fall-prevention sensors" is a desirable and promising approach for decreasing falls and injuries in the NH setting. Such programs will be most effective if they are targeted to NH residents who are at high risk of falling. Table 14–3 lists the characteristics of NH residents that are strongly associated with recurrent falls.

ASSESSMENT AND MANAGEMENT

Assessment

As with any acute or chronic disease, the first steps in caring for fallers involve establishing the cause or causes for falling and setting treatment goals. Ideally, the risk of falling should be minimized without compromising mobility or functional independence. After identifying and treating injuries,

Table 14-3   Characteristics of NH residents at high risk for falling

Female
Older than 75
Newly admitted
Previous fall within a year
Dementia
Diminished safety awareness
Gait instability, poor balance
Multiple physical disabilities
Inability to carry out more than two basic activities of daily living
Poor vision ($<20/40$)
Muscle weakness (hip, ankle dorsiflexors)
More than four prescription medications
Routine psychotropic drug use
Postural hypotension
Urinary incontinence

a thorough assessment should be undertaken. Recalling that the accumulated effects of multiple diseases and disabilities—as well as the environment—predispose an elderly individual to falling, a fall evaluation should identify all potential contributing factors. Intrinsic risk factors (including sensory impairment, neurological, musculoskeletal, and systemic diseases) should be identified. Specific assessment techniques targeted at these risk factors are outlined in Table 14–4. As for almost all geriatric conditions, a review of medications is an important part of the assessment. A wide variety of medications, especially cardiovascular and psychotropic agents, can contribute to falls. The environment should be evaluated for potential hazards related to the fall. A careful history should be obtained from the resident (if possible), witnesses, and NH staff. Table 14–5 outlines the key points of the history.

A very useful technique in the assessment of NH residents who fall is a systematic evaluation of balance and gait. Tinetti has developed an excellent "performance-based" balance and gait evaluation (Table 14–6). The overall score on this evaluation is not as important as the identification and description of *specific* aspects of balance and gait that are abnormal and that might be amenable to rehabilitation or other interventions. We recommend that such a systematic gait evaluation be performed on NH residents who recurrently fall, as well as at the time of admission and at least annually thereafter, so that balance and gait abnormalities can be detected early and intervention implemented (see Chaps. 3 and 4).

Based on the results of the assessment, a wide variety of medical, rehabilitative, or environmental interventions might be appropriate (Table 14–4). Residents with sensory impairments should be referred for appropriate evaluation and intervention (e.g., refraction, cataract extraction, fitting of hearing aid). Vestibular problems are managed by avoiding ototoxic drugs if possible, providing habituation exercises, and identifying and avoiding problem maneuvers. Those with proprioceptive deficits contributing to instability should be evaluated to exclude vitamin B_{12} deficiency and diabetes. Rehabilitative approaches include balance exercises, assistive devices for walking, appropriate footwear (e.g., firm soles provide better proprioceptive input than bare feet or slippers). Any central nervous system process can contribute to instability and falling. A neurologic examination is therefore an important component of the evaluation of instability and falling. The focus should be on mental status, strength, sensation, tone, and coordination. A formal gait and balance assessment can be done utilizing the Tinetti scale mentioned above (Table 14–6). The goal of this evaluation is to reproduce the positional changes and gait maneuvers used during the resident's daily activities, especially those that have been associated with falls. The evaluation can be used to determine the rehabilitative and environmental interventions that may improve gait and mobility and decrease the risk of falling.

Table 14-4 Assessment and intervention techniques for risk factors for falls among NH residents

Factor	Assessments	Interventions
Vision	Near and distant visual acuity Visual fields Dark adaptation	Appropriate refraction Prescription or adjustment of medications Appropriate lighting
Vestibular	Nystagmus Ear, nose, and throat examination	Avoidance of toxic drugs Surgery if indicated Balance exercises Appropriate lighting
Peripheral nerves and spinal cord	Motor and sensory examination Vitamin B_{12} level if indicated Blood glucose	Treat underlying disease Adequate lighting Appropriate walking aids and footwear
Cervical	Motor and sensory examination for signs of radiculopathy (e.g., clumsiness with fine motor tasks, mild spastic quadriparesis)	Balance exercises Surgery
Central nervous system disorder	Mental status examination to assess judgment (see Chap. 9) Neurological examination to identify focal deficits	Supervised, structured, safe environment
Musculoskeletal		
Arthritides, especially of lower extremities	Joint and periarticular muscle examinations Range of motion	Medical and/or surgical treatment of underlying disease
Muscle weakness, contractures	Strength testing Range of motion	Strengthening exercises; balance and gait training; appropriate adaptive devices
Foot disorders	Podiatric evaluation	Treatment for bunions, calluses, deformities, etc. Appropriate footwear
Systemic diseases		
Postural hypotension	Postural vital signs	Hydration, lowest effective dose of necessary medications, reconditioning exercises, stockings (see Chap. 19)
Cardiac, respiratory, metabolic disease	Thorough physical and laboratory evaluation	Optimal medical management
Depression	Psychiatric or psychologic evaluation Depression scale	Nonpharmacologic and pharmacologic treatment (see Chap. 10)
Medications	Medication review Evaluate side effects (e.g., postural hypotension, visual disturbance)	Reduce or eliminate dose when possible
Environmental	Environmental assessment	Appropriate modifications where feasible (see Table 14-2)

Table 14-5   Evaluating falls: key points in the history

General medical history focusing on risk factors (see Tables 14-1 and 14-3)

History of previous falls

Medications (especially antihypertensive and psychotropic agents)

Resident's thoughts on the cause of the fall
    Was resident aware of impending fall?
    Was it totally unexpected?
    Did resident trip or slip?

Circumstances surrounding the fall
    Location and time of day
    Resident's position before fall (standing, wheelchair, bed)
    Witnesses' accounts
    Relationship to changes in posture, turning of head, cough, urination

Premonitory or associated symptoms
    Light-headedness, dizziness, vertigo
    Palpitations, chest pain, shortness of breath
    Sudden focal neurological symptoms (weakness, sensory disturbance, dysarthria, ataxia, confusion, aphasia)
    Aura
    Incontinence of urine or stool

Loss of consciousness
    What is remembered immediately after fall?
    Could the resident get up? If so, how long did it take?
    Could loss of consciousness be verified by a witness?

Source: Kane RL, Ouslander JG, Abrass IB: *Essentials of Clinical Geriatrics,* 2d ed. New York, McGraw-Hill, 1989, p 202.

Rehabilitative recommendations for residents with proximal muscle weakness, commonly associated with arthritis or deconditioning, include strengthening exercises and the use of firm high chairs and a raised toilet seat. For residents with a balance problem, bright lights, night lights, and an appropriate walking aid should be considered. For residents with abnormal gait patterns such as decreased step height or step length, gait training by a physical therapist should be recommended, as well as an environmental assessment to eliminate tripping hazards. Environmental assessment in NHs should be an ongoing process and should be targeted particularly to residents at risk (see Tables 14–2 and 14–3). Potential hazards to look for include cords and wires, inadequate lighting, slippery floors, inadequate or missing grab bars, and inaccessible switches and call buttons. Closet shelves and drawers should be designed so that they are reachable without forcing unsteady residents to stand on tiptoe or on chairs to reach them.

The value of this type of fall assessment for the frail institutionalized

Table 14-6   Tinetti balance and gait evaluation[a]

BALANCE

Instructions: The subject begins this assessment seated in a backless (or straight-backed), armless, firm chair. A *walking aid* is defined as a cane or walker. Circle the appropriate score.

1. *Sitting balance*

Leans or slides down in chair	= 0
Steady, stable, safe	= 1

2. *Rising from chair*

Unable without human assistance	= 0
Able but uses arms (on chair or walking aid) to pull or push up	= 1
Able to rise in a single movement without using arms on chair or walking aid (Note: use of arms on subject's own thighs scores a 2)	= 2

3. *Attempts to rise*

Unable without human assistance	= 0
Able but requires multiple attempts	= 1
Able to rise with one attempt	= 2

4. *Immediate standing balance (first 3–5 s)*

Any sign of *unsteadiness* (defined as grabbing at objects for support, staggering, moving feet, or more than minimal trunk sway)	= 0
Steady but USES WALKING AID or grabs other object for support	= 1
Steady without holding onto walking aid or other object for support	= 2

5. *Standing balance*

Any sign of unsteadiness regardless of stance, or holds onto object	= 0
Steady but *wide stance* (defined as medial heels more than 4 in. apart) or USES WALKING AID or other support	= 1
Steady with *narrow stance* (defined as medial heels less than 4 in. apart) and without holding onto any object for support	= 2

6. *Nudge on sternum* (with subject standing with feet as close together as possible, examiner pushes with light even pressure over sternum three times; reflects ability to withstand displacement)

Begins to fall or examiner has to help maintain balance	= 0
Needs to move feet but able to maintain balance (e.g., staggers, grabs, but catches self)	= 1
Steady, able to withstand pressure	= 2

7. *Balance with eyes closed* (with subject standing with feet as close together as possible with arms at sides, examiner counts out 5 s)

Any sign of unsteadiness or needs to hold onto an object	= 0
Steady without holding onto any object with feet close together	= 1

Table 14-6 (*Continued*)   Tinetti balance and gait evaluation[a]

8. *Turning balance (360°)* (from a standing still position, have
   the subject turn around in a 360° circle; demonstrate this
   first and give the subject one chance to practice)
   Steps are *discontinuous* (defined as subject puts one foot   = 0
   completely on the floor before raising the other foot)
   Steps are *continuous* (defined as the turn is a flowing   = 1
   movement)
   Any sign of unsteadiness or holds onto an object   = 0
   Steady without holding onto any object   = 1

9. *Sitting down*
   Unsafe (falls into chair, misjudges distances, lands off-center)   = 0
   Needs to use arms to guide self into chair or not a smooth   = 1
   movement
   Able to sit down in one safe, smooth motion   = 2

                                                                    Balance Score: /16

GAIT

Instructions: The subject stands with the examiner. They walk down the hallway or across a
room (preferably where there are few people or obstacles). The subject should be told to
walk at his/her "usual" pace using his/her usual walking aid. Circle the appropriate score.

10. *Initiation of gait* (subject is asked to begin walking down the
    hallway immediately after being told to "go")
    Any hesitancy, multiple attempts to start, or initiation of gait   = 0
    not a smooth motion
    Subject begins walking immediately without observable   = 1
    hesitation and initiation of gait is a single, smooth motion

11. *Step length and height* (Observe distance between toe of
    stance foot and heel of swing foot, observe from the side, do
    not judge first few or last few steps, observe one foot at a
    time)
    Right swing foot does *not* pass left stance foot with each step   = 0
    Right swing foot passes left stance foot with each step   = 1
    Right swing foot does *not* clear floor completely with each   = 0
    step (may hear scraping) or is raised markedly high (e.g., due
    to drop foot)
    Right swing foot completely clears floor but is not markedly   = 1
    high
    Left swing foot does *not* pass right stance foot with each step   = 0
    Left swing foot passes right stance foot with each step   = 1
    Left swing foot does *not* clear floor completely with each step   = 0
    (may hear scraping) or is raised markedly high (e.g., due to
    drop foot)
    Left swing foot completely clears floor but is not markedly   = 1
    high

12. *Stem symmetry* (observe distance between toe of each stance
    foot and heel of each swing foot, observe from the side, do
    not judge first few or last few steps)

Table 14-6 (*Continued*)   Tinetti balance and gait evaluation[a]

Step length varies between sides or resident advances with same foot with every step	= 0
Step length same or nearly same on both sides for most step cycles	= 1
13. *Step continuity*	
Steps are *discontinuous* (defined as subject places entire foot, heel and toe, on floor before beginning to raise other foot) or subject stops completely between steps	= 0
Steps are *continuous* (defined as subject begins raising heel of one foot as heel of other foot touches the floor) and there are no breaks or stops in subject's stride	= 1
14. *Path deviation* (observe in relation to floor tiles or a line on the floor, observe one foot over several strides—about 10 ft of path length, observe from behind; difficult to assess if subject uses a walking aid)	
Marked deviation of foot from side-to-side or toward one direction	= 0
Mild/moderate deviation, or subject USES A WALKING AID	= 1
Foot follows close to a straight line as subject advances	= 2
15. *Trunk stability* (observe from behind)	
Marked side-to-side trunk sway or subject USES A WALKING AID	= 0
No side-to-side trunk sway, but subject flexes knees or back or subject spreads arms out while walking	= 1
Trunk does not sway, knees and back are not flexed, arms are not abducted in an effort to maintain stability	= 2
16. *Walk stance* (observe from behind)	
Feet apart with stepping	= 0
Feet should almost touch as one foot passes the other	= 1
	Gait score: /12
	Total score: /28

[a] Reprinted with permission from M. Tinetti.

elderly has been demonstrated in a prospective randomized clinical trial that included a detailed postfall assessment. Many remediable problems (for example, weakness, environmental hazards, orthostatic hypotension, drug side effects, gait dysfunction) were detected. At the end of a 2-year follow-up period, the intervention group had 26 percent fewer hospitalizations and a 52 percent reduction in hospital days compared with controls. Residents in the intervention group also had 9 percent fewer falls and 17 percent fewer deaths than controls after 2 years (the latter trends were not, however, statistically significant).

ADMINISTRATIVE CONSIDERATIONS

A careful assessment of NH residents with gait instability and falls can reduce morbidity and, in turn, reduce health care costs. Clinicians practicing in NHs—as well as the administrator—should become familiar with the problem, so that strategies can be developed to deal with the prevention of falls and to avoid potential undesired consequences, such as citations by regulatory agencies or legal action by residents and their families.

A fall that results in injury is an incident reportable to the health department. This requires a systematic approach to falls in each institution that will stand the scrutiny of medical standards as well as administrative survey. Most NHs use a generic "incident report form" that provides information on the time, outcome, and corrective action or other interventions (i.e., resident education, medication change, or environmental modification) for falls. This form can provide epidemiological data on the frequency, timing, and factors associated with and outcomes of falls in the institution. This information may then be used by administration for quality-assurance and risk-management purposes. For example, comparing trends of falls with staffing ratios or time of day may help pinpoint specific problems that may play a role in causing falls. Since falls tend to occur in times of peak activity when most staff is on duty, effective utilization of staff at peak periods is essential for resident safety. Information gathered via other established mechanisms, such as drug regimen review, may also provide data pertinent to the risk and prevention of falls. For example, residents on a high number of medications or who frequently use hypnotics or other psychotropics are at high risk. These data may be used to modify clinical practice and potentially prevent falls. Resident case mix may play a role, since falls are more likely in a predominantly ambulatory NH resident population than among those who are predominantly bed-bound.

The administrator should use specific epidemiological and quality-assurance data in decisions related to safety measures. For example, a predominantly ambulatory demented NH population may require more sensor devices (Fig. 14–2) than a physically disabled but cognitively intact population. Similarly, a population with the majority of residents ambulatory and eating in a main dining room requires more staff at meals and thereafter to assist with transfers than does a population of predominantly bed-bound residents.

Policies related to restraints, such as side rails or "postural supports," should be consistent with regulations contained in OBRA (see Appendix). Keeping safety at the top of the agenda of staff meetings is also part of an effective fall-prevention program. Gathering information on how well the staff is complying with policies and procedures, offering them feedback, and letting them know how their compliance affects outcomes are critical to successful quality-assurance activities related to the prevention of falls and injuries.

SUGGESTED READINGS

Robbins A, Rubenstein LZ, Josephson K, Schulman B, Osterweil D: Predictors of falls among elderly people. *Arch Intern Med* 149:1628–1633, 1989.

Rubenstein LZ, Robbins A, Josephson K, Schulman B, Osterweil D: The value of assessing falls in an elderly population: A randomized clinical trial. *Ann Intern Med* 113:308–316, 1990.

Rubenstein LZ, Robbins AS, Schulman B, et al: Falls and instability in the elderly. *J Am Geriatr Soc* 36:266–278, 1988.

Sudarsky L: Gait disorders in the elderly. *N Engl J Med* 322:1441–1445, 1990.

Tideiksaar R: Alarm systems, in *Falling in Old Age.* Springer Publishing Co, 1989, pp 175–177.

Tideiksaar R, Osterweil D: Prevention of bed falls: The Sepulveda GRECC method. *Geriatr Med Today* 8:70–78, 1989.

Tinetti ME: A performance-oriented assessment of mobility problems in the elderly. *J Am Geriatr Soc* 34:119–126, 1986.

Tinetti ME, Williams TF, Mayewsky R: Fall risk index for elderly patients based on number of chronic disabilities. *Am J Med* 80:429–434, 1986.

Wolfson LI, Whipple R, Amerman P, Kleinberg A: Stressing the postural response: A quantitative method for testing balance. *J Am Geriatr Soc* 34:845–850, 1986.

FIFTEEN

SENSORY DEPRIVATION

We live in an environment in which our senses are constantly being bom-
barded by a series of stimuli. Woodburn Heron demonstrated that when col-
lege students were placed in an environment devoid of sensory stimuli, their
cognitive abilities deteriorated within 24 h. The students were also more
likely to accept the arguments of others. By 48 h they developed hallucinations and perceptual distortions in this environment. Even the best of
long-term-care institutions tend to promote states of inactivity that can interact with age-related perceptual changes to result in the development of a
sensory deprivation syndrome. Table 15-1 lists the major features of the
sensory deprivation syndrome, which occurs because of lack of stimulation
of one or more of the senses—hearing, vision, touch, kinesthesis, smell, and
taste. Loss of these senses is often coupled with forced physical inactivity
or excessive dependence on others to carry out activities of daily living.

Little formal information is available on the sensory deprivation syndrome in nursing homes (NHs). Oster developed a program that included
brief psychotherapy focused on the prevention of regression and development of increasing independence. The program included reality orientation,
enhanced environmental stimuli, ludotherapy (therapy to promote group
cohesiveness and interpersonal relations), proprioceptive stimulation, musi-
cal therapy for auditory stimulation, bedside visiting, a fiscal responsibility
program, intensive concentration on improving activities of daily living, and
an active resident council. This comprehensive intervention subjectively
improved cognition, memory, attention span, and orientation; it also

Table 15-1 Features of the sensory deprivation syndrome

Decreased quality of life	Inappropriate sexual behavior
Decreased cognition	Withdrawal
Hallucinations	Altered body image
Perceptual distortions	Agitation
Delusions	Incontinence
Emotional lability	Muscle atrophy
Submissiveness	Constipation
Dependent behavior	Osteopenia
Decreased attention span	Decreased immune system responsiveness
Decreased sociability	Fear of abandonment and death

enhanced interpersonal interactions and increased critical and challenging behaviors by the resident.

In this chapter the major sensory impairments that affect NH residents will be discussed. Taste and its effects on nutritional status are discussed briefly in Chap. 11.

HEARING

Approximately one in four persons over the age of 65 suffers from hearing impairment. Ninety percent of persons over 90 years of age have a hearing deficit. The reported prevalence of hearing impairment in NHs varies from 46 percent to 100 percent. Hearing impairment has been associated with significant emotional, social, and communication deficits as well as with social isolation. Cognitive impairment may be identified when mental status tests are administered verbally to hearing-impaired individuals. Hearing loss can result in irritable or unsociable behavior and apparent inattentiveness. Paranoid ideation has also been associated with hearing loss.

The common causes of hearing loss in older NH residents are listed in Table 15-2. There is no change in cerumen production with advancing age. Cerumen impaction occurs in older persons because of a decrease in the cerumen-producing glands, which results in a reduction in moisture in the external auditory canal. In men, large vibrissae (hairs) may also become entangled with the wax. Cerumen impaction can be prevented by regularly placing mineral oil or 6.5 percent carbamide peroxide drops in the ear. This approach is contraindicated when there is a history of tympanic membrane perforation or chronic ear disease.

Middle ear diseases such as otitis media occur no more commonly in older than in younger individuals. Arthritic changes of the ossicular chain are extremely common in persons over age 70 but have not been shown to correlate with conductive hearing loss.

Table 15-2   Causes of hearing loss in the nursing home

Conductive	Sensorineural
External auditory canal	Presbycusis
Cerumen impaction	Vascular insufficiency
Foreign bodies	Meniere's disease
Otitis externa	Acoustic neuroma
Tumors	Hypothyroidism
Middle ear	Collagen-vascular disorders
Otitis media	Ototoxicity
Tympanic membrane perforation	Aminoglycoside antibodies
Otosclerosis	Nonsteroidal anti-inflammatory drugs
Cholesteatoma	Salicylates
	Quinine
	Quinidine
	Furosemide, ethacrynic acid, and bumetanide
	Topical aural antibiotics

Major causes of inner ear hearing loss in the older population include presbycusis, vascular insufficiency, neoplasms, Meniere's disease, and ototoxicity. Presbycusis is the most common cause of hearing loss with advancing age. It primarily affects high tones and is bilateral. Asymmetric sensorineural hearing loss should be evaluated in order to exclude an acoustic neuroma. Sudden sensorineural hearing loss is usually vascular in origin and should be treated as an emergency with a combination of histamine, niacin, propantheline bromide, and prednisone; this regimen may sometimes preserve some hearing. Full evaluation is then carried out after 2 weeks of steroid therapy. This saves an extensive workup in those who have either mild vascular disease or who recover spontaneously. Those who have previously undergone stapes surgery require exploration for a perilymphatic fistula.

Two tools are available for identifying hearing-impaired older persons: the Hearing Handicap Inventory for the Elderly (HHIE) and the Welch-Allyn audioscope. We have adapted the HHIE for use in the NH (Table 15-3). A score of 0 to 4 suggests an extremely low likelihood of hearing impairment, while a score above 13 suggests a very high probability of hearing impairment. The hand-held Welch-Allyn audioscope (Fig. 15-1) is an excellent instrument with which to screen for hearing impairment. It delivers a 40 dB tone at frequencies of 500, 1000, 2000, and 4000 Hz. Hearing impairment can be defined as a 40 dB loss at the 1000 or 2000 Hz frequency in both ears or a 40 dB loss at the 1000 and 2000 Hz frequencies in one ear. The audioscope has approximately a 94 percent sensitivity and a 72 percent specificity for the detection of hearing loss when it is used in a quiet room.

A screening program utilizing the Welch-Allyn audioscope in a VA NH yielded the following results: hearing was found to be impaired in 38 percent

Table 15-3   Hearing handicap inventory for the elderly (adapted for nursing home residents)

Does a hearing problem cause you to feel embarrassed or upset when you meet new people?
Does a hearing problem cause you to feel frustrated when you are talking?
Do you have difficulty in hearing when someone speaks in a whisper?
Do you feel handicapped by a hearing problem?
Does a hearing problem cause you difficulty when you are talking to friends, family, or staff?
Does a hearing problem cause you to go to religious services less often than you would like?
Does a hearing problem cause you to have arguments?
Does a hearing problem cause you difficulty when you are listening to television or radio?
Do you feel that any difficulty with your hearing limits or hampers your social life with other residents?
Does a hearing problem cause you difficulty when you are in the nursing home dining room?

Note: All responses can be scored "yes" (2 points), "sometimes" (1 point), or "no" (0 points). A score of 13 suggests hearing impairment.

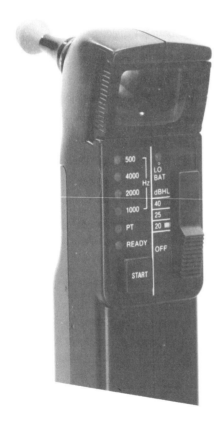

Figure 15-1, The Welch-Allyn audioscope. This device delivers a 400 dB tone at frequencies of 500, 1000, 2000, and 4000 Hz. It is useful in screening for hearing impairment.

of the residents screened; of these 25 percent had cerumen impaction. After removal of cerumen, 47 percent had improved hearing. Morale scores were increased in 65 percent of the residents after removal of the cerumen. These data illustrate the importance of regular hearing evaluations and wax removal in the NH setting.

All residents with hearing impairment should be evaluated for the potential to benefit from hearing aids. There are three basic types of hearing aids: canal, in-the-ear, and behind-the-ear. In general, the worse the hearing, the larger the hearing aid needed. Some residents will do very well with a simple amplification device (e.g., a Pocketalker). Those with profound hearing impairment may benefit from cochlear implants.

Table 15-4 lists examples of assistive devices that may be useful in the NH. A telephone should be available in the NH with a handset amplifier, and hearing impaired residents should be instructed in its use. Classes in speech-reading may be helpful for some NH residents. Table 15-5 provides suggestions for improving communication in the hearing-impaired NH resident.

VISION

Changes in vision do not cause as great a decrease in social interaction as do hearing impairments. Nevertheless, vision impairment does increase feelings of vulnerability and social isolation. Legal blindness is defined as a corrected visual acuity in the better eye of 20/200 or worse or when vision is restricted to 20° in its widest diameter. Three percent of persons over the age of 85 in the United States are blind. In NHs approximately 25 percent of the residents are legally blind.

Table 15-4   Assistive devices for the hearing impaired

Telephone handset amplifiers
Television
   Television caption units
   Infrared sensor with individual volume control (Sennheiser, Sound Plus; resident wears
      headset that picks up sound anywhere in the room; no connection to TV set)
   TV listening loop (allow individual to plug in listening device at different parts of room)
   Direct audio input connection (connected directly to TV)
   Dynamic pillow speaker
Personal amplification devices
   Electronic stethoscopes
   Pocket talker
   Direct audio input
   Multipurpose communicator (for group meetings)
   Hand-held communicator (allows directional input)

Table 15-5 Improving communication for hearing-impaired nursing home residents

Between resident and caregiver
   Screen all residents for hearing impairment.
   Reduce or eliminate background noise. Close doors and turn off TV or running water.
   Face the listener. Keep your face at the level of the listener's eyes. Maintain eye contact.
   Allow adequate light to fall on your face.
   Give the listener a clear view of your face. Keep hands or other objects down. Avoid chewing gum. Beards or mustaches should be well trimmed so as not to interfere with speech reading.
   Use facial expressions and gestures to convey meaning.
   Avoid talking while writing or walking around the room.
   Gain the person's attention before beginning to speak.
   Speak in a normal tone of voice or slightly louder.
   Shouting does not help because hearing loss is not simply a reduction in loudness. Making voice slightly deeper sometimes improves hearing.
   Speak clearly, a little more slowly, in short sentences, using simple words.
   Because the person may not admit to a handicap, have the person repeat to be sure the message was understood.
   Be redundant: repeat or rephrase in a different way. Write key words if the person can read.
   If the individual has a hearing aid, learn how to help him or her with it.
   Learn how to use assistive listening devices. Have an amplifier available for important communications.
   Arrange for the individual to have a vision exam.
   Teach lip reading.

In the environment
   Consult with your audiologist for evaluation of background noise in social gathering areas and request ideas on how to reduce or eliminate competing noise.
   Arrange seating in small groups, preferably in circles or at round tables.
   In large meetings, have speakers provide outlines for residents to review.
   Seek help from outside resources such as a local SHHH (Self-Help for Hard-of-Hearing People, Inc.).[a]

---

[a] These groups encourage identification of persons with hearing losses, provide education, foster public programs, engage hearing-impaired participants in communication, urge participation in daily activities, and help hearing-aid users cope because hearing aids do not do the entire job.
Source: Voeks et al: *J Am Geriatr Soc* 38:141, 1990, with minor modifications.

Presbyopia is the commonest eye complaint of older persons. Presbyopia is the inability to focus clearly at normal reading distances due to thickening of the anteroposterior diameter of the lens. Some persons with presbyopia may be able to read again without bifocals ("second sight"). This is due to the development of myopia, which is often related to the development of cataracts.

Sudden visual loss is an ophthalmic emergency. Individuals with sudden visual loss will have a Marcus-Gunn pupillary response (i.e., illumination of the nonblind eye will result in bilateral pupillary constriction, while illumination of the blind eye immediately thereafter will result in apparent bilateral pupillary dilatation). If this is not present, hysterical blindness is a possibility. The causes of sudden visual loss are listed in Table 15-6. Care should be taken not to use topical steriods in patients with red eyes. Examples of other common visual complaints of NH residents and their causes are listed in Table 15-7.

The major causes of gradual visual loss in older people are cataracts, glaucoma, macular degeneration, and diabetic retinopathy. Individuals with cataracts complain of generalized blurred vision; those with glaucoma have blurred peripheral vision; and those with macular degeneration have blurred central vision.

The diagnosis of glaucoma is made by the combination of an increased intraocular pressure (greater than 23 mmHg), an increase in the optic cup-to-disk ratio, and the presence of visual field defects. All NH residents should have their intraocular pressure measured on a yearly basis with a Schiotz indentation tonometer after the eye has been anesthetized with a local anesthetic. The vast majority of individuals with glaucoma have the open-angle version, which is best treated with a combination of eye drops (e.g., timolol, which decreases aqueous humor formation, and/or pilocarpine, a miotic which decreases resistance to the outflow of aqueous humor). Systemic medications that include carbonic anhydrase inhibitors are also sometimes used. It should be remembered that instillation of eye drops into the conjunctival sac is the equivalent of an intravenous infusion of the drug and can result in systemic side effects such as bradycardia. Paresthesias, anorexia, confusion, depression, and drowsiness can all be side effects of carbonic anhydrase inhibitors.

Age-related macular degeneration is diagnosed by the presence of macular degeneration and multiple pale-yellow spots (drusen). Residents with

Table 15-6   Causes of sudden visual loss

Monocular loss
  Painless
    Subretinal hemorrhage (macular degeneration)
    Occlusion of central retinal artery or vein
    Retinal detachment
    Ischemic optic neuritis
    Vitreous hemorrhage (diabetic retinopathy)
  Painful
    Glaucoma (angle-closure)
    Temporal arteritis

Binocular loss
  Bilateral occipital lobe infarcts

Table 15-7 Potential causes of common visual complaints in nursing home residents

Blepharoptosis
  Myasthenia gravis
  Horner's syndrome (Pancoast tumor or
    tuberculosis)
  Hyperthyroidism
  Normal aging

Periocular pain
  Sinusitis
  Herpes zoster
  Tic douloureux
  Migraine
  Intracranial aneurysm

Painful red eye
  Angle-closure glaucoma
  Bacterial corneal ulcers
  Herpes simplex (may not be painful)

Painless red eye
  Viral conjunctivitis
  Chlamydial conjunctivitis
  Bacterial conjunctivitis
  Allergy
  Subconjunctival hemorrhage

Diplopia
  III, IV, VI cranial nerve palsies
  Cataracts (monocular diplopia)
  Vertebrobasilar artery insufficiency
  Myasthenia gravis
  Eaton-Lambert syndrome

Flashing lights/floaters
  Vitreous detachment
  Retinal tear

Visual hallucinations
  Brain tumor
  Cortical ischemia
  Sensory deprivation
  Schizophrenia

Purulent discharge
  Bacterial conjunctivitis

macular degeneration should be referred to an ophthalmologist, as some may benefit from laser photocoagulation. Although there is some controversy, it appears that the rate of deterioration of macular degeneration may be slowed by the administration of zinc sulfate 220 mg three times per day.

Visuospatial abnormalities and the inability to distinguish moving objects clearly have been identified in patients with Alzheimer's disease. These deficits can result in startle reactions. Following stroke, the presence of homonymous hemianopsia may be associated with hemineglect. Hemineglect may result in behaviors such as failing to shave one side of the face. Hemineglect may also lead to falls due to ignoring objects in the way of the neglected side. NH residents with hemineglect require intensive stimulation, frequent reminders, and occupational therapy to help restore care for the neglected side.

Age-related changes in the lens (yellowing and opacity) and diabetes mellitus may result in problems with color vision. This can cause residents to dress in poorly coordinated clothes. Changes in color vision with age can also interfere with the ability of NH residents to follow simple color codes.

Cataracts can result in severe glare in bright light, which may further impair color vision.

A number of strategies that may help to compensate for visual problems among NH residents are outlined in Table 15-8. Table 15-9 lists some of the adaptive devices that may be useful to the visually impaired.

THE SKIN SENSES

Development of sensory neuropathies can decrease the individual's awareness of the environment. NH residents with neuropathies may benefit from utilizing highly textured objects. Rubber thimbles or rubber-tipped pencils may help these people to turn pages. Increased intensity of touch may be necessary when residents have lost deep touch. Vigorous massage may also restore a sense of adequate tactile sensation. The resident's response to a handclasp can identify the need for touch. The person who clings is clearly

Table 15-8   Adaptive strategies to compensate for visual problems in the nursing home

Object placement
  Avoid a cluttered environment.
  Keep furniture in same placement. If changes are made, inform residents.
  Place food and utensils in the same place on the tray every day.
  Keep clothes and objects in the resident's room in the same place.

Lighting
  Make sure light is consistent throughout the building and evenly distributed throughout
    each room.
  Use increased bulb wattage.
  Have dimmer switches in rooms for residents with cataracts.
  Use window blinds to control light.
  Have night lights available.
  Use fluorescent or brightly colored tape around electrical outlets, light switches, and
    doorknobs.
  Use cups and glasses with a contrasting rims.

Color
  Light objects should be placed on dark surfaces, and vice versa.
  Contrasting color coding may be useful (use distinctly different colors).

Other
  Offer residents repeated and unhurried orientation to surroundings.
  Identify yourself when you are approaching the resident.

Source: Adapted from Hooyman NR, Lustbader W: *Taking Care of Your Aging Family Members.* New York, The Free Press, 1986.

Table 15-9 Adaptive devices available for residents with visual impairments

Magnifying glasses
Large-print books and newspapers
Magnifying television screen systems
Talking books[a]
Computer-operated voice synthesizers that read from books
Audiotape cassettes for correspondence
Radio stations with special programming for the visually impaired
Large-print telephone directories
Self-threading needles
Adaptive clothing—zippers, Velcro openers, large buttons
Braille watches/talking clocks
Adapted games
Telephone adaptations for the visually impaired (e.g., giant push-button adapters or call makers)
Braille or other coded markings at entrances to commonly used rooms

[a] Available from the Library of Congress; the National Federation of the Blind; or Books on Tape, Newport Beach, CA 92660.

seeking increased touch. Touch can decrease anxiety, increase self-esteem, create a trusting relationship, and express caring and concern.

KINESTHESIS

Kinesthesis is the ability to recognize the position and movements of body parts without visual aid. Advancing age is associated with cerebellar dysfunction and a resultant failure to allow adequate discrimination of body movements. Passive movements for NH residents who are bed-bound or have had a stroke can help to maintain kinesthetic sense. Upright posture using a tiltboard or waist support can also help to maintain the sense of equilibrium. Regular walking for chairbound residents or water exercises (where a pool is available) can serve a similar function.

SUGGESTED READINGS

Sensory Deprivation

Oster C: Sensory deprivation in geriatric patients. *J Am Geriatr Soc* 24:461, 1976.

Hearing

Lichtenstein MJ, Bess FM, Logan SA: Validation of screening tools for identifying hearing-impaired elderly in primary care. *JAMA* 259:2875, 1988.

Mhoon E: Otology, in Cassel CK, Riesenberg DE, Sorensen LB, Walsh JR (eds): *Geriatric Medicine*, 2d ed. New York, Springer-Verlag, 1990, p 403.

Mulrow CD, Aguilar C, Endicott JE, et al: Association between hearing impairment and quality of life of elderly individuals. *J Am Geriatr Soc* 38:45, 1990.

Mulrow CD, Aguilar C, Endicott JE, et al: Quality-of-life changes and hearing impairment: A randomized trial. *Ann Intern Med* 113:188–194, 1990.

Voeks SV, Gallagher CM, Langer EH, Drinka PJ: Hearing loss in the nursing home. *J Am Geriatr Soc* 38:141, 1990.

Vision

Hooyman NR, Lustbader W: *Taking Care of Your Aging Family Members*. New York, The Free Press, 1986.

Kollarits CR: The aging eye, in Calkins E, Davis PJ, Ford AB (eds): *The Practice of Geriatrics*. Philadelphia, Saunders, 1986, p 268.

Mehelas TJ, Kliess RD, Kollarits CR, et al: Visual loss in geriatric residents of northwestern Ohio nursing homes. *Ohio State Med Assoc J* (March Issue):235, 1984.

SIXTEEN

ENDOCRINE AND METABOLIC PROBLEMS

Endocrine and metabolic problems are not rare among nursing home (NH) residents. This chapter will briefly discuss the practical considerations of managing these problems in the NH setting.

THYROID DISORDERS

A number of studies have demonstrated a fairly high prevalence of hypo- and hyperthyroidism in older individuals with medical illnesses. The prevalence of overt hypothyroidism ranges from 0.7 percent to 9.4 percent and of overt hyperthyroidism from 0.3 percent to 3.0 percent. Hypothyroidism has also been found to occur in up to 5 percent of patients with dementia. Based on these data, screening for thyroid disease would appear to be appropriate in all new admissions to a NH and thereafter on a yearly basis.

Clinical acumen plays no role in the diagnosis of hypo- or hyperthyroidism in the frail, older NH resident. Many NH residents suffer from the classical signs and symptoms of hypothyroidism due to the interaction of disease and aging processes rather than from true hypothyroidism. In addition, hyperthyroidism may present in an apathetic manner, with blepharoptosis instead of exophthalmos, anorexia instead of hyperphagia, depression instead of anxiety or agitation, weight loss, proximal muscle myopathy, heart failure, and atrial fibrillation. For these reasons we recommend regular biochemical screening for thyroid disease in the NH setting.

Figure 16-1 summarizes the approach to screening for thyroid dysfunc-

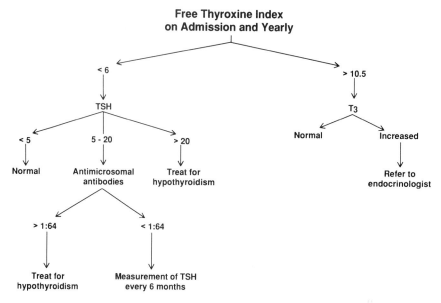

Figure 16-1 Approach to screening for thyroid dysfunction in the nursing home.

tion in the NH. Initial biochemical screening consists of thyroxine (T_4) and a triiodothyronine uptake (T_3U). When the T_3U uptake is normalized and multiplied by the T_4, a free thyroxine index is generated. For screening purposes, a narrower range of normal than reported by the laboratory is recommended (i.e., 6 to 10.5). When the value is greater than 10.5, a free triiodothyronine (T_3) level should be obtained to exclude T_3 toxicosis. When the value is below 6, a thyroid stimulating hormone (TSH) level should be obtained. If the TSH level is greater than 20 mIU/ml, the diagnosis of hypothyroidism is made and treatment should be instituted. Values between 5 and 20 mIU/ml are in a borderline zone and may revert to normal. In these cases antimicrosomal thyroid antibodies should be obtained. If the titer is 1:64 or less, the resident can be followed with TSH levels every 6 months. If the titer is greater than 1:64, the resident should be started on thyroid replacement, because individuals with the titer above this level have a higher probability of becoming hypothyroid. The supersensitive TSH assay is not recommended for this purpose, as illnesses and circulating antibodies decrease its sensitivity and specificity, making it less cost-effective for screening for thyroid dysfunction in the NH setting.

A major problem in the diagnosis of thyroid dysfunction in sick persons is the development of the "euthyroid sick syndrome." Illness can generate thyroid function tests similar to those seen in hypothyroidism. Table 16-1 distinguishes between the euthyroid sick syndrome and hypothyroidism.

Table 16-1   Comparison of thyroid function tests in the euthyroid sick syndrome, hypothyroidism, and the sick hypothyroid patient

	Euthyroid sick syndrome	Hypothyroid	Sick hypothyroid
Thyroxine (T_4)	Normal or decreased	Decreased	Decreased
Triiodothyroxine (T_3)	Very low (<25 ng/dl)	Low normal	Very low
T_3 uptake (T_3U)	Increased	Decreased	Normal
Thyrotropin (TSH)	Normal, increased, or decreased	Increased	Increased or high normal

Acute psychiatric illnesses can result in elevated thyroxine and/or triiodothyroxine levels. Depression may be associated with low thyroid hormone levels. A variety of drugs can also interfere with thyroid function tests. Beta blockers can produce an elevated free thyroxine index. Phenythoin, salicylates, and furosemide can result in a spuriously low free thyroxine index. Iodine-containing cough mixtures can result in suppressed thyroid function. Radioiodine contrast agents can result in an elevation in thyroxine and in an older person who is iodine-deficient, leading to iodine-induced thyrotoxicosis. The antiarrhythmic agent amiodarone (an iodine-containing drug) has both induced thyrotoxicosis and produced thyroid function tests consistent with hypothyroidism.

When thyroxine-binding globulin levels are abnormal, the free thyroxine index is usually normal because of the T_3 uptake value. A rare dysalbuminemia syndrome, which results in albumin with an abnormal avidity for binding thyroxine, may cause an elevated free thyroxine index in the presence of a normal triiodothyronine level.

Isolated T_4 toxicosis can occur in some older persons whose concomitant illness has suppressed their ability to convert T_4 to T_3. The TSH response at 30 minutes to 500 μg of thyrotropin-releasing hormone (TRH) may be helpful in this situation. If the TSH is greater than 5 mIU/ml at 30 minutes, thyrotoxicosis is not present. A flat TSH response to TRH, however, does not necessarily indicate thyrotoxicosis, because aging, illness, and depression can all result in a flat response.

Treatment of hypothyroidism in the older individual involves slowly increasing L-thyroxine dosage from 25 μg per day by 12.5 μg every week to a dose between 50 and 100 μg (0.05 to 0.10 mg) per day. Overreplacement of thyroid hormone may temporarily increase alertness but in the long run leads to an increased propensity for osteoporosis and muscle weakness. Thyroid extract should not be used because of poor standardization from batch to batch. A TSH should be measured every 8 weeks until the TSH is below 5 mIU/ml. At this stage a thyroxine level should be checked and the resident should be maintained on 6 to 8 mg/dl. The supersensitive TSH assays are expensive and do not appear to have a major advantage in this situation.

Older individuals with hyperthyroidism should be treated with radioactive iodine. Beta blockers can be used to give temporary symptomatic relief. Some individuals with apathetic hyperthyroidism benefit symptomatically from treatment with an antidepressant. Goiter (an enlarged thyroid gland) is often seen in older individuals, particularly in those who were not exposed to sufficient iodine in the diet when they were growing up (i.e., those from some areas of the Midwest and Appalachian regions). If the individual is not biochemically hyperthyroid, the goiter is multinodular, and no symptoms of tracheal compression are present, the goiter should be ignored. With a large goiter and dyspnea, a CT scan of the trachea to demonstrate narrowing or a ventilation flow-loop study may be useful.

Solitary thyroid nodules are at risk for being malignant. Approximately 5 percent of females over 50 years of age have a solitary nodule. The incidence of thyroid cancer falls rapidly after the age of 50 and most nodules are adenomas or cysts. Most thyroid cancers are of the follicular or papillary type and have a relatively benign course, though they tend to behave more aggressively in older individuals. Anaplastic thyroid carcinomas increase in prevalence with advancing age such that, by 80 years of age, half of the thyroid cancers are anaplastic.

Given these facts, how should one treat the solitary thyroid nodule in a NH resident? If, on admission to the NH, a solitary thyroid nodule is found, it should be observed at 3 and 6 months. If it is enlarging, the resident should be referred for a fine needle aspiration. If a *new* thyroid nodule is detected, fine needle biopsy is indicated because of the higher possibility of anaplastic cancer. It is, therefore, important that on admission to the NH the presence or absence of thyroid nodules be carefully documented.

DIABETES MELLITUS

Diabetes mellitus occurs commonly in older individuals. Approximately 20 percent to 30 percent of NH residents have diabetes mellitus. In addition, diabetes mellitus often leads to NH admission at a younger age. Major factors resulting in the increased admission of diabetics to NHs are blindness and amputations.

The increased propensity of older individuals to develop dehydration due to failure to perceive thirst puts the NH resident at particular risk of developing hyperosmolar coma. Minor infections (urinary tract, respiratory, sinuses) can often precipitate a rapid increase in blood glucose levels. For this reason, special attention must to be paid to the hydration of diabetic NH residents. The outcome for hyperosmolar coma is particularly poor among those hospitalized from NHs. Some older diabetics with type II diabetes mellitus develop pancreatic exhaustion and can develop diabetic ketoacidosis.

Hypoglycemia is an ever-present problem in NH residents receiving treatment for their diabetes. However, recent studies have suggested that if the physician aims generally to maintain the blood glucose between 100 to 200 mg/dl, hypoglycemia is rarely a problem in the NH. NH staff should be instructed to pay special attention to behavior changes (lethargy or agitation) in diabetic residents. Diabetic residents with abrupt behavioral changes should immediately receive sugar and the blood glucose level should be checked. Where possible, nursing staff should be allowed to administer 50 ml of 50 percent dextrose when starting an intravenous line on a diabetic resident suspected of being hypoglycemic. In addition, diabetic NH residents should have a standing order for 1 mg of glucagon intramuscularly in case of hypoglycemia associated with confusion and/or lethargy.

Table 16-2 lists the reasons for maintaining relatively good glucose control among diabetic NH residents. Blood glucose should be controlled before using pentoxifylline (Trental) to treat intermittent claudication in diabetics. It should be remembered that to see improvement in the symptoms of intermittent claudication, treatment for hyperglycemia must have been instituted for at least 120 days. Recent studies have suggested that depression may occur more commonly in older persons with diabetes mellitus, and the presence of depression may be directly related to poorer outcomes in diabetics. A number of studies have demonstrated that diabetics are more likely to complain of pain. This appears to be due to elevated glucose levels, which prevent a normal interaction of beta-endorphin with the opioid receptor.

Diabetics appear to be more likely to develop infections and, in particular, unusual infections. Tuberculosis should always be considered in the older diabetic with chest disease. Malignant otitis externa due to *Pseudomonas aeruginosa* is another example of an unusual infection seen in diabetics.

Table 16-2 Reasons for maintaining good glucose control in diabetic nursing home residents

Reduced incontinence due to diuretic effect of elevated glucose
Improved vision
Decreased platelet adhesiveness (reduces chance of myocardial infarction or stroke)
Improved outcome if a stroke should occur
Decrease in intermittent claudication
Improved cognitive function
Decreased pain perception
Decreased infection (possible)

Diabetic amyotrophy is a progressive, painful proximal myopathy with minimal sensory changes. Diabetic neuropathic cachexia is a severe form of this disorder, which is associated with anorexia and extreme weight loss. Both of these conditions can lead to NH admission, and both often resolve spontaneously within 6 months to 2 years.

Diabetics often have hyperzincuria, which can lead to borderline zinc status. Zinc deficiency can lead to immune deficiency. All diabetic NH residents with ulcers related to peripheral vascular disease or pressure sores should receive zinc supplementation (220 mg three times a day with meals) to promote wound healing.

Table 16-3 outlines an approach to the management of diabetes mellitus in the NH. Chlorpropamide should never be used in the NH, because its long half-life can lead to prolonged hypoglycemia and it has a propensity to produce hyponatremia. The second-generation oral sulfonylureas are probably superior to the first-generation agents because of the decreased chances of drug-drug interactions. The choice of an oral agent should include consideration of the cost of the drug. When Metformin becomes available in the

Table 16-3   Approach to management of diabetes mellitus in the nursing home

Diagnosis
  Two fasting blood glucoses >140 mg/dl or
  Two random blood glucoses >200 mg/dl

Initial management
  Drug therapy
    Low dose second generation agent (e.g., glyburide 2.5 mg daily or glipizide 5 mg daily)
    Increase dose twice weekly until glucoses are consistently 100–200 mg/dl
  Diet
    No added free sugar (ADA diabetic diet unnecessary unless resident has been on it long-term)
  Exercise program compatible with resident's abilities

If inadequate response to maximal doses of oral agents (i.e., glyburide 10 mg daily or glipizide 20 mg daily)
  Institute insulin therapy
    NPH in the morning
    Regular or NPH later in day if necessary

Monitor glucose daily until stable with values >70 mg/dl and <200 mg/dl

Monitor glucose at least weekly by finger stick when resident is stable

Having standing orders for
  Giving Glucola for glucose <50 mg/dl
  Giving Glucagon 1 mg IM if glucose <30 mg/dl or if acute confusion or delirium occurs

When acute illnesses intervene, monitor glucose more frequently to detect stress-induced hyperglycemia

United States, it would appear reasonable to avoid its use in the NH because it can cause anorexia and lactic acidosis.

There appears to be little advantage to using ADA diabetic diets for NH residents. Most diabetic NH residents should be on a regular diet with no added free sugar. Diabetic NH residents need to be carefully observed for weight loss, as this may necessitate a reduction in the dose of insulin or of the oral sulfonylureas. All diabetics should receive a snack before going to sleep (the amount eaten recorded) and be on a regular exercise program (including those who are chair-bound).

When a diabetic NH resident is stabilized on an oral agent or insulin, measurement of a fasting glucose and at least two glucoses 2 to 3 h after meals by a finger-stick technique once a week should be sufficient. When diabetic residents are begun on a new treatment (insulin or oral agent), values should be monitored at least three times per week. Among residents who are difficult to control, a glucose between 2 and 3 a.m. should be measured to check for the Somogyi effect (hypoglycemia in the early hours of the morning, resulting in daytime hyperglycemia). Adequate diabetic control can, in many cases, result in improved quality of life for NH residents.

ADDISON'S DISEASE AND HYPOPITUITARISM

Addison's disease and hypopituitarism are rare but treatable conditions that are easily missed in the NH resident. Addison's disease should be suspected in the resident with postural hypotension, unexplained hyperkalemia and/or hyponatremia, fatigue, and in some cases difficulty in maintaining diabetic control because of hypoglycemia. The diagnosis of adrenal insufficiency is made by administering 250 μg of synthetic 1-39 ACTH (cosyntropin) intramuscularly after obtaining a basal cortisol level. Cortisol levels are then obtained at 30 and 60 min. Failure of cortisol levels to increase by at least 8 μg/dl or to a level greater than 25 μg/dl makes the diagnosis of adrenal insufficiency. Replacement treatment is with hydrocortisone 25 mg in the morning and 12.5 mg at lunchtime. Do not give steroids in the evening, as this may cause sleep disturbances. Doses should be doubled if the resident becomes infected.

Hypopituitarism should be suspected in the resident who is generally doing poorly and has borderline low thyroid function and in male residents with low testosterone levels. The diagnosis is often difficult to make, but an elevated prolactin level may be helpful. Computed tomography may demonstrate a pituitary tumor.

Low levels of dehydroepiandrosterone sulfate (DHEA-S) have been demonstrated in the male NH population. Very low levels seem to be correlated with poor functional status. Because DHEA-S has been shown to improve cognitive function in animals, it has been suggested that the low levels of

DHEA-S may play a causative role in deteriorating functional status. However, at present this is highly speculative, and testosterone replacement is not indicated to improve functional status.

Low levels of somatomedin-C (insulin growth factor-I) are also seen in the NH population. The decrease in somatomedin-C appears to be greater than that normally seen with aging. The low levels of somatomedin-C in NH residents appear to be predominantly an indicator of protein-energy malnutrition. They also are predictive of death in the NH. Patients with low somatomedin-C levels may, in the future, be candidates for replacement with recombinant growth hormone.

VITAMIN D DEFICIENCY

Exposure of the skin to sunlight is necessary in order to obtain adequate amounts of vitamin D. Many NH residents have inadequate sunlight exposure and also ingest too few calories to obtain adequate amounts of vitamin D in the diet. In addition, with aging there is decreased conversion of 25(OH) vitamin D to $1,25(OH)_2$ vitamin D (the active form). In addition, when older people go out of doors they often cover up sun-exposed areas, and those with skin cancer may use sunblock lotions to prevent exposure to ultraviolet light. This combination of factors causes many NH residents to develop borderline vitamin D status.

Vitamin D deficiency should be suspected in any resident who has a low or low-normal calcium and elevated alkaline phosphatase. Vitamin D deficiency is present in up to 50 percent of individuals with hip fracture. Diagnosis can be made either by measuring 25(OH) vitamin D levels or giving a therapeutic trial of vitamin D. Treatment of vitamin D deficiency consists of giving 400 IU of vitamin D daily or 50,000 IU of vitamin D twice a year. Some older individuals develop vitamin resistance and require higher doses of vitamin D (e.g., 50,000 IU of vitamin D twice a week). When higher doses of vitamin D are given, calcium needs to be closely monitored.

HYPONATREMIA

Hyponatremia is present in up to 20 percent NH residents at any one time; up to 50 percent of all NH residents have a single episode of hyponatremia in a given year. In most cases the hyponatremia is mild and has no obvious symptomatic consequences. However, residents with mild hyponatremia are at increased risk of developing severe hyponatremia when they receive intravenous fluids. Limitation of fluids in residents with mild hyponatremia can prevent precipitation of severe hyponatremia (Table 16-4).

Table 16-4   Causes of hyponatremia in the nursing home

Tube feeding with inadequate salt
Syndrome of inappropriate antidiuresis (SIADH)
CNS disorders
Lung disease
Hypothyroidism
Drugs
Phenothiazines
Carbamazepine
Ectopic ADH production
Oat cell cancer of lung
Lymphoma
Pancreatic cancer
Idiopathic hyponatremia
Psychogenic polydipsia
Drugs, e. g., thioridazine (Mellaril)
Psychiatric disorders
? Inappropriate atrionaturetic factor (ANF) release
Congestive heart failure
Liver disease

Note: ? = possible.

Two major causes of hyponatremia among NH residents have been identified. The first is tube feeding with inadequate salt loads. The majority of non-tube-fed residents with hyponatremia have the syndrome of inappropriate antidiuretic hormone secretion (SIADH). Major causes include phenothiazines, central nervous system disorders, pulmonary disease, hypothyroidism, and ectopic production of ADH by oat cell carcinoma of the lung. When a resident consistently has serum sodium levels less than 120 meq/liter, treatment with demeclocycline (600 to 1200 mg/dl) may be necessary. NH residents receiving the antipsychotic agent thioridazine (Mellaril) may develop psychogenic polydipsia, which can result in hyponatremia. The role of the newly identified atrionaturetic factor (ANF) in the hyponatremia seen among NH residents is uncertain.

SUGGESTED READINGS

Mooradian AD, Morley JE, Korenman SG: Endocrinology in aging. *Disease-a-Month* 34:395–461, 1988.
Mooradian AD, Osterweil D, Petrosek D, Morley JE: Diabetes mellitus in elderly nursing home

patients: A survey of clinical characteristics and management. *J Am Geriatr Soc* 36:391–396, 1988.

Morley JE: A place in the sun does not guarantee adequate vitamin D. *J Am Geriatr Soc* 37:663–664, 1989.

Morley JE: Geriatric endocrinology, in Mendelsohn G (ed): *Diagnosis and Pathology of Endocrine Disorders.* Philadelphia, JB Lippincott Co, 1988, pp 603–617.

Morley JE, Mooradian AD, Rosenthal MJ, Kaiser RD: Diabetes mellitus in elderly nursing home patients: Is it different? *Am J Med* 83:533–544, 1987.

SEVENTEEN

INFECTIONS AND INFECTION CONTROL

Infections are among the most common medical conditions encountered in the nursing home (NH) setting, and in several studies, they have been the most common reason for the acute hospitalization of residents. The Centers for Disease Control estimate that close to 1.5 million infections occur annually in NHs, which averages out to almost one infection per year per resident. With regard to nosocomial infections, point prevalence surveys (which overestimate chronic infections) have demonstrated a prevalence of 3 percent to 18 percent, which is comparable to the rate in acute care hospitals.

Several factors make NH residents susceptible to infections, including age-related changes in immunity, impaired functional status (especially urinary and fecal incontinence), and the high prevalence of chronic medical conditions, such as diabetes mellitus, chronic obstructive pulmonary disease, cancer, and peripheral vascular disease. All these conditions predispose NH residents to a variety of infections. A majority of infections in NHs are endemic, but many epidemics of respiratory infections (influenza, tuberculosis) and gastroenteritis have been reported. The relatively closed environment of the NH in which regular interaction among residents and staff is encouraged, increases susceptibility to epidemic infections.

Three-quarters or more of all infections in the NH come from three sources: the urinary tract, the respiratory tract, and the skin and soft tissues. But infections among NH residents may be difficult to recognize and localize. Like other medical conditions, infections often present atypically in the frail, functionally impaired geriatric population. Fever and localizing signs of infection may be completely absent. Acute changes in functional status, decreased food and fluid intake, increased confusion or delirium, and falls may be the manifestations of an infectious process. Thus, when these conditions are reported, an infection should be considered. Although empiric antimicrobial therapy may be warranted in some situations, an attempt should be made to localize an infection by means of appropriate diagnostic studies. The overuse of empiric antimicrobial therapy can lead to the development of a variety of resistant organisms within the facility.

Despite the prevalence, morbidity, and costs associated with NH infections, several surveys have suggested that infection control policies and procedures are poorly developed in many NHs. In addition, many unnecessary cultures are probably performed, and antimicrobials are often administered inappropriately. The purpose of this chapter is twofold: to give the primary physician a perspective on the management of common infections in the NH and to provide an overview of appropriate infection control practices for the NH setting.

MANAGEMENT OF COMMON INFECTIONS IN THE NH

In general, the approach to treating infections in the NH depends on three factors:

1. Characteristics of the resident (underlying diseases, functional status, quality of life, and preferred intensity of treatment)
2. Nature and severity of the infection
3. Resources available within the NH

Table 17-1 lists infections that occur commonly in the NH. Each of these will be discussed briefly, emphasizing what is important in the NH setting.

Table 17-1 Common infections in the nursing home

Urinary tract	Skin and soft tissues
Noncatheterized residents	Conjunctivitis
Asymptomatic bacteriuria	Cellulitis
Symptomatic infection/urosepsis	Infected pressure sores
Catheterized residents	Herpes zoster
Asymptomatic bacteriuria	Tetanus
Symptomatic infection/urosepsis	Gastrointestinal tract
Respiratory tract	Gastroenteritis/infectious diarrhea
Upper respiratory tract infections	Antibiotic-associated enterocolitis
Bronchitis	Other
Influenza	Appendicitis
Pneumonia	Diverticulitis
Tuberculosis	Cholecystitis
	Hepatitis

Readers should refer to textbooks of medicine and infectious disease for more detailed information on these conditions.

Urinary Tract Infections

The approach to managing urinary tract infections (UTI) in the NH setting should take into account two fundamental considerations:

1. Residents with indwelling bladder catheters should be considered separately from those without them.
2. There is a high prevalence of "asymptomatic" bacteriuria. If it is truly asymptomatic, it should not generally be treated.

Table 17-2 lists key principles of managing UTI in noncatheterized NH residents. In most NHs, the prevalence of bacteriuria, defined as growth of more than 10^5 colony forming units per milliliter of urine, is between 30 percent and 50 percent in women and slightly lower in men. Epidemiological studies have clearly shown that this bacteriuria comes and goes without treatment.

The relationship of chronic or intermittent bacteriuria to morbidity and mortality among NH residents is controversial. Several studies have suggested, however, that attempts to eradicate asymptomatic bacteriuria do not have a prominent influence on morbidity and mortality and can lead to the development of resistant organisms. Thus, it is clear that true asymptomatic bacteriuria should not be treated in the NH. An important caveat, however, lies in the definition of *asymptomatic*. Because symptoms and signs of infection may be nonspecific, there should be a high index of suspicion for infection when acute or subacute changes in status occur. As discussed in Chap. 13, otherwise asymptomatic bacteriuria should be eradicated in the course of evaluating and initiating therapy for urinary incontinence, at least until better data become available.

If infection is suspected, a good clean specimen of urine for urinalysis and culture is necessary. It is difficult if not impossible to collect a midstream "clean catch" specimen from a functionally impaired NH resident. Thus, most women will require an in-and-out catheterization if an accurate specimen is to be obtained. The morbidity associated with this procedure is less than that which might result from treatment based on an inaccurate bladder specimen. Among functionally capable men, especially those who are circumcised, an accurate specimen can often be obtained from an uncleansed, freshly voided specimen. In functionally or cognitively impaired men, an accurate bladder specimen can be obtained by cleaning the penis with an antiseptic solution, applying an external catheter, and rapidly processing the first voided specimen. Other laboratory studies should also be done to determine the severity of illness (Table 17-2).

NH residents who appear clinically unstable and possibly septic should be transferred to an acute care hospital (or "subacute" unit if available) for

Table 17-2   Management of urinary tract infections in noncatheterized nursing home residents

Do not routinely treat asymptomatic bacteriuria
    If significant pyuria is present with bacteriuria in a catheterized specimen, have a high index of suspicion for nonspecific manifestations of UTI.
    Though the issue remains controversial, it is suggested that asymptomatic bacteriuria be eradicated when one is evaluating and initiating therapy for urinary incontinence (see also Chap. 13)
Clinical manifestations of UTI may be nonspecific
    High fever ($>101°F$), dysuria, and hematuria are less common than nonspecific symptoms, such as new or worsening incontinence, anorexia, mental status changes
When UTI is suspected, a basic evaluation should include
    A clean urine for urinalysis and culture
        In the majority of functionally and cognitively impaired females, this will require in-and-out catheterization
        For functionally or cognitively impaired men, an accurate bladder specimen can be obtained by cleaning the penis with an antiseptic, and applying an external catheter
            An accurate specimen from functional, circumcised men can generally be obtained by an uncleansed first voided specimen
    Blood work to determine severity of illness
        Complete blood count
        Glucose, electrolytes, BUN, creatinine
        Blood cultures (if resident is very ill)
If resident is clinically unstable with high fever, delirium, or dehydration, hospitalization (or transfer to a subacute-care unit if available) for parenteral antimicrobial therapy and hydration is usually indicated
If resident is clinically stable, begin oral antimicrobial therapy
    Choice of antimicrobial depends on facility resistance patterns
    In the absence of a history of recurrent UTI or recent antimicrobial therapy, trimethoprim-sulfamethoxazole or amoxicillin-clavulanic acid are adequate initial therapy
    With a history of recurrent UTI or recent antimicrobial therapy, initial therapy should include a quinolone (norfloxacin, ciprofloxacin) until culture and sensitivity data are available
    Treat women for 7–10 days, men for 10–14
If symptomatic UTI recurs
    A urologic evaluation to exclude urinary retention or structural abnormality is indicated
    In the absence of correctable genitourinary pathology, suppressive therapy (e.g., $\frac{1}{2}$ tablet of single-strength trimethoprim-sulfamethoxazole nightly) is indicated to prevent reinfection

parenteral antimicrobial therapy, intravenous hydration, and close monitoring. If such residents are clinically stable and taking oral fluids, oral antimicrobial therapy can be initiated. The selection of an antimicrobial should take into account resistance patterns noted at the facility. In the absence of a history of recurrent UTI or recent antimicrobial therapy, trimethoprim-sulfamethoxazole or ampicillin-clavulanic acid would be adequate initial therapy. If the resident has a history of recurrent UTI or was recently treated with an antimicrobial, a quinolone (norfloxacin, ciprofloxacin) should be prescribed until sensitivity data become available.

Residents who have recurrent symptomatic UTI should be evaluated urologically in order to exclude correctable genitourinary pathology. In the absence of such pathology, suppressive therapy is a reasonable approach. This is generally done by administering one-half tablet of single-strength trimethoprim-sulfamethoxazole or a similar agent nightly.

Table 17-3 lists key principles of managing UTI in residents with indwelling bladder catheters. The basic approaches are similar to those outlined for catheter-free residents, but several points should be emphasized. As noted in Chap. 13, significant bacteriuria is universal in NH residents with chronic indwelling bladder catheters. The bacteriuria is generally polymicrobial and changes frequently. When a symptomatic UTI is suspected, it is best to

Table 17-3   Management of urinary tract infections in nursing home residents with indwelling bladder catheters[a]

Do not treat asymptomatic bacteriuria
　With an indwelling catheter, urine always has significant bacteriuria
　Bacteriuria is generally polymicrobial
　Organisms change frequently, so that routine cultures in the absence of symptoms are
　　unnecessary and may be misleading
Clinical manifestations of symptomatic UTI are often nonspecific
　Fever in a catheterized resident should not automatically be attributed to UTI
　A high index of suspicion of UTI is appropriate when there are unexplained nonspecific
　　symptoms, such as acute or subacute changes in mental status, functional abilities, food
　　and fluid intake
When UTI is suspected, a basic evaluation should include
　A urinalysis, culture, and sensitivity *after* the catheter is changed
　Blood work to determine severity of illness
　　Complete blood count
　　Glucose, electrolytes, BUN, creatinine
　　Blood cultures (if resident is very ill)
If resident is clinically unstable with high fever, delirium, or dehydration, hospitalization (or
　transfer to a "subacute" unit if available) for parenteral antimicrobials and hydration is
　usually indicated
　Initial empiric therapy
　　Coverage of Group D enterococci (e.g., ampicillin or amoxicillin, vancomycin,
　　　imipenem/cilastin)
　　Gram-negative coverage (e.g., third-generation cephalosporins, aztreonam, quinolones)
　Continue parenteral therapy for 3 to 7 days depending on clinical response; therapy
　　beyond 10 to 14 days not indicated
If resident is clinically stable, oral therapy can be initiated
　If resident has not recently been on antibiotics, trimethoprim-sulfamethoxazole or
　　amoxicillin-clavulanic acid can be initial therapy
　If resident has recently been on antibiotics or has a history of recurrent UTI, initial therapy
　　should include a quinolone (norfloxacin, ciprofloxacin) until culture data are available
If symptomatic UTI recurs frequently, a urological evaluation is indicated to identify
　genitourinary abnormalities that may predispose to recurrences (e.g., periurethral abscess,
　stone)

[a] See also Table 13-11.

change the catheter before obtaining a urine specimen, because cultures taken from catheters that are already in place may reflect colonization of the catheter rather than the pathogen in the bladder. Initial empiric antimicrobial coverage should include Group D enterococci as well as gram-negative organisms (Table 17-3), which generally require parenteral therapy. Parenteral therapy should continue for 3 to 7 days, depending on the clinical condition. Therapy beyond 10 to 14 days is not indicated. If symptomatic UTI recurs frequently, a urological evaluation is indicated to identify genitourinary abnormalities, such as periurethral abscess or bladder calculi—which may predispose to recurrent episodes.

Respiratory Tract Infections

Three types of respiratory tract infections will be discussed in some detail because of their prevalence and associated morbidity and mortality: influenza, bacterial pneumonia, and tuberculosis. Upper respiratory infections—including viral nasopharyngitis, bacterial sinusitis, and acute viral and bacterial tracheobronchitis are also common in the NH—but the principles of managing these conditions do not differ substantially from those for the community-dwelling geriatric population. The overprescription of antimicrobials for what are predominantly viral illnesses should be avoided so as not to promote the development of resistant organisms. On the other hand, NH residents with significant chronic lung disease are susceptible to decompensation from acute bronchitis; antimicrobial therapy is appropriate for these residents when they become symptomatic, producing purulent sputum in the absence of signs of pneumonia.

Epidemics of influenza can be devastating in the NH setting. Table 17-4 lists some general principles regarding influenza in the NH. A vigorous attempt should be made to vaccinate all residents as well as direct-care staff annually, between late October and early December. There should be a high index of suspicion for an early outbreak if there is an outbreak in the community or if residents and/or staff begin to develop symptoms (Table 17-4). If this occurs, throat cultures should be obtained to determine if the outbreak represents type A influenza, because amantadine prophylaxis may be useful in preventing infection due to this virus (but not to type B influenza). Serological testing is not necessary unless an epidemic is being investigated. If amantadine prophylaxis is used, the dose must be adjusted for age and renal function. The standard dose of 200 mg/day should be reduced to 100 mg/day or less in NH residents because of their reduced renal excretion and propensity to develop side effects, especially delirium. Recurrent fever or signs of respiratory distress suggest superimposed bacterial pneumonia.

Pneumonia, known as the "old person's friend," is one of the most common causes of hospitalization and death among NH residents if not *the* most common. Pneumonia should be at the top of the differential diagnosis list

Table 17-4   Influenza in the nursing home

Influenza, especially type A, is a major cause of preventable morbidity and mortality in the NH setting

All residents and staff providing direct care should be immunized annually, between late October and early December

A high index of suspicion for an influenza outbreak is necessary during winter months when
  An outbreak occurs in the community
  Staff are absent with respiratory illnesses
  Residents begin to develop clinical manifestations
    Fever, headache, malaise, myalgias, arthralgias
    Rhinorrhea, nasal congestion, cough

Symptomatic residents and staff should have throat cultures early in the course of a suspected outbreak of type A influenza
  Once a case is confirmed by culture, all similar illnesses should be considered influenza
  Serological testing is not necessary unless an epidemic is under investigation

Amantadine is useful for prophylaxis for type A influenza (but not type B)
  If given within 24 to 48 h of the onset of illness, it may reduce the severity of symptoms
  Should be given to vaccinated residents and staff only if outbreak occurs within 2 weeks of vaccination (antibody protection takes about 2 weeks to develop)
  May be given to asymptomatic unvaccinated residents and staff as prophylaxis throughout a severe outbreak
  The usual dose of 200 mg/day must be reduced to 100 mg or less in residents over age 65 and reduced further if renal function is impaired
  NH residents are susceptible to side effects of amantadine, especially delirium

Recurrent fever, tachypnea, or other signs of respiratory distress may indicate superimposed bacterial pneumonia

for any NH resident who has an acute or subacute change in mental or functional status or in food or fluid intake. Typical symptoms are frequently absent, although tachypnea is an especially important sign and is easily missed by nursing staff. Table 17-5 lists several key principles of managing pneumonia in the NH, and Table 17-6 lists antimicrobials that are appropriate for the therapy of NH-acquired pneumonia. In general, NH residents should be treated in an acute care hospital or subacute unit where adequate staff and diagnostic capabilities are present because of the high incidence of concomitant conditions such as hypoxia, dehydration, metabolic disturbances, and cardiac decompensation. Antimicrobial therapy should generally be administered parenterally for at least 7 days. Because adequate sputum specimens are difficult to obtain from NH residents, antimicrobial therapy is most often empiric. It should cover organisms that are known to cause NH-acquired pneumonia, including gram-negative rods (especially *Klebsiella*), *Streptococcus pneumoniae, Hemophilus influenza,* and *Staphylococcus aureus.* Excellent supportive care is also essential for the successful treatment of pneumonia and the prevention of iatrogenic complications (Table 17-5).

Table 17-5   Management of pneumonia in nursing home residents

Fever and pulmonary symptoms are often absent in NH residents with pneumonia
  High index of suspicion for pneumonia if there are acute or subacute changes in mental
  status, functional status, food and fluid intake
Most NH residents with pneumonia should be hospitalized (or transferred to a "subacute"
  unit if available) for parenteral antimicrobial and fluid administration
Initial diagnostic evaluation should include
  Complete blood count
  Glucose, electrolytes, BUN, creatinine
  Blood cultures
  Chest film
  Arterial blood gas
  Electrocardiogram (if indicated)
  Gram stain and culture of sputum if obtainable
  Diagnostic thoracentesis (if indicated)
Life-threatening conditions (e.g., hypotension, hypoxia, severe anemia, dehydration, cardiac
  arrhythmias) should be stabilized
Antimicrobials should generally be administered parenterally for 7 days more, depending on
  the clinical condition
  Antimicrobial therapy should cover organisms frequently isolated in NH-acquired
    pneumonia (see Table 17-6)
    Gram-negative organisms (especially *Klebsiella*)
    Streptococcus pneumoniae
    Haemophilus influenza
    Staphylococcus aureus
  When resident is clinically stable, oral antimicrobial therapy can be initiated and continued
    for 7 to 10 days (see Table 17-6)
Excellent supportive care is essential
  Proper hydration
  Adequate nutrition
  Adequate oxygenation
  Pulmonary care
  Management of other medical illnesses
  Skin care
  Mobilization to prevent complictions from immobility

Source: After Yoshikawa TT: Pneumonia, UTI, and decubiti in the nursing home: Optimal management. *Geriatrics* 44:32–43, 1989.

Tuberculosis, though relatively uncommon, is very important in the NH population for several reasons. First, NH residents are especially susceptible to the reactivation of *Mycobacterium tuberculosis.* Second, like bacterial pneumonia, pulmonary tuberculosis is difficult to recognize but curable if appropriate treatment is instituted. Third, unrecognized tuberculosis can result not only in the death of the resident but also in an epidemic within the facility. Finally, in many areas of the country a substantial proportion of the staff are immigrants who may have an increased susceptibility to tuberculosis.

Table 17-6 Empiric antimicrobial therapy for nursing-home-acquired pneumonia

Drug	Dose[a]
Parenteral	
Second-generation cephalosporins	
Cefuroxime	1.5 g q 8–12 h
Cefoxitin	2 g q 6 h
Cefotetan	1–2 g q 12 h
Third-generation cephalosporins	
Ceftriaxone	1–2 g q 12–24 h
Cefoperazone	1–2 g q 12 h
Ticarcillin (3 g)-clavulanate (0.1 g)	3.1 g q 4–8 h
Ampicillin (1 g)-sulbactam (0.5 g)	1.5–3 g q 6–12 h
Oxacillin plus aztreonam	2 g q 6 h (oxacillin) 1–2 g q 8–12 h (aztreonam)
Cefazolin plus aminoglycoside	1 g q 8–12 h (cefazolin) 1.5 mg/kg q 8–12 h (gentamicin)
Oral therapy[b]	
Known organism	Treat on the basis of susceptibility
Unknown organism	Amoxicillin-clavulanic acid Cefuroxime-axetil Ciprofloxacin (with or without penicillin G or ampicillin) Trimethoprim-sulfamethoxazole (with clindamycin or another agent)

[a] Doses are based on absence of significant renal dysfunction.

[b] Initiate after 7 or more days of parenteral therapy when resident is clinically stable; total duration of therapy should be 14 to 21 days.

Source: After Yoshikawa TT: Pneumonia, UTI, and decubiti in the nursing home: Optimal management. *Geriatrics* 44:32–43, 1989.

Table 17-7 provides a detailed outline of the principles of managing tuberculosis in the NH. These recommendations are straightforward and consistent with recommendations published elsewhere. Although it is not mandatory in all areas, we recommend that residents and staff have a tuberculin skin test annually. Further details on the management of tuberculosis can be found in some of the suggested readings, and an example of a policy for NHs is included in the Appendix.

Infections of Skin and Soft Tissues

A wide variety of infections of the skin and soft tissues occur among NH residents, including conjunctivitis, cellulitis, herpes zoster (shingles), and infected ulcers and pressure sores. Although it is very rare, tetanus is always

Table 17-7 Principles of managing tuberculosis in the nursing home setting

All staff should have tuberculin skin testing at the time of employment and annually with intermediate-strength (5 tuberculin units) purified protein derivative (PPD) antigen

All new admissions to the facility should have an intermediate-strength PPD placed *unless* they have had a well-documented and evaluated positive skin test in the past

    If the initial test is negative (less than 10 mm of induration at 48 h), they should be *retested* within 2 weeks with PPD and dermal control antigens (*Candida, Trichophyton,* mumps) in order to detect the "booster" phenomenon as well as cutaneous anergy

All residents with a positive PPD (including booster) should have a chest film and careful evaluation to determine if active disease may be present

Although not mandatory, annual skin testing of all residents is recommended

Chemoprophylaxis should be administered to residents with

    Close contact with an infected person

    History of tuberculosis *not* previously treated with INH

    Conversion to a positive PPD within 2 years

    Positive PPD and

        Diabetes mellitus

        Silicosis or other chronic lung disease

        End-stage renal disease

        Under- or malnutrition

        Prolonged corticosteroid therapy (e.g., 15 mg or more of prednisone daily for more than 2 weeks)

        Other immunosuppressive therapy

        Hematogenous or reticuloendothelial malignancy

        AIDS or positive HIV serology

Chemoprophylaxis includes

    INH 300 mg and pyridoxine (B6) 50 mg for a minimum of 6 months if chest film is normal

    If chest film is abnormal (stable lesion, negative mycobacteriology) or resident has HIV infection, 12 months of therapy is recommended

For *active* pulmonary tuberculosis

    Nine months of therapy

        INH 300 mg/day

        Rifampin 600 mg/day

        Pyridoxine (B6) 50 mg/day

All residents treated with INH should have liver function tests *every 3 months*

    If the SGOT increases more than threefold, therapy should be stopped

    If indicated, after normalization of liver function tests, rechallenge with 50 mg/day, increasing by 50 mg at weekly intervals (up to 300 mg) may be attempted while following liver function tests carefully

        If liver function tests deteriorate again, do not rechallenge

        If prophylaxis absolutely necessary, ethambutol plus rifampin may be tried

---

a concern, because many NH residents have not had adequate immunization.

In some point prevalence surveys, conjunctivitis is among the most common infections identified in the NH setting. The predominant symptoms and signs are conjunctival erythema and a purulent discharge. Most conjunctivitis is bacterial; it should be treated with a topical antimicrobial solution and warm compresses (the latter if a lot of discomfort is present). Cultures are not necessary. When conjunctivitis is recurrent, regular attention should be given to the cleanliness of the eyelids in order to help prevent recurrences.

Bacterial cellulitis most commonly affects the lower extremities. An obvious source of the cellulitis, such as an ulcer or abrasion, is found in only half or less of cases. Cultures are only indicated if there is a lesion; attempts to get cultures by needle aspiration do not generally yield clinically useful information. Culture results may be helpful if there is a poor response to initial therapy, if there is an outbreak of skin infections in the facility, or if isolation is a consideration for staphylococcal infections. Cellulitis of the lower or upper extremities is treatable in the NH. An oral or parenteral semisynthetic penicillin or cephalosporin, erythromycin, or clindamycin are reasonable initial therapy. The affected area should be observed carefully for the first 24 to 48 h; if there is no improvement or the condition becomes worse, hospitalization for parenteral therapy should be considered. It is helpful to mark the borders of the cellulitis to document improvement or progression. Cellulitis involving the face or neck should generally be treated with parenteral therapy in an acute care setting.

Bacterial cellulitis should be differentiated from two other skin infections in the NH: candidiasis and scabies. NH residents, especially diabetics and those who have been on broad-spectrum antibiotics, are susceptible to mucocutaneous candidiasis. The most common manifestation is acute intertriginous infection of the perianal skin, perineum, and genitalia and macerated skin surfaces under breasts or skin folds. The diagnosis can be confirmed by observing the fungus microscopically in a skin scraping exposed to potassium hydroxide. Treatment includes good hygiene and a topical antifungal agent. Scabies is caused by a mite that burrows under the skin. It can become epidemic in the NH if not diagnosed and managed properly. Residents with excoriated pruritic papules should be suspected of having scabies. The excoriations can become severe and be complicated by cellulitis. The diagnosis is made by observing the mite microscopically in a skin scraping. All affected residents and their contacts should be treated with an antiscabetic solution and antipruritic agents as needed. All clothing and linens should be thoroughly laundered, and residents should be reevaluated in 3 to 6 weeks if pruritus persists.

Herpes zoster, generally known as shingles, results from a reactivation of latent varicella-zoster virus. This virus is also responsible for chickenpox, and 95 percent of adults have had a primary infection. The incidence of shingles increases with advancing age. A prodrome of fever, malaise, or pain (which may be severe and can mimic many conditions) may precede the eruption of skin lesions by a few days. Early skin lesions are grouped vesicles on a red base in a specific dermatome, which does not cross the midline. The lesions become pustular in 3 to 4 days, crust within 7 to 10 days, and generally disappear within 2 to 3 weeks. The management of shingles involves the prevention of complications, the relief of acute symptoms, and the treatment of chronic complications. The major complications of herpes zoster are dissemination and chronic pain or postherpetic neuralgia. Dissemination is extremely rare in people who are not immunosuppressed. In the presence of significant immunosuppression (hematological or reticuloendothelial malignancy, cancer chemotherapy, chronic steroid treatment), intravenous acyclovir 500 mg/m^2 of body surface area should be administered every 8 h for 7 days in order to prevent dissemination (pneumonia, myelitis, paralysis, ocular complications). Ten to 15 percent of patients have cranial nerve involvement, most often the ocular branch of the trigeminal nerve. Because of the risk of ocular complications, those with cranial nerve involvement should be treated with oral acyclovir 600 mg five times per day for 10 days.

The pain during the acute phase of shingles may be severe and often requires narcotic analgesics, even among those with a high tolerance for pain. Postherpetic neuralgia, defined as pain lasting longer than a month, is the most common complication of shingles and can last months or even years. The use of corticosteroids to prevent chronic pain is controversial. Many clinicians favor its use despite a lack of convincing evidence of effectiveness from controlled trials. If steroids are used, they should be started as early as possible and tapered over 3 to 4 weeks. Management of postherpetic neuralgia is difficult. A wide variety of measures have been used with variable and limited success including amitriptyline, carbamazepine, transcutaneous electrical stimulation, nerve blocks, and capsaicin, a new topical cream.

During the acute phase of shingles, the skin vesicles contain infectious material. Staff, children, and other individuals who have not had chickenpox should not come in contact with the affected resident until all the lesions are crusted and dry. Although gowns, gloves, and masks are not necessary, proper handwashing techniques should be used after contact with an affected resident. Residents with shingles do not have to be isolated but should not be in the same room with residents who are immunosuppressed.

The basic principles of managing infected pressure sores are outlined in Table 17-8. The approach to infected ulcers and other skin wounds are basically the same. Several points should be emphasized. As in the case of urine in residents with chronic indwelling catheters, bacterial colonization without evidence of infection is the rule. Growth of organisms on a culture is *not* in itself an indication for antimicrobial therapy, which should be reserved for specific indications, including cellulitis, osteomyelitis, or signs of sepsis without another source. When antimicrobial therapy is indicated, it should be based on *properly collected* cultures. Surface swabs of pressure ulcers and other skin wounds are of no value and may be misleading.

Table 17-8   Principles of managing infected pressure sores in the nursing home

Bacterial colonization without clinical evidence of infection is common—analogous to catheter-related bacteriuria
  Growth of organisms on culture is not in itself an indication for treatment
Cultures must be done properly in order to determine the cause of deep tissue infection
  Surface swabs are of no value and may be misleading
  Cultures of purulent drainage and/or debrided necrotic tissue are more predictive of causative organisms
  If osteomyelitis is suspected based on radiology and/or bone scan, a bone biopsy for culture is necessary to identify the pathogen(s)
  If systemic infection is suspected, blood cultures should be obtained
  Anaerobic as well as aerobic cultures should be done
Pathogens in deep tissue infections are generally polymicrobial
  In stage 1 and 2 sores, gram-positive cocci and aerobic gram-negative rods are common
  In stage 3 and 4 sores, a mixture of aerobic gram-negative rods and anaerobes is common
Antimicrobial therapy should be reserved for specific indications
  Cellulitis (not just erythema of healing tissue)
  Osteomyelitis
  Clinical signs of sepsis in the absence of another source
Antimicrobial therapy should be based on culture results whenever possible
  Unless a superficial cellulitis is being treated, initial antimicrobial therapy should generally be parenteral
  Anaerobic coverage should be included for deep tissue infections
  Appropriate antimicrobials include (not in order of preference):

Ampicillin-sulbactam	Cefotetan
Cefoxitin	Chloramphenicol
Clindamycin	Metronidazole
Piperacillin (or mezlocillin)	Ticarcillin-clavulanate

  In case of severe infection or sepsis, one of the above should be combined with aztreonam or an aminoglycoside to adequately cover gram-negative bacilli

Cultures should be taken from purulent drainage, debrided necrotic tissue, or bone biopsy. Anaerobic cultures should be done in addition to standard aerobic cultures because of the prevalence of anaerobic pathogens in deep tissue infections. When such infection is present, antimicrobial therapy should be parenteral and should include adequate anaerobic coverage. Table 17-8 contains a list of antimicrobials that would be appropriate in this situation.

Tetanus is a rare disease, but it is serious and preventable. Most elderly people except those who served in the armed forces, have either never had a primary series of immunizations or have not had a booster shot in many years, which may make a single booster at the time of injury ineffective in achieving sufficient protection from subsequent wounds. The method of immunization depends on the nature of the wound and the immunization status of the resident. If the resident has had three or more doses of tetanus-diphtheria toxoid (Td) with the last being within the previous 5 years, no immunization is necessary. For clean, minor wounds, Td should be administered. Consideration should be given to giving a primary series of three Td injections (at the time of injury, 4 to 6 weeks later, and 6 to 12 months after the second dose) to residents who have never been immunized or had their last dose many years earlier. For deep and contaminated wounds, tetanus immune globulin, 250 to 500 units, should be administered (by a separate syringe at a different site) in addition to Td.

Gastrointestinal Tract Infections

Though not as prevalent as the infections already discussed, infections in the gastrointestinal tract are relatively common and are an important source of morbidity and mortality in the NH population. In addition, some of these infections can cause serious epidemics in an institutional setting.

In most cases of acute diarrheal illness or gastroenteritis, a pathogen is not identified and the illness is generally attributed to a virus. All NH residents with the new onset of diarrhea should, however, have a stool specimen collected and sent for examination for leukocytes and culture for pathogens. The absence of fecal leukocytes suggests a viral etiology or a toxin-induced illness (e.g., staphylococcal or clostridial food poisoning). Fecal leukocytes are present when there is tissue invasion or inflammation of the intestinal mucosa, as can be seen in bacterial or parasitic infection, toxin-induced illness, or inflammatory bowel disease (i.e., Crohn's). Infectious agents can come from a human reservoir (e.g., *Salmonella typhi, Shigella, Giardia*) or from food or water (e.g., nontyphoid *Salmonella, Yersinia* spp., *Campylobacter, E. coli* 0157:H7). *E. coli* 0157:H7 has been responsible for epidemics associated with the eating of undercooked beef.

Treatment of acute gastroenteritis with antimicrobials is generally limited to residents with severe bacterial dysentery, systemic infection, or parasitic infection. NH residents with profuse diarrhea should be hospitalized for management of fluid and electrolyte balance. Enteric precautions should be instituted for all residents with an acute gastroenteritis and prolonged diarrhea.

Diarrhea occurs commonly during or just after antibiotic therapy. This, due to changes in intestinal flora, is often mild and self-limited. In many cases, however, diarrhea can lead to intestinal inflammation and damage. This entity is generally termed "antibiotic-associated enterocolitis." Its signs and symptoms usually develop within a week after a course of antibiotics is initiated but may occur as long as a month later. A high index of suspicion for this disorder is necessary for any NH resident who develops diarrhea and/or other gastrointestinal symptoms within a month after a course of antibiotics. Diarrhea in this situation should *not* automatically be attributed to other factors common in this population, such as enteral feedings, nutritional supplements, or laxatives. Although the precise frequency is not known, a majority of studies suggest that most antibiotic-associated entero-colitis is caused by *Clostridium difficile.* Some NH residents may be colo-nized with C. *difficile* without symptoms, and in such instances it may be difficult to attribute the illness to this organism. Many cases of antibiotic-associated enterocolitis are severe enough to cause pseudomembranous colitis. This entity can be diagnosed by the detection of C. *difficile* toxin in the stool and characteristic intestinal mucosal changes will be seen on endoscopy. Other organisms (e.g., *Pseudomonas aeruginosa*) can also cause pseudomembranous colitis. If the clinical picture is consistent with antibiotic-associated enterocolitis, all NH residents with positive stool assays for C. *difficile* toxin should have antibiotics discontinued and be treated with either oral vancomycin (125 mg four times per day) or metronidazole (500 mg four times per day) for 5 days. Enteric precautions should be insti-tuted for all residents with antibiotic-associated enterocolitis.

Other infections of the gastrointestinal tract also occur in the NH pop-ulation. Acute appendicitis, cholecystitis, and diverticulitis should always be considered in the differential diagnosis of an infection in a NH resident. As with other infections, the clinical manifestations may be minimal, nonspe-cific, or deceiving. A careful abdominal examination is essential in any NH resident with a fever or unexplained gastrointestinal symptoms, no matter how vague. Although leukocytosis may be absent, a white blood cell count and differential should be ordered. Unexplained leukocytosis or a left shift should make an intra-abdominal infection a strong consideration, even in the absence of localizing signs or symptoms. Surgical consultation should be obtained early in the course of any suspected intra-abdominal infection.

Hepatitis is an important infection in the NH, not so much because of its prevalence but because of its potential to cause an epidemic in an insti-tutional setting. Any NH resident or staff suspected of having hepatitis should have appropriate blood studies performed. If hepatitis is diagnosed, it is imperative to identify a source whenever possible in order to prevent a potential epidemic within the institution.

AIDS

We would be remiss if we did not at least mention one last infection that may assume growing importance in NHs over the next several years: acquired immunodeficiency syndrome (AIDS). With the increasing preva-lence of this disorder and the potential for those afflicted with AIDS to develop dementia and other functional disabilities, there will be an increas-ing need for institutional care for this population. NHs should develop edu-cational programs and policies and procedures about AIDS, so that these individuals can be properly cared for and will pose no threat to other resi-dents and staff.

INFECTION CONTROL

All NHs are required to have an infection control program. This requirement has been reinforced by the OBRA 1987 legislation (see Appendix). The broad goals of such a program are to provide a sanitary and comfortable environment and to prevent the development and transmission of infection whenever possible. Infection control activities range from the development of policies and procedures to screening and preventive activities for residents and staff to ongoing surveillance to determine the incidence of infection and identify outbreaks.

Table 17-9 lists several key aspects of an infection control program for the NH setting. The program is best overseen by a multidisciplinary infection control committee that should meet at least quarterly. In addition to reviewing surveillance data, this committee should be involved in the development of a number of different policies and procedures that are relevant to infection control (see Table 17-9). The committee should be chaired by a physician or nurse with a special interest and experience in infectious diseases whenever possible. In addition, a staff person, usually a nurse, should be designated as the infection control practitioner. A defined proportion of this individual's time (the amount depending on the size of the facility) should be dedicated to surveillance and other infection control activities.

It is beyond the scope of this chapter to discuss all aspects of infection control. The Suggested Readings contain sources of more detailed information about infection control for NHs. In addition, the Appendix contains some examples of specific definitions, policies, and procedures relevant to infections in the NH setting. A few points are worthy of emphasis. Because of the nature of documentation in NH records, the laboratory resources available, and the clinical presentation of infectious diseases already discussed, it is generally not possible to apply standard definitions of infections used in hospitals. Standard definitions recommended by the Centers for Disease Control should be modified for surveillance procedures (see Appendix for examples). Proper techniques to prevent the spread of infections in an institutional setting are critical. In addition to universal precautions, these techniques include handwashing, aseptic techniques for handling sterile equipment (such as catheters), proper care and cleaning of equipment (such as respiratory equipment and whirlpools), explicit procedures for isolation and waste disposal when contagious diseases are identified (e.g., infectious diarrhea, herpes zoster, hepatitis, tuberculosis), thorough laundering of bed linens soiled by incontinent urine or stool, and proper pest control whenever this is a problem.

Screening and preventive activities are essential components of any infection control program. These activities should extend to staff as well as residents. As noted earlier in this chapter, NH residents should receive proper immunizations to help prevent influenza, pneumococcal pneumonia,

Table 17-9 Key aspects of an infection control program in a nursing home[a]

The goal of the infection control program is to provide a sanitary and comfortable environment and to prevent the development and transmission of infections whenever possible

The facility should have an infection control committee
    Members should include representatives of multiple departments, including nursing, medical, dietary, pharmacy, housekeeping, maintenance, and laundry
    Meetings should be quarterly, with minutes kept for each meeting

Written policies and procedures should be developed for the prevention and control of infections and the maintenance of a sanitary environment, including
    Definitions of various infections
    Reporting procedures
    Universal precautions
    Handwashing and aseptic techniques
    Isolation and disposal procedures
    Immunizations
        Influenza
        Pneumococcal infection
        Tetanus
    Tuberculosis
        Skin testing of residents and staff
        Prophylaxis
    Employee health
        Preemployment immunizations and infectious disease history
        Tuberculosis skin testing
        Screening of dietary personnel
    Processing laundry
    Pest control
    Cleaning and care of equipment

Surveillance should be ongoing
    Regular reporting of all infections
    Collation of culture results
    Review of susceptibility patterns
    Review of antibiotic usage
    Quarterly summary to identify trends
    Potential epidemics should be continuously considered
        Respiratory illness
        Gastroenteritis
        Skin and soft tissue infections

[a] The Appendix contains several examples of materials useful for infection control.

and tetanus. All residents should be tested for tuberculosis and an appropriate policy of prophylaxis for skin-test converters should be developed (see Appendix for an example). Employees should also be screened for tuberculosis, and their immunization and infectious disease histories should be recorded at the time of employment. Proper screening of dietary personnel is especially important because of their potential to spread contagious diseases. Employees should also be encouraged to report any potentially contagious conditions, such as diarrhea and respiratory illness, and not to report to work during such episodes.

Although standard software packages are available for infection control, any simple spreadsheet program can be utilized to enter and analyze the incidence of various infections. An example of a reporting format is included in the Appendix. In addition to the incidence of infections, ongoing surveillance should include examination of culture results, sensitivity patterns of cultured organisms, and antibiotic usage. In many areas, clinical laboratories and pharmacies can provide valuable assistance in accumulating these data. Surveillance results are generally examined quarterly to identify trends and potential problem areas; it is extremely important, however, to identify potential outbreaks early in their course so that appropriate measures can be instituted to manage the outbreak and prevent an epidemic in the facility.

SUGGESTED READINGS

Centers for Disease Control: Recommendations of the Immunization Practices Advisory Committee, Centers for Disease Control: Prevention and control of influenza. *J Am Geriatr Soc* 36:963–968, 1988.

Crossley K, Henry K, Irvine P, and Willenbring K: Antibiotic use in nursing homes: Prevalence, cost and utilization review. *Bull NY Acad Med* 63:510–518, 1987.

Crossley KB, Irvine P, Kaszar DJ, and Loewenson RB: Infection control practices in Minnesota nursing homes. *JAMA* 254:2918–2921, 1985.

Finucane T: The American Geriatrics Society statement of two-step PPD testing for nursing home patients on admission. *J Am Geriatr Soc* 33:77–78, 1988.

Irvine PW, Van Buren N, and Crossley K: Causes for hospitalization of nursing home residents: The role of infection. *J Am Geriatr Soc* 32:103–107, 1984.

Patriarca PA, Arden NH, Koplan JP, and Goodman RA: Prevention and control of type A influenza infections in nursing homes. *Ann Intern Med* 107:732–740, 1987.

Smith PW (ed): *Infection Control in Long Term Care Facilities.* New York, Wiley, 1984.

Stead WW, and To T: The significance of the tuberculin skin test in elderly persons. *Ann Intern Med* 107:837–842, 1987.

Stead WW, To T, Harrison RW, and Abraham JH: Benefit-risk considerations in preventive treatment for tuberculosis in elderly persons. *Ann Intern Med* 107:843–845, 1987.

Thomas DR, Bennett RG, Laughon BE, et al: Postantibiotic colonization with *Clostridium difficile* in nursing home patients. *J Am Geriatr Soc* 38:415–420, 1990.

Verghese A and Berk LS (eds): *Infections in Nursing Homes and Long Term Care Facilities.* Karger, New York, 1990.

Yoshikawa TT: Pneumonia, UTI, and decubiti in the nursing home: Optimal management. *Geriatrics* 44:32–43, 1989.

Yoshikawa TT and Norman DC: *Aging and Clinical Practices: Infectious Diseases—Diagnosis and Treatment.* New York, Igaku-Shoin, 1987.

Zimmer JG, Bentley DW, Valenti WM, and Watson NM: Systemic antibiotic use in nursing homes: A quality assessment. *J Am Geriatr Soc* 34:703–710, 1986.

EIGHTEEN

CHRONIC NEUROLOGICAL CONDITIONS

STROKE

The most common chronic neurological condition in nursing homes (NHs) is cerebrovascular accident or stroke. Stroke often results in major impairment of quality of life. Stroke can result not only in impaired ability to walk and to utilize an upper limb but also in the inabilities to communicate, think, or see adequately. The different causes of stroke are outlined in Table 18-1. Recognition of these is important to allow both the diagnosis of treatable causes of stroke and intervention to prevent a recurrence of stroke.

When a stroke victim is admitted to the NH, the physician should make sure that the resident has had a platelet count, Westergren sedimentation rate (looking for vasculitis), CT scan (to distinguish hemorrhage from ischemia), and electrocardiogram. Where embolus is suspected, echocardiography can be performed. A two-dimensional echocardiogram is, however, only 50 percent sensitive for mural thrombi in individuals with atrial fibrillation, and it provides poor images of mechanical prosthetic valves. It should be recognized that the presence of mural thrombi does not predict embolic risk in dilated cardiomyopathy. The presence of cardiolipin antibodies may indicate vasculitis, but aging per se may also increase titers of these antibodies.

Up to 25 percent of residents will have another stroke within a year of their first one. The risk of another stroke is increased in residents with any of the conditions outlined in Table 18-2. Control of blood glucose levels to under 150 mg/dl in residents with diabetes mellitus may not only prevent the recurrence of stroke but also result in improved rehabilitation potential.

Table 18-1   Causes of stroke

Ischemic (82%)
  Thrombosis
  Embolus
    cardiac
    carotid
  Hypotension
    myocardial infarction
    other
  Vasculitis
Hemorrhage (18%)
  Intracerebral
    hypertension
    A-V malformations
    metastatic tumors
    iatrogenic coagulopathy
    congophilic angiopathy
  Subarachnoid
    Berry aneurysms
    A-V malformations
    coagulopathies
    infectious endocarditis
    vasculitis
    idiopathic hemorrhage

Diastolic blood pressure should be kept to between 90 to 95 mmHg to prevent recurrence of stroke .

The use of anticoagulation or antiplatelet therapy in ischemic stroke depends on the general health status of the resident and the history of previous bleeds. In the short-term stayer admitted for acute rehabilitation, low-dose aspirin should be used on a daily basis. Anticoagulation with coumadin, making sure that the prothrombin time is maintained at 13 to 15 s (i.e., just above control levels), should be used for cariogenic embolism and possibly also for artery-to-artery thromboembolism. This appears to give maximum protection with minimum bleeding. Our experience has suggested that in the very frail resident, anticoagulation greatly increases the potential

Table 18-2   Factors predisposing to stroke

Cardiac disease
Hypertension
Diabetes mellitus
Peripheral vascular disease
Cervical bruit
Transient ischemic attacks

---

of gastrointestinal bleeding. Thus, decisions on the use of aspirin or antico-agulation must be individualized. The combination of low-dose aspirin and a nonsteroidal anti-inflammatory agent makes little sense and may potenti-ate bleeding. Some of the general principles of rehabilitation are discussed in Chap. 22. The success of rehabilitation in residents with stroke is improved by early intervention (within 48 h). In addition, it is important to ensure that there is no hiatus in rehabilitation when transfer to the NH occurs. Range-of-motion exercises are extremely important, and each affected extremity should be moved through the complete range of motion with five repetitions twice daily. Stretching should be done with care and overstretching avoided. Foot boards and splints for wrists and fingers can help to maintain these parts of the extremities in a functional position. Flac-cid extremities should be kept in the neutral position and the shoulder should be abducted for some period each day. Hands should be elevated if edema is present. Subluxation of the shoulder can occur, and use of a sling, pillow, or wheelchair board may be necessary in order to prevent its occur-rence in a flaccid limb. A painful shoulder may respond to hot packs or ultrasound, though local or systemic corticosteroids may be necessary. Spasticity can be treated by diazepam (though with careful dosing in older individuals) or by baclofen. Biofeedback may also help. Judicious use of adaptive devices may result in major functional improvement. Residents should be taught how to use paralyzed extremities in order to passively assist in activities of daily living.

For mobility, the resident must regain balance. Standing in parallel bars is helpful in this regard. Most residents with stroke will require a hemiwalker or quad cane to allow mobility in the early phase after a stroke. Braces too can play an important part in allowing full mobility. Therapy focusing on completing tasks necessary for dressing and grooming is also critical. In many NHs, the failure of nursing staff to be prepared to wait a sufficient period of time for the resident to complete a task is a major hindrance to rehabilitation. It can take a resident with a stroke up to 2 h to complete bathing, brushing teeth, combing hair, shaving, and dressing. With patience, this time can be reduced within 1 to 2 months to less than a half hour.

Residents with nondominant frontoparietal infarcts often have hemine-glect. This can cause them to bump into objects on the neglected side and fail to be able to read half of a page. Such residents often have problems not only in dressing but also in shaving on the affected side. Figure 18-1 shows an example of a drawing made by a resident with hemineglect.

Problems with speech are common following stroke. Dysarthria (diffi-culty in pronouncing words) can be due to involvement of either the periph-eral or central nervous system. Involvement of Wernicke's area (anterior lesions) leads to a fluent speech defect that often includes "nonsense" words. These residents also tend to find word or sentence substitutions for the word they wish to use and can have impaired understanding of verbal

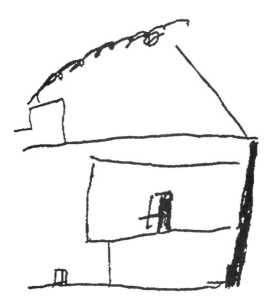

Figure 18-1 Picture of a house drawn by a man with a severe left hemineglect.

commands. Involvement of Broca's area, on the other hand, leads to a "non-fluent" speech (expressive aphasia). The resident may be able to pronounce the nouns and verbs but leaves out the in-between words. Aphasia following stroke can take up to a year to resolve maximally. All residents with speech problems can benefit from a consultation with a speech pathologist. Residents with speech defects should be formed into groups to facilitate communication and social support.

Residents with lesions in the supplementary motor area supplied by the anterior cerebral artery may develop impairment of carrying out automatic movements such as those used for brushing their teeth, despite having the necessary motor function to carry out the task. Such residents require painstaking retraining to reestablish the necessary motor patterns.

Approximately one-third of residents will develop a major depressive episode within 2 years of a stroke. Residents should be screened for depression at 3-monthly intervals following a stroke. Stroke may also result in a reduced attention span and cognitive dysfunction. Emotional lability and inappropriate emotional responses are also seen in residents who have had strokes.

The resident who has had a stroke requires special attention to a number of syndromes. Lack of awareness of the syndromes associated with stroke can cause frustration for both NH residents and staff. Table 18-3 summarizes the common conditions associated with stroke and some of the available management approaches. It is important to involve the resident's

Table 18-3   Common syndromes associated with stroke and approaches to their management

Syndrome	Management
Painful shoulder	Hot packs or ultrasound
Hemineglect	Occupational therapy concentrating on neglected side
Speech problems dysarthria aphasia	Speech pathologist Communication groups
Impairment of automatic movements	Recognition and retraining
Dysphagia	Speech pathologist Special foods Enteral tube feeding if necessary
Spasticity/cramping	Baclofen Diazepam (low-dose) Biofeedback
Depression	Low-dose antidepressant Group therapy
Reduced attention span	Limited activity sessions
Cognitive problems	Memory aids Memory retraining
Emotional lability	Staff awareness that this is related to stroke
Incontinence	Frequent toileting Exclude urinary retention, urinary tract infection Consider pharmacologic treatment for urge incontinence (see Chap. 13)
Shoulder subluxation	Sling may help

family members in the understanding of the various syndromes associated with stroke. Involvement in family counseling may be necessary to allow family members to deal with their own psychological stress associated with a stroke occurring in a family member.

PARKINSON'S DISEASE

Parkinson's disease occurs in 1 percent of persons over the age of 65. Parkinson's disease is characterized by tremor, difficulty in initiating movement (akinesia), and slowness in movement (bradykinesia). Cognitive impairment can occur in up to 20 percent of residents with Parkinson's disease, and depression can be present in up to 40 percent. Visual hallucinations and illusions can also occur, sometimes as a result of antiparkinsonian medication.

Several complications of immobility are common in residents with Parkinson's disease. Ankle and pedal edema can be limited by increased exercise of the lower extremities. Incontinence, usually of the urge type, can be managed behaviorally and/or pharmacologically (see Chap. 13). Constipation is related to decreased movement, inability to develop adequate abdominal pressure when straining at stool, and decreased bowel mobility (due to both the disease and its therapy). Thus, residents with parkinsonism should be on some type of bowel regimen that includes stool softeners and regular toileting after breakfast in order to "train" the bowel habit and prevent fecal impaction. Orthostatic hypotension can be particularly troublesome in residents with Parkinson's disease (see Chap. 19).

Weight loss is common in Parkinson's residents. This may be associated with difficulties in swallowing, particularly when the head can no longer be maintained in an erect position. It is often associated with sialorrhea. The major cause of weight loss in many parkinsonian residents, however, is the energy expended by the incessant tremors at rest.

Residents with Parkinson's disease often show poor motivation to maintain an exercise program. Group sessions may help provide peer pressure to keep residents in such a program. Exercise sessions for these residents should be limited to 10 min at a time and repeated three to four times per day. Full range-of-motion exercises for those muscle groups necessary for activities of daily living should be carried out at each session. Exercises to prevent stooped posture and leaning to one side are important. Leg-raising exercises may reduce the accumulation of edema. Placing objects on the ground and making the resident step over them can improve gait speed and possibly help prevent tripping due to the typical shuffling gait. The resident with Parkinson's disease and poor balance requires a wheeled walker. Nonwheeled walkers can cause these residents to fall backwards when they lift the walker off the ground.

The drug therapy of choice for Parkinson's disease is a combination of L-dopa and carbidopa (Sinemet). Sinemet should be taken 30 to 60 min before meals to enhance absorption. However, if nausea develops, it may have to given with meals. Excessive protein intake should be avoided in residents with Parkinson's disease because it may interfere with the brain's uptake of L-dopa. Some residents develop abnormal movements 3 h after taking Sinemet. They may benefit from the addition of a direct dopamine agonist such as bromocriptine (Parlodel) or pergolide (Permax). Usually the dose of Sinemet is not reduced when these agents are added. Deprenyl, a monoamine B oxidase inhibitor, may enhance the effect of Sinemet by 20 percent to 30 percent, improve the longevity of residents with Parkinson's disease, and enhance mental functioning. Anticholinergic drugs are usually not useful in NH residents because of side effects. Anticholinergic drugs should be tapered slowly, as they may otherwise result in a withdrawal syndrome consisting of 2 to 3 days of worsening parkinsonian symptoms. Amantadine at 200 mg/day or less may result in some improvement. Side effects include hallucinations, purple mottling of the skin, and ankle swelling. In residents with end-stage Parkinson's disease, tapering of drugs can be tried, but this needs careful monitoring for increased rigidity and immobility, which can, in turn, lead to complications such as pressure sores and aspiration.

Table 18-4 summarizes the major modalities useful for management of the resident with Parkinson's disease.

TREMORS

A number of drugs may cause tremors in NH residents. These include anticholinergic drugs, neuroleptics, lithium, adrenergic agonists, theophylline, corticosteroids, and thyroid hormone (given in excessive amounts for replacement). Pathological causes of tremor include anxiety, hyperthyroidism, cerebellar disease, Parkinson's disease, alcoholism, and alcohol withdrawal. Essential tremor is extremely common with advancing age. Beta blockers (e.g., propranolol 240 mg/day) are partially effective at controlling tremors, but in older individuals they may cause serious side effects (e.g.,

Table 18-4 Modalities useful to manage residents with Parkinson's disease

---

Leg exercises four times per day for 3 to 5 min at a time if edema is present.
Range-of-motion exercises three to four times per day for 5 min at a time. Usually better
  compliance if carried out in groups.
Exercises to correct stooped posture and leaning to one side.
Regular walking using a wheeled walker.
Training to step over real or imaginary objects to help initiate gait.
Support the neck muscles with exercise; a soft cervical collar may be helpful.
Limit protein intake to 40 g per 70 kg of body weight in diet. (Resident may need increased
  calories because of energy expenditure due to tremors.)
Adequate fluid intake.
Train resident to push on abdomen when straining at stool. (For this purpose a soft cushion
  pushed into the abdomen may help.)
Screen regularly for depression and treat when present.
Assess and treat incontinence when present.
Medications
  Avoid anticholinergics in the older NH resident.
  Sinemet (L-dopa and carbidopa)
  Dopamine agonists: bromocriptine, pergolide
  Deprenyl (monamine oxidase B inhibitor)—expensive, but may improve mental function
  Amantadine, low-dose (100–200 mg/day)

---

heart failure, bronchospasm, fatigue, limb "heaviness"). Primidone (start at 62.5 mg and increase to 250 mg three times per day over 3 weeks) has been suggested, but its severe side effects, including vomiting, ataxia, and headache, make it a poor choice for NH residents. Drug therapy of essential tremor in NH residents is justified only when the tremor interferes substantially with the resident's ability to carry out activities of daily living.

EPILEPTIC SEIZURES

There is little information on the management of epileptic seizures in NH residents. New-onset seizures in any person over age 60 should be investigated to rule out the possibility of tumor or subdural hematoma. Many residents are placed on antiepileptic therapy at the time of a single seizure associated with a stroke, hypoxia, or neurosurgery. Many of these residents do not need this treatment long-term and the medication can be discontinued 6 weeks following the event with no adverse consequences. There are also many NH residents who are on anticonvulsant medication for unclear reasons. In view of the severity of side effects of these medications, these residents are deserving of a trial off medication. This is also true of residents who have had a single seizure at some time in the past. Of individuals with a single seizure, 60 percent will not have a repeat seizure within 5 years.

MULTIPLE SCLEROSIS

Multiple sclerosis is a common cause of institutionalization, especially among those suffering from the chronic progressive form. Institutionalized residents with multiple sclerosis are often much younger than the majority of residents in a NH. Symptoms are commonly worse in the afternoon and when the temperature increases. Keeping the temperature low, use of swimming therapy and vigorous therapy of elevated temperatures with acetaminophen and external cooling may all play a useful role in limiting symptomatology.

Infections may trigger an exacerbation of the underlying disease. Even in young persons with multiple sclerosis, infections often present atypically either with delirium or a failure to see the expected fever normally associated with infection. Any NH resident with multiple sclerosis who has a change in functional mental status, even if it is subtle, should be evaluated to exclude a treatable infection.

Spasticity is a common problem in advanced multiple sclerosis and may respond to baclofen or diazepam in addition to range-of-motion exercises. Incontinence is also very common and is generally associated with detrusor hyperreflexia. Individuals with multiple sclerosis can, however, develop a wide variety of lower urinary tract dysfunctions, including detrusor-sphincter dyssynergy and acontractile bladder. For these reasons, residents with multiple sclerosis who develop new or worsened incontinence should have a careful urodynamic evaluation (see Chap. 13).

Many residents with multiple sclerosis also develop some degree of cognitive dysfunction. Depression is very common and requires active therapy. Sexual dysfunction may be a major concern among younger males with multiple sclerosis. Vacuum tumescence devices or penile prostheses may be a reasonable therapy for some of these residents. Physicians should be supportive of residents with multiple sclerosis and be optimistic concerning the possibility of improved treatments. The length of exacerbations may be shortened by treatment with methylprednisone or ACTH. Experimental therapies include cyclosporine, cyclophosphamide, and plasmapheresis.

HUNTINGTON'S CHOREA

Huntington's chorea is a dominant disorder associated with a gene on chromosome four. It involves degeneration of the caudate nucleus and the putamen of the basal ganglia and is associated with a selective loss of γ-aminobutyric acid.

Huntington's chorea presents in the fourth or fifth decades of life, and those afflicted generally develop disabilities severe enough to need NH care at a young age. Residents with this disorder will typically survive 10 to 20 years in the NH. These residents have a cognitive disturbance predominantly involving the ability to carry out complex processes and to maintain good judgment. The ability to maintain long-term memory and speech functions often remains intact until late in the disorder. The major debilitating feature is the abnormal choreiform movements that involve both upper and lower limbs, the face, and the trunk. These movements often respond well to baclofen. However, as the disease progresses, extremely high doses of neuroleptics may be necessary to maintain the abnormal movements at an acceptable level—one that allows the staff to care for the resident. Abnormal movements are worse when the resident is disturbed and flailing motions can injure staff. Staff need to be warned that the resident understands what is being said. It is important to provide support for the resident's family and provide sensory stimulation for the resident.

MEIGS SYNDROME (BLEPHAROSPASM AND OROFACIAL CERVICAL DYSTONIA)

This disorder usually presents after the age of 60. It consists of blepharospasm, abnormal movements of the mouth, clenching of the jaw, lip smacking, and occasionally spasms of cervical muscles. Dysarthria and swallowing difficulties may also be associated with this syndrome. Meigs syndrome may be confused with tardive kinesia secondary to neuroleptic use. When blepharospasm interferes with function, it may be controlled by injecting botulinum toxin into the eyelid muscle or by surgery.

SUGGESTED READINGS

Stroke

Kelly JF and Winograd CH: A functional approach to stroke management in elderly patients. *J Am Geriatr Soc* 33:48–60, 1985.
Nadeau SE: Stroke. *Med Clin North Am* 73:1351, 1989.
Sarno MT: Communication disorders in the elderly, in T. Franklin Williams (ed): *Rehabilitation in the Aging.* New York, Raven Press, 1984, p. 161.
Yibson CJ, Caplan BM: Rehabilitation of the patient with stroke, in T. Franklin Williams (ed): *Rehabilitation in the Aging.* New York, Raven Press, 1984, p. 165.

Parkinson's Disease

Cote LJ, Henly M: Parkinson's disease, in Hazzard WR, Andres R, Bresman EL, Blass JP (eds): *Principles of Geriatric Medicine and Gerontology.* New York, McGraw-Hill, 1990, p. 954.

Tremor

Cleaves L, Findley LJ: Tremors. *Med Clin North Am* 73:1307, 1989.

Multiple Sclerosis

Rosenthal MJ: Chronic care issues in multiple sclerosis. *Geriatric Med Today* 7(4):73, 1988.

NINETEEN

SELECTED MEDICAL CONDITIONS

The purpose of this chapter is to briefly review the management of several common clinical disorders in nursing home (NH) residents that are not covered in other chapters of this text. We do not mean to imply that conditions discussed are unimportant; we have tried to focus on conditions that are most common and treatable in the NH population.

ANEMIA

Anemia (a hemoglobin below 12 g/dl) is present in 30 percent to 50 percent of institutionalized older persons. In approximately 30 percent of these individuals, the anemia will be unrecognized; in another 30 percent, it will be recognized but not treated. The causes of anemia are outlined in Fig. 19-1. In a NH population, the major cause of a hemoglobin between 10 and 12 g/dl will be an anemia of chronic disease and/or malnutrition. It is important, however, to distinguish the treatable anemias from the anemia of chronic disease. It is also critical to recognize that NH residents with acute blood loss or dehydration may have anemia in the presence of a normal hemoglobin.

The first step in diagnosing the cause of an anemia is to obtain a reticulocyte count and calculate the reticulocyte index (Table 19-1). If the reticulocyte index is greater than 3 percent, the anemia is due either to hemorrhage or hemolysis. In these residents the stool should be checked for blood and medication lists reviewed to exclude drugs (e.g., methyldopa) that may cause an autoimmune hemolytic anemia or gastrointestinal bleeding (e.g.,

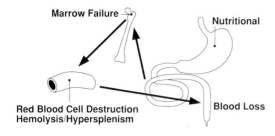

Figure 19-1 Basic causes of anemia in the nursing home population.

nonsteroidal anti-inflammatory agents). If blood loss cannot be identified, the next step is to obtain a Coombs test to rule out the presence of auto-immune hemolytic anemia, which is the most common cause of hemolysis in older persons. Table 19-2 lists the most common causes and the treatment options for autoimmune hemolytic anemia. Microangiopathic hemolytic anemias associated with neoplasms or severe infection are not uncommon in older individuals. Diagnosis is made by finding decreased platelet levels, a prolonged partial thromboplastin time, hemosiderin in the urine, and red cell fragments on the smear.

When the reticulocyte index is less than 3 percent, the next step is to determine whether the red cell indices are micro-, normo-, or macrocytic. Normocytic indices may suggest a combination of vitamin B_{12} and iron deficiency. Currently it is recommended that these residents undergo further investigation only when the hemoglobin is below 11 g/dl. Multiple myeloma can occur in this population. If it is suspected, a serum and urine protein electrophoresis should be obtained. Residents with microcytic anemia should undergo iron studies, including iron transferrin saturation, total iron binding capacity, and ferritin (Table 19-3). This should allow the diagnosis of either iron-deficiency anemia or the anemia of chronic disease to be made. When the results are equivocal, a bone marrow biopsy may be necessary to make the final diagnosis. Iron-deficiency anemia is often over-treated. To correct an iron-deficiency anemia, approximately 20 mg of iron

Table 19-1   Reticulocyte index (RI)

$$RI = \text{reticulocyte count} \times \frac{\text{resident's HCT}}{\text{normal HCT}} \times \frac{1}{\text{maturation time}}$$

Maturation time	HCT, %
1.0	45
1.5	35
2.0	25
2.5	15

Note: HCT = hematocrit. Normal RI is 73 percent.

Table 19-2   Common causes and treatment of hemolytic anemias in nursing home residents

Causes
   Mycoplasma infections (bilateral infiltrate on chest x-ray)
   Chronic lymphocytic leukemia
   Non-Hodgkin's lymphoma
   Collagen vascular disorders

Drugs
   Methyldopa
   Quinine
   Quinidine
   Salicylates
   Penicillins

Treatment
   Ig/G red cell antibodies: steroids and possibly splenectomy
   Ig/M red cell antibodies: refractory to treatment

per day for 7 weeks is needed, and 300 mg of iron sulfate contains 60 mg of iron (325 mg of iron gluconate contains 37 mg of iron). Thus one tablet of iron a day is sufficient to correct the anemia. A reticulocyte count should be obtained after 1 week of therapy with iron to check for an adequate response. Residents with a normal transferrin saturation (>20 percent) should be worked up for hypothyroidism, Addison's disease, protein-energy malnutrition, or a hemoglobinopathy. When iron deficiency is diagnosed, the resident should have at least three stools collected for occult blood. If any of these stools contains blood, both a lower and upper GI endoscopy should be performed (Table 19-4).

   Sideroblastic anemia is a disorder of older persons. Iron is deposited in the mitochondria of normoblasts, resulting in the presence of ringed sidero-

Table 19-3   Differential diagnosis of iron-associated anemias

	Iron deficiency	Anemia of chronic disease	Sideroblastic anemia
Iron	Low	Low	High
Transferrin saturation	$<20\%$	$<20\%$	High
Ferritin	<20 ng/dl	<100 ng/dl	20–100 ng/dl
Total iron-binding capacity	>375	<250	250–375
Bone marrow	Absent iron stores	Normal or increased iron stores	Ringed sideroblasts

blasts in the marrow. The peripheral smear is dimorphic, with both macrocytes and normocytes being present and approximately 50 percent of them showing hypochromia. The reticulocyte count may be normal or increased and there is often a mild neutropenia. Clinically, in addition to symptoms of anemia, residents may have a lemon-yellow hue to their skin, hepatosplenomegaly, and anorexia. Sideroblastic anemia occurs more commonly in residents with diabetes mellitus or congestive heart failure. Residents with sideroblastic anemia have an increase in serum iron and transferrin saturation, normal total iron binding capacity and ferritin, and an increased free erythrocyte protoporphyrin. Most sideroblastic anemias are idiopathic, and approximately 10 percent of these will respond to 200 mg of pyridoxine three times per day. Sideroblastic anemias are occasionally associated with drug administration (e.g., isoniazid, pyrazinamide, chloramphenicol) or with lead toxicity or chronic neoplastic or inflammatory disease. Drug-associated sideroblastic anemia may also respond to pyridoxine. Residents with sideroblastic anemias are at increased risk for developing acute myelogenous leukemia.

Macrocytic anemias are due either to vitamin B_{12} or folate deficiency. Pernicious anemia occurs in 3 percent of females and 1 percent of males

Table 19-4 Causes of anemias associated with low serum iron in older subjects

Blood loss
  Gastrointestinal
    Gastritis
    Esophagitis
    Ulcers
    Neoplasia
    Angiodysplasia
    Diverticular disease
    Aspirin and nonsteroidal anti-inflammatory drugs
    Alcohol
  Epistaxis
  Hemoptysis
  Hematuria
  Hematoma (especially after hip fracture)
  Coagulation disorders
  Coumadin

Anemia of chronic disease
  Infections
  Neoplasia
  Pressure sores
  Collagen vascular disorders
  Rheumatoid arthritis
  Polymyalgia rheumatica

over the age of 60. It is associated with a lack of intrinsic factor, which binds the vitamin B_{12} to allow its absorption in the small intestine. A blood smear demonstrates macrocytosis, pancytopenia, and hypersegmented polymorphonuclear leukocytes. The resident may have increased indirect circulating bilirubin levels and an increased lactic dehydrogenase. Besides anemia, residents with pernicious anemia may have dementia, ataxia, posterior column abnormalities (loss of position sense), and glossitis. Residents with pernicious anemia have increased risk of developing hypothyroidism, diabetes mellitus, Addison's disease, and nontropical sprue. Vitamin B_{12} deficiency may also be due to ileal disease or to protein-energy malnutrition. Serum vitamin B_{12} levels below 200 pg/ml are considered low. Residents with values between 200 to 400 pg/ml should have their serum B_{12} level measured at 6-monthly intervals. The definitive diagnosis of vitamin B_{12} deficiency can be made by demonstrating deficient vitamin B_{12} absorption with the Part I Schilling test; the diagnosis of pernicious anemia is made by demonstrating that this malabsorption corrects when radiolabeled vitamin B_{12} is coadministered with intrinsic factor. Treatment of vitamin B_{12} deficiency is by biweekly injection of 100 μg of vitamin B_{12} until the anemia corrects and then monthly injections. For Medicaid reimbursement, the full diagnostic workup generally must be completed.

Some elderly NH residents develop severe anemia due to bone marrow failure. This is generally associated with one or more chronic diseases. In some cases, the marrow contains an increased number of blast cells, but not enough to make the diagnosis of leukemia. These residents may require repeated blood transfusions to maintain their hemoglobin values above the range of 7 to 8 g/dl.

CARDIOVASCULAR DISORDERS

Cardiovascular disease is the major cause of death in older persons, accounting for nearly half the deaths in those over age 75. Digoxin, diuretics, beta blockers, calcium channel blockers, nitrates, and angiotensin converting enzyme inhibitors are among the most common drugs utilized in the NH. A full discussion of cardiovascular disease is beyond the scope of this chapter. Only a few points of special importance to NH residents will be highlighted.

Myocardial Infarction

In older persons, myocardial infarction often presents without chest pain. The new onset of dyspnea is the most common presentation of myocardial infarction in institutionalized elderly individuals. Myocardial infarction should also be suspected in any NH resident who has acute onset of confusion. The incidence of syncope as a presentation of myocardial infarction doubles in institutionalized individuals. Syncopal episodes should, therefore, arouse suspicion of an acute myocardial infarction in a NH resident.

Cardiac Amyloidosis

Cardiac amyloidosis is a disease of older persons. It may cause heart failure and angina (when the coronary arteries are involved). Diagnosis should be considered when the resident has a restrictive cardiomyopathy with an electrocardiogram demonstrating low-voltage left axis deviation and a pseudoinfarct pattern (decreased R waves in the precordium and Q waves anteriorly). An echocardiogram demonstrates "granular speckling." Residents with amyloidosis may be especially likely to develop digoxin toxicity.

Digoxin Use and Arrhythmia Treatment

Digoxin is a dangerous drug in older persons and it is greatly overused in NHs. Many residents receive digoxin because of lower extremity edema, which is due to stasis, varicose veins, and decreased serum albumin rather than heart failure. Digoxin can cause protein-energy malnutrition in as many as 25 percent of older residents receiving this drug, because it causes anorexia. Digoxin can also produce dementia and depression in a substantial number of residents. In NH residents, digoxin use should probably be limited to those with atrial fibrillation and a ventricular response greater than 100 beats per minute or a history of other recurrent symptomatic supraventricular arrhythmias. Digoxin can, however, precipitate heart block in individuals with sick sinus syndrome, and 24-h monitoring should be used to exclude this diagnosis. Contraindications to digoxin include idiopathic hypertrophic subaortic stenosis and ventricular diastolic dysfunction, which are being increasingly recognized in the geriatric population. These conditions are better treated with calcium channel blockers.

Management of ventricular arrhythmias should initially ensure that potassium and magnesium values are normal. The incidence of ventricular arrhythmias, even among elderly individuals without symptomatic cardiac disease, is high. No studies have documented improved outcomes resulting from treatment of these arrhythmias, and antiarrhythmic drugs have numerous serious side effects. In most cases, the advantages of drug therapy for ventricular arrhythmias is offset by these side effects. Therefore we rarely use antiarrhythmics in NH residents unless a resident is bothered by palpitations or treatment is strongly recommended by a cardiologist. Automatic implantable defibrillation systems are available for recurrent ventricular tachycardia or fibrillation, but they are extremely expensive.

Hypertrophic Obstructive Cardiomyopathy

The diagnosis of hypertrophic obstructive cardiomyopathy should be considered in residents with heart failure, angina, and syncope. Echocardiography demonstrates septal hypertrophy. Like heart failure associated with ventricular diastolic dysfunction, this disorder responds specifically to beta blockers and calcium channel blockers. Digoxin is not indicated for congestive heart failure associated with hypertrophic obstructive cardiomyopathy and may exacerbate this condition.

Aortic Stenosis

Aortic stenosis is common in the very old and may progress to cause syncope, heart failure, and angina. NH residents who are suspected of having aortic stenosis and who are candidates for surgical interventions should be followed with periodic (6 to 12 months) echocardiography with Doppler flow to detect progression. Clinically, aortic stenosis of increasing severity presents with dyspnea. This worsening dyspnea must be distinguished from that due to coexistent chronic obstructive pulmonary disease. Properly timed valve replacement surgery can preserve several years of life. For some residents who are too ill to undergo valve replacement, balloon valvuloplasty may provide at least temporary relief of disabling symptoms. Residents with aortic stenosis are also at greater risk of having gastrointestinal bleeds from angiodysplasia.

Hypertension

Hypertension is present in approximately 40 percent of individuals over age 65. The European multicenter study has demonstrated that there is a U-shaped mortality curve associated with diastolic blood pressure, with blood pressures below 90 mmHg being as liable to result in death as those over 100 mmHg. For this reason, it is recommended that blood pressure control in NH residents aims at a diastolic blood pressure between 90 and 95 mmHg. Where possible, monotherapy should be attempted. Costs suggest that thiazide diuretics are the drugs of choice to treat hypertension in this population. The dose should be limited to 25 mg daily of hydrochlorothiazide. Only when potassium depletion is demonstrated should potassium supplementation or triamterene be added. Hyperkalemia is more likely than hypokalemia to cause sudden death without prior symptoms. Triamterene can be associated with triamterene kidney stones, particularly in dehydrated residents. If a thiazide diuretic fails, an angiotensin converting enzyme inhibitor as monotherapy can be tried. New central acting agents (e.g., quanfacine HCl) may also be effective. Many NH residents have concomitant disorders that may guide drug therapy (e.g., a calcium channel blocker may be appropriate in residents with angina and hypertension, and nitrates may be appropriate in those with concomitant heart failure). Classical step therapy can be tried if these approaches fail. Weight loss in NHs often results in improvement in the resident's blood pressure; hence the need for antihypertensive medications should be regularly reevaluated. In addition, the possibility that the resident is suffering from side effects of antihypertensive therapy should regularly be reviewed. While hypertension is often responsive to low-salt diets in NH residents, we do not recommend this approach routinely because it may unnecessarily interfere with the resident's dietary satisfaction and result in the potential for producing protein-energy malnutrition through dietary manipulation.

Pseudohypertension

A small percentage of older persons (less than 5 percent) have "pseudohypertension" due to rigidity of the arteries. This should be suspected when the radial artery is palpable while the blood pressure cuff is inflated above the systolic blood pressure. Care should be taken not to overtreat if such an individual is to be considered for antihypertensive therapy.

Meal-Associated Hypotension

A number of older NH residents have been found to have declines in mean blood pressure of between 5 to 20 mmHg following ingestion of a meal. The blood pressure drop may last for 2 to 3 h. This drop in blood pressure has been correlated with an increased prevalence of falls following a meal in the NH population. The fall in blood pressure is predominantly related to the carbohydrate content of the meal. It can be ameliorated by giving meals with a higher fat content or by giving multiple small meals. A somatostatin analog has been shown experimentally to prevent the meal associated fall in blood pressure and is available in the United States for treatment of acromegaly.

Orthostatic Hypotension

Postural hypotension (a drop of 10 mmHg in systolic blood pressure or 5 mmHg in diastolic blood pressure within 2 min after arising from the recumbent position) has been reported to be present in 8 percent to 11 percent of NH residents. Old age alone is not a sufficient reason for postural hypotension, and the cause of postural hypotension should be documented in all NH residents in whom it is present. The major causes of postural hypotension are outlined in Table 19-5. When a full-blown autonomic neuropathy is sus-

Table 19-5   Causes of postural hypotension

Medications	Autonomic neuropathy
Diuretics	Diabetes mellitus
Antidepressants	Amyloidosis
Neuroleptics	Alcoholism
Antihypertensives	Central nervous system
Antianginals	Parkinson's disease
Antiparkinsonians	Stroke
Anticholinergics	Peripheral nervous
Hypovolemia	Guillain-Barré
Dehydration	Familial dysautonomia (Riley-Day)
Blood loss/anemia	Cardiovascular
Malnutrition	Hypertrophic cardiomyopathy
Prolonged recumbency	Venous insufficiency (varicose veins)
	Baroreceptor destruction/dysfunction
Endocrine	Idiopathic
Adrenal insufficiency	Multisystem atrophy (Shy-Drager)
Hypoaldosteronism	Idiopathic orthostatic hypotension
Pheochromocytoma	

pected, the diagnosis can be confirmed by demonstrating the presence of one or more of the following:

1. Failure of the diastolic blood pressure to increase by 10 mmHg during isometric hand grip
2. The absence of sinus arrhythmia
3. Demonstration that, during Valsalva maneuver, the ratio of the R-R interval during the bradycardia phase to the R-R interval during the tachycardia phase is less than 1.3

The first approach to the management of orthostatic hypotension should be nonpharmacological (Table 19-6). The use of support hose is controversial. If they are to be of any use, support hose must extend to the level of the groin and be put on before the resident gets out of bed. The major pharmacological treatment of postural hypotension is the mineralocorticoid 9-alpha fludrocorticosterone. The starting dose should be 0.1 mg a day, and the maximum dosage should be 1 mg/day. This agent can precipitate hypokalemia, supine hypertension, and congestive heart failure and thus must be used cautiously in residents with cardiovascular disease. Other drugs that may be helpful in treating postural hypotension are listed in Table 19-7. Xamoterol, a beta-1 agonist and beta-2 antagonist, appears to be a useful drug for treating hypotension in residents with cardiac or respiratory disease. In those residents with CNS involvement, desmopression and/or

Table 19-6   Nonpharmacological management of postural hypotension

---

Teach patient to get up slowly
Teach prestanding exercises
Supply bedside urinal/bedpan
Have walker or rail next to bed
Raise head of bed
Ensure adequate fluid intake
Ensure adequate salt intake
Provide support hose (thigh high)
Stop or decrease medication dose of implicated medicines
Treat electrolyte disturbances

---

the somatostatin analog (now experimental) may prove to be useful. Figure 19-2 outlines an approach to the management of orthostatic hypotension.

RHEUMATOLOGICAL CONDITIONS

Table 19-8 lists the major diagnostic criteria for different rheumatological conditions seen in NH residents.

Arthritis is the most prevalent chronic disorder, afflicting almost half the population over 75 years of age. The most common form of arthritis in older individuals is osteoarthritis. The approach to management of this disorder is outlined in Table 19-9. Recent studies have suggested that the more potent nonsteroidal anti-inflammatory agents may accelerate the progression of the disease. For this reason the lowest dose that gives adequate pain relief should be prescribed. While the prostaglandin analog misoprostol has been shown to be protective against nonsteroidal anti-inflammatory drug-induced bleeding, NH residents can rarely tolerate the dosages needed for

Table 19-7   Drugs used to treat postural hypotension

Fludrocortisone (0.1 to 1 mg/day)
Prostaglandin synthetase inhibitors
Somatostatin analog (experimental)
Xamoterol (better than prindolol)
Alpha-adrenergic agonists
Vasopressin
Dehydroergotamine
Caffeine
Dopamine antagonists
Desmopressin

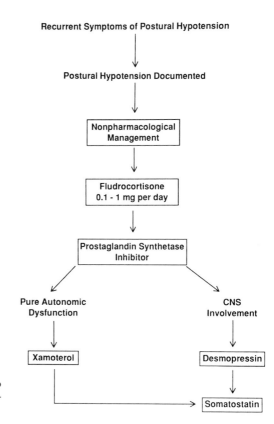

Figure 19-2 Basic approaches to the management of postural hypotension.

Table 19-8 Common manifestations of rheumatological conditions in nursing home residents

	Osteoarthritis	Rheumatoid arthritis	Polymyalgia	Gout	Pseudogout
Onset	Gradual	Gradual	Gradual	Acute	Acute
Early morning symptoms	0	+	±	0	±
Joint pain	+++	+++	+	+++	+++
Joint swelling	++	+++	+	+++	+++
Muscle pain	±	±	+++	0	0
Westegren sedimentation rate	Normal	Elevated	Elevated	Normal	Normal
Rheumatoid factors	0	Positive	Positive	0	0
Synovial fluid crystals	0	0	0	Yellow, needle-shaped, negatively birefringent (monosodium urate)	Weakly positive birefringent rhomboid crystals (calcium pyrophosphate dihydrate crystals)

Note: 0 = none; varying numbers of + related to greater frequency of event.

Table 19-9   Approach to the management of osteoarthritis in nursing home residents

Provide adequate analgesia
  Enteric-coated aspirin
  Nonsteroidal anti-inflammatory agents
  Acetaminophen
  Codeine
Weight reduction if greater than 130% of average body weight
Regular exercise programs
Application of heat to joints, particularly prior to exercise
Use of cane or other walking aides to relieve weight bearing
Consider prosthetic joint replacement
Screen for and treat depression when present

cytoprotection. The common side effects of anti-inflammatory agents are listed in Table 19-10. Systemic steroids have no place in the management of osteoarthritis. Enteric-coated aspirin and ibuprofen are the cheapest anti-inflammatory agents available and are a reasonable choice for initial therapy.

Polymyalgia rheumatica is not rare in older females. Muscle aching, muscle weakness and fatigue are the common features. The Westergren erythrocyte sedimentation rate is greater than 40 mm/h. Treatment is with steroids. Polymyalgia rheumatica may be associated with temporal arteritis, which can cause blindness. Temporal arteritis should be suspected when the resident complains of unilateral headache or visual changes. Diagnosis is made by temporal artery biopsy. If temporal arthritis is suspected, this should be treated as a medical emergency with high-dose steriods.

Soft tissue rheumatism (fibrositis) is associated with aching, stiffness (especially early morning stiffness), fatigue, anorexia, and sleep distur-

Table 19-10   Potential side effects of nonsteroidal anti-inflammatory agents

Gastrointestinal bleeding
Platelet inhibition
Cognitive problems
Depression
Dizziness
Water retention
Hyperkalemia
Acute renal failure
Nausea and vomiting
Hepatotoxicity

bances. Passive range of motion is usually not restricted. There are usually tender areas which, when pressed, reproduce the pain (trigger points). Laboratory tests are all normal. Treatment includes antidepressants, local heat, direct pressure to trigger points, and local anesthetic or steroid injections.

Inflammation of a bursal sac is a common problem in NH residents. Figure 19-3 shows locations of bursal sacs that commonly become inflamed. Bursitis involving the anserine or one of the peripatellar bursae is a common cause of knee pain, which responds to local injection of lidocaine into the bursa. One to four local injections with corticosteroids is generally curative. Trochanteric bursitis may mimic hip pain. The diagnosis is made by eliciting the pain when pressure is applied over the bursa. Again, local injection of lidocaine and a corticosteroid may provide dramatic relief. NH residents are also prone to other disorders, such as bicipital tendinitis (which can occur as a result of pushing the wheels of a wheelchair). It may respond well to local injections.

Another disorder that is relatively common in the NH population is carpal tunnel syndrome. This generally presents as pain and/or paresthesias in the hands and should not be confused with more typical degenerative joint disease. Symptoms often begin with paresthesias at night and a feeling of clumsiness of the hand. The diagnosis can be made clinically by reproducing the symptoms by compressing the median nerve (this can be done by flexing the wrist for a prolonged period) and by documenting neurological deficits in the first four digits. The primary therapy is immobilization with a splint. If this fails and symptoms are disabling and/or weakness develops, surgical relief of pressure on the nerve should be considered.

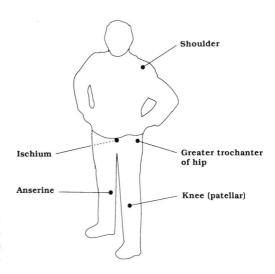

Shoulder

Ischium

Greater trochanter of hip

Anserine

Knee (patellar)

Figure 19-3 Common sites of bursal inflammation. Bursitis in these areas can mimic other conditions and often responds to local injections (see text).

SUGGESTED READINGS

Anemia

Kushner JP, Lee GR, Wintrobe MM, Cartwright GE: Idiopathic refractory sideroblastic anemia: Clinical and laboratory investigation of 17 patients and review of the literature. *Medicine* 50:139, 1971.

Lipshitz DA, Mitchell CO, Thompson C: The anemia of senescence. *Am J Hematol* 11:47, 1981.

McLennan WJ, Andrews GR, Macleod C, Caird FI: Anemia in the elderly. *Q J Med* 52:1, 1973.

Cardiovascular Disorders

Ahmad RAS, Watson RDS: Treatment of postural hypotension. *Drugs* 39:74, 1990.

Morley JE, Reese SS: Clinical implications of the aging heart. *Am J Med* 80:77, 1989.

Rheumatological Disorders

Baum J: Rehabilitation aspects of arthritis in the elderly, in Williams TF (ed): *Rehabilitation in the Aging*. New York, Raven Press, 1984, p 177.

Kantrowitz FG, Munoz G, Roberts N, et al: Rheumatology in geriatrics, in Gambert SR (ed): *Contemporary Geriatric Medicine* (Vol. 2). New York, Plenum Press, 1986, p 183.

TWENTY

GASTROINTESTINAL DISORDERS

The major gastrointestinal problems in nursing home (NH) residents are dysphagia, gastrointestinal bleeding, and constipation. These conditions will be discussed in some detail in the sections that follow. In addition, a number of other gastrointestinal disorders can interfere with quality of life in NH residents. These conditions will also be discussed briefly in this chapter.

XEROSTOMIA

Xerostomia, or dry mouth, is present in 40 percent to 50 percent of NH residents. Classical presentations of xerostomia include difficulty in swallowing, inability to speak clearly, difficulty in maintaining dentures in the mouth, hypogeusia, lips sticking to teeth, and dental caries. The major causes of xerostomia are listed in Table 20-1. Management of xerostomia includes, whenever possible, discontinuing drugs that may be contributing, ensuring adequate hydration, and providing artificial saliva, such as carboxymethylcellulose. If the resident still has teeth, the synthetic saliva chosen should contain fluoride. Squeeze bottles which the resident can use to squirt saliva into the mouth are the cheapest delivery system. In some residents, ease of delivery may be improved by a pump spray bottle or aerosol spray. Care should be taken to see that the resident maintains a good hydration status. Residents with teeth should brush with toothpaste before going to bed, and, after rinsing the mouth, apply 0.4 percent stannous fluoride by brushing again with a toothbrush. They should then spit the fluoride out without further rinsing to obtain full protection throughout the night.

Table 20-1   Causes of xerostomia

Drugs
   Antidepressants
   Other psychotropic drugs
   Anticholinergics
   Calcium channel blockers
Radiation therapy
Sjögren's syndrome
Dehydration
Systemic illnesses

ORAL MUCOSAL DISORDERS

Approximately 60 percent of NH residents have oral mucosal lesions. Hyper-plasia and stomatitis of the tongue are the commonest lesions. Ulcerations are usually associated with dentures. Other oral conditions seen in the NH population include hyperkeratotic lesions, fistulas, and angular cheilitis. Pain associated with these lesions is present in approximately 12 percent. Leu-koplakia and carcinoma are rare oral lesions. Regular examination of the oral cavity, inquiry concerning oral pain, and periodic evaluation by a dentist experienced with the geriatric population are an important part of the care of NH residents.

DYSPHAGIA

Dysphagia is a relatively common and potentially life-threatening condition in the NH. It is associated with aspiration pneumonia, excessive expectora-tion of saliva, weight loss, heartburn, laryngeal irritation, and Zenker's diver-ticulum. In persons over the age of 80, there are decreased esophageal peri-staltic waves, increased nonperistaltic waves, and delayed relaxation of the esophageal sphincter, all of which, physiologically, can lead to mild dyspha-gia and/or aspiration. Residents with achalasia can have nocturnal aspira-tion, with coughing spasms that wake them. The major causes of dysphagia in NH residents are listed in Table 20-2. Severe dysphagia is almost always due to an organic cause, and the cause should be documented in all NH residents. The evaluation should include an assessment by a speech thera-pist trained to evaluate swallowing disorders and a barium swallow under observation of an experienced radiologist and/or speech therapist. NH resi-dents with dysphagia should have such an evaluation before a permanent or temporary enteral feeding tube is placed.

   Up to one-third of older persons have some degree of cricopharyngeal

Table 20-2   Causes of dysphagia in nursing home residents

Preesophageal	Esophageal
Neuromuscular	Neuromuscular
Pseudobulbar palsy	Cricopharyngeal muscle dysfunction
Myasthenia gravis	Achalasia
Parkinson's disease	Diffuse esophageal spasm
Multiple sclerosis	Diabetes mellitus
Amyotrophic lateral	Structural—intrinsic
sclerosis	Esophageal ring
Diabetes mellitus	Peptic stricture
Structural—intrinsic	Candidal esophagitis
Pharyngitis due to	Herpes simplex esophagitis
moniliasis	Carcinoma
Structural—extrinsic	Structural—extrinsic
Oropharyngeal abscess	Aortic aneurysm
Neoplasm	Peritracheal lymph node enlargement
Diverticulum	Bronchogenic carcinoma
	Enlarged left atrium

dysfunction, making this a potentially important cause of dysphagia in the NH. Cricopharyngeal muscle dysfunction leads either to failure to swallow food or to the trapping of food at the entrance of the esophagus. Solids are easier than liquids for residents with this disorder to swallow. The treatment is cricopharyngeal myotomy.

Not only does esophageal spasm cause dysphagia, but it can also produce chest pain, which is often confused with angina. Treatment consists of nitroglycerin before meals, isosorbide dinitrate, or calcium channel blockers. Occasionally, dilatation of the esophagus may be necessary.

UPPER GASTROINTESTINAL HEMORRHAGE

Upper gastrointestinal hemorrhage is a major problem in NH residents. The most common causes of upper gastrointestinal bleeding in older persons are duodenal ulcer, gastric erosions, gastric ulcer, hiatal hernia associated esophagitis, and carcinoma of the stomach. Mallory-Weiss tears can also be seen in older persons after repeated retching or vomiting. Drugs are a common precipitating factor in gastrointestinal bleeding. Drugs associated with bleeding include aspirin, nonsteroidal anti-inflammatory drugs, steroids, warfarin, and alcohol. Enteric-coated drugs reduce the possibility of bleeding. While misoprostol, a prostaglandin analog, can reduce the possibility of bleeding associated with the use of nonsteroidal anti-inflammatory drugs, diarrhea usually limits its effectiveness in the NH resident. NH residents on any of these drugs should have their hemoglobin levels checked periodically (e.g., every 1 to 2 months).

Peptic ulcer disease increases in prevalence in older persons despite the age-related decrease in the secretion of gastric acid. Recently, the bacterium *Helicobacter pylori* has been demonstrated to play a role in the pathogenesis of ulcers and gastritis. This organism increases in frequency with advancing age due to achlorhydria and mucosal damage. All older persons with a gastrointestinal bleed due to ulcers or gastritis may benefit from 14 days of treatment with amoxycillin and metronidazole in an attempt to eradicate this bacterium.

Management of acute or chronic gastrointestinal bleeding in older persons involves a choice of H_2 blockers (cimetidine or ranitidine) or sucralfate. Antacids often cause diarrhea, are difficult to administer regularly at 3-h intervals (which is necessary for optimum effects), alter absorption of drugs, and may cause magnesium or aluminum toxicity in the presence of renal disease. Omperazole's safety is yet to be established in older persons. The side effects of H_2 blockers are listed in Table 20-3. The ideal dose of cimetidine in a 90-year-old is 100 mg daily and in an 80-year-old 200 mg twice daily. This reduced dosage decreases the risk of toxicity. Sucralfate has virtually no systemic side effects but needs more frequent administration than H_2-receptor antagonists. H_2-receptor antagonists are often misused in NH residents when they are given chronically in an attempt to prevent bleeding.

Table 20-3   Side effects of H_2-receptor antagonists

Mental confusion[a]
Diarrhea
Myalgias
Rashes
Hypotension
Bradycardia
Impotence
Neutropenia
Renal dysfunction
Drug interactions[b]
    Diazepam
    Warfarin
    Theophylline
    Phenytoin
    Propranolol
    Metronidazole

[a] Worse in presence of renal or hepatic disease.
[b] Cimetidine reduces the hepatic metabolism of these drugs.

There is little evidence that this practice is useful, and it increases the possibility of side effects, as well as drug-drug interactions.

HEPATOBILIARY DISORDERS

Gallstones are common in older persons, particularly females. Emergency surgery carries a 10 percent mortality rate, compared to less than 2 percent for elective surgery. The availability of extracorporeal shock-wave lithotripsy has further enhanced the safety of gallstone treatment. Abdominal pain is present in most NH residents with acute cholecystitis, but fever and peritoneal signs are absent in half or more. Jaundice, which may be painless, occurs in one-third. Gallbladder disease may mimic myocardial infarction, with referred chest pain and Q waves on electrocardiography. Complications of acute cholecystitis that occur commonly in older persons are perforation, empyema, emphysematous cholecystitis, and ischemic necrosis of the gallbladder with gangrene. NH residents with symptoms or signs consistent with gallbladder disease should undergo abdominal ultrasonography as a first diagnostic step.

Hepatitis (especially non-A non-B hepatitis) is not rare in older persons. It is often transient, presenting with right-upper-quadrant pain, fever, mild jaundice, and changes in liver function tests. It may mimic gallbladder disease. Treatment is observation. Acetaminophen should be avoided in these residents. All NH residents suspected of having hepatitis should have serologic studies because of the risks of spread throughout the NH and the need for proper infection control precautions (see Chap. 17).

MESENTERIC VASCULAR OCCLUSION

Acute intestinal infarction is a life-threatening condition in older persons. Surgery may be lifesaving. This condition may present with relatively few signs or may be manifested by periumbilical pain or symptoms suggestive of intestinal obstruction. Approximately 30 percent of NH residents may have an acute confusional episode associated with this disorder. Mesenteric occlusion is often accompanied by severe acidosis, elevated white blood cell count, and fever. Any NH resident with a sudden mental status change, leukocytosis, and acidosis should be suspected of having acute intestinal infarction even in the absence of gastrointestinal signs or symptoms.

Chronic intestinal ischemia or "abdominal angina" is often missed in older NH residents. This condition may present with midabdominal pain that is often worse after eating or with early satiety. Diarrhea and chronic weight loss are also common. Treatment is with nitrates or calcium channel antagonists.

APPENDICITIS

Older persons who have appendicitis have a high mortality rate. On admission to the NH, previous appendectomy should be documented. If the appendix is still intact, the physician should always include appendicitis in the potential diagnosis of abdominal disease. As in most other intra-abdominal conditions, localizing symptoms and signs may be absent, requiring a high index of suspicion. This is especially important, because perforation occurs in approximately 50 percent of older persons with appendicitis and early diagnosis can be lifesaving. When appendicitis is suspected, modern ultrasound techniques are usually diagnostic.

DIVERTICULAR DISEASE

Diverticula are present in 50 percent of persons over 80 years of age. While diverticula are generally asymptomatic, approximately one-fourth of NH residents who have them are at risk for diverticulitis, intestinal obstruction, perforation, or gastrointestinal bleeding. Older persons are more likely than younger individuals to have more extensive colonic involvement, including both left and right sides of the colon. In younger persons, fever, leukocytosis, and rebound tenderness are commonly associated with acute diverticular disease. However, these findings are much less common in older persons. The signs and symptoms of diverticular disease are outlined in Table 20-4. Residents with any of the symptoms listed and unexplained fever and/or leukocytosis should arouse suspicion for diverticulitis even in the absence of suggestive abdominal signs.

DIARRHEA

Diarrhea in NH residents can be either acute or chronic. Acute diarrheas are usually associated with an infectious process, dietary change, ingestion of

**Table 20-4 Signs and symptoms
of diverticular diseases**

Symptoms	Signs
Abdominal pain	Bleeding
Constipation	Left ileal fossa mass
Rectal bleeding	Abscess
Flatulence	Perforation
Vomiting	Fistula
Diarrhea	Peritonitis
Urinary complaints	Obstruction

milk by those with lactose deficiency, or tube feeding. Infectious diarrheas are discussed in some detail in Chap. 17. Chronic diarrheas are either secretory or nonsecretory. Secretory diarrheas continue after a 24-h fast, whereas nonsecretory diarrheas are dependent on food to stimulate the process. The most common causes of chronic diarrhea are fecal impaction, malabsorption syndromes, chronic intestinal ischemia, laxative abuse, neoplasms, and anorectal incontinence. All NH residents with diarrhea should be checked for fecal impaction, which is probably the most common cause of diarrhea in this population. Fecal impaction can also cause fecal incontinence. (The causes and management of fecal incontinence are discussed in Chap. 13.) If diarrhea persists for more than 2 or 3 days or if it occurs in several residents simultaneously, an infectious cause should be considered. Stool should be sent for a culture for pathogens as well as for *Clostridium difficile* toxin. Antibiotic-associated diarrhea or enterocolitis should be suspected in residents who develop diarrhea while on or within 2 to 4 weeks of treatment with antibiotics (see Chap. 17).

CONSTIPATION

Constipation, either real or imagined, is a major problem in NH residents. It should be remembered that normal bowel function ranges from three times per day to three times per week. With advancing age and immobility, there is a tendency for stools to occur less often. A major cause of constipation in NH residents is the "terminal reservoir syndrome." This syndrome occurs because the gastrocolic reflex needs physical activity for its initiation. In addition, in NH residents who require help with toileting, there is often failure to respond to the gastrocolic reflex at the appropriate time. The major causes of constipation in older NH residents are listed in Table 20-5. The

Table 20-5   Causes of constipation in nursing home residents

Immobility (the terminal reservoir syndrome)
Poor hydration
Fecal impaction
Depression (tricyclics may make constipation worse)
Drugs (Table 20-6)
Organic causes
   Hypothyroidism
   Hypercalcemia
   Intestinal obstruction
   Hypomagnesemia
   Other electrolyte disorders
   Parkinsonism
Laxative abuse (Table 20-9)
High-fiber diet in immobile resident

Table 20-6   Drugs commonly associated with constipation

Antacids
Anticholinergics
Calcium
Iron
Opiates
Calcium channel antagonists
Antidepressants
Antiparkinsonian drugs
Ephedrine
Terbutaline
Nonsteroidal anti-inflammatory drugs
Neuroleptics

new onset of constipation should prompt a search for treatable causes. Several drugs commonly prescribed for NH residents can also cause or aggravate constipation (Table 20-6). It should be noted that fiber, often used to treat constipation, may actually cause constipation in residents who are immobile, because the gastrocolic reflex is necessary to move fiber through the gastrointestinal tract. A high tea intake may also aggravate constipation. Major complications of constipation include megacolon, volvulus, and fecal incontinence (Table 20-7).

An overview of the approach to the management of constipation in the NH is illustrated in Fig. 20-1. The first step is to make sure that the resident is adequately hydrated. A BUN-to-creatinine ratio of 20:1 or greater is suggestive of poor hydration. Treatment is 4 to 8 glasses (1 to 2 liters) of fluid daily unless contraindicated by severe heart or renal failure or hyponatremia. The second step is to use fiber in the mobile resident. Psyllium (in Metamucil) at 20 g/day (10 g twice daily) generally works well. Alternatively, a cup of bran will give approximately the same amount of fiber. The third

Table 20-7   Complications of constipation

Megacolon
Sigmoid volvulus
Fecal impaction
Fecal incontinence
Rectal prolapse
Refactory straining
   Syncope
   Arrhythmias
   Transient ischemic attacks

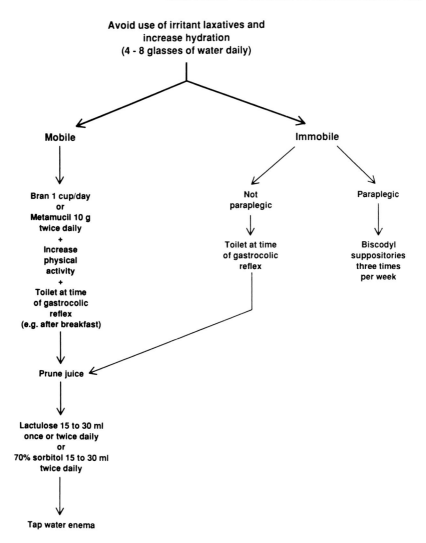

Figure 20-1 Approach to chronic constipation in nursing home residents.

step is to increase physical activity after meals and attempt to toilet the resident at the time of the gastrocolic reflex. We do not use stool softeners in the majority of residents. Many are marketed with irritant laxatives, may be hepatotoxic, and may be aspirated in those residents with swallowing problems. Discontinuation of stool softeners coupled with adequate hydration has produced no complaints in our NH residents. When the above measures fail, a subgroup of residents may need osmotic diuretic therapy (e.g., lactulose 15 to 30 ml once or twice per day or 70 percent sorbitol 15 to 30 ml twice a day). Prune juice is cheap and may be an excellent agent in some residents who insist on a laxative. Sorbitol is cheaper when it is prepared in bulk quantities in the institution. Tap water enemas distend the rectum and colon and produce reflex evacuation. Regular enema use can lead to fecal incontinence (Table 20-8). Biscodyl suppositories (Dulcolax) 10 mg three times per week are necessary in some residents with paraplegia or significant immobility who cannot take advantage of the gastrocolic reflex. In addition, residents with lax abdominal muscles may benefit from pushing with their hands on the lower abdomen at the time of toileting.

Irritant laxatives and stool softeners (Table 20-9) are overprescribed for NH residents. Up to three-quarters of NH residents are prescribed a laxative "as needed," and 50 percent receive daily scheduled laxatives. The prescribing of multiple laxatives for the same resident is also very common. Although prune juice can often be substituted for irritant laxatives, nurses tend to strongly prefer the use of the latter—especially Dulcolax suppositories and milk of magnesia with cascara. Chronic use of irritant laxatives can lead to severe constipation (so-called laxative colon). There is much mythology concerning laxatives among NH staff, and physicians need to be aware that many residents will not need irritant laxatives if they are managed by the strategy outlined above.

Table 20-8   Causes of fecal incontinence

Fecal impaction with overflow

Altered reservoir capacity
   Irradiation
   Surgery

Neuronal damage
   Local
     Laxative abuse
     Diabetes mellitus neuropathy
   Spinal cord
     Autonomous or reflex colon
   Surgery

Functional impairment
   Dementia
   Delirium
   Depression
   Immobility
   Poor access to toilet facility

Diarrhea

Table 20-9   Irritant laxatives and stool softeners[a]

Generic name	Trade name	Side effects
Bisacodyl	Dulcolax Carter's Little Pills	Gastric irritation
Anthraquinone (senna)	Senokot Perdiem (with psyllium) Fletcher's Castoria (with alcohol)	Degeneration of Meisner's and Auerbach's plexus
Phenolphthalein	Correctol[b] Ex-Lax Doxidan[b] Feen-A-Mint[b] Laxative mints[b]	Rashes
Casanthrol	Dialose Plus[b] Peri-Colace	Rashes
Magnesium hydroxide	Milk of magnesia Haley's MO (with mineral oil)	Magnesium toxicity
Docusate sodium	Colace Dialose DOSS	Rashes

[a] These drugs should be avoided in most NH residents (see text).
[b] Also contains docusate.

SUGGESTED READINGS

Altman DF: Gastrointestinal diseases in the elderly. *Med Clin North Am* 67:433, 1983.

Castle SC: Constipation: Endemic in the elderly. *Med Clin North Am* 73:1497, 1990.

Ekelund R: Oral mucosal disorders in institutionalized elderly people. *Age Ageing* 17:193, 1988.

Finucane PM, Arunachalum T, O'Dourd J, Pathy MSJ: Acute mesenteric infarction in elderly patients. *J Am Geriatr Soc* 37:355, 1989.

Goldstein MK, Brown EM, Holt P, et al: Fecal incontinence in an elderly man. *J Am Geriatr Soc* 37:991, 1989.

Shamburek RD, Farrar JT: Disorders of the digestive system in the elderly. *N Engl J Med* 322:438, 1990.

Wald A: Constipation and fecal incontinence in the elderly. *Gastroenterol Clin North Am* 19:605, 1990.

GENERAL MANAGEMENT ISSUES

Quality of Life

To live or not to live, that is the question.
    Whether 'Tis nobler to suffer slings and
Arrows of old age, or being warehoused in a nursing home,
    Opposing the years and praying not to end up on a peripad.

To sleep a drugged sleep, to awake confused,
    And end the thousand thoughts the mind is heir to.
"Mama, where is my doll? What happened to my quality of life?"
    'Tis a consummation devoutly to be avoided.

To feed oneself, to bathe, to walk perchance
    To fall and break a hip, Ay there's the rub.
For in those simple skills, what peace of mind may come,
    To avoid the calamity of so long a life.

For who can bear the whips and scorns of bureaucrats
    Who have never suffered the burning of an N/G tube.
They mean full well—they want us all to die in good health.
    May they be spared the torture of such assaults.

Nature calls at last, so please don't let them
    Subject my tired body to a gastrostomy tube.
Oh, here they come with enemas and catheters.
    My bed sores scream in stench and pain.

Look! The Pearly Gates have come into view.
    Relief is finally within my grasp.
The bitter battle has been won.
    Nature will give me rest at last.

I hear a siren. An ambulance is on its way!
    Oh no! My doctor forgot to document my plea for no heroics.
I struggle to escape. A needle is my reward.
    Even the ambulance ride I can't enjoy.

In the E.R., the interns and nurses grunt and sweat.
    They start IV's and respirators and even intubate.
The Pearly Gates soon fade from view.
    Have I no right to decide my fate?

But I am not made of immortal stuff,
    My worn out body can't even cry.
They have wasted their priceless resources,
    And plans of great pitch and moment go awry.

The Health Department has new rules which no one knows thereof
    Soon the ECF will not have to bear the inspector's wrong.
They don't have to hydrate, just let us go in peace.
    Soft you now—my final sleep cometh.

The late Phillip L. Rossman, M.D.
Los Angeles, California

TWENTY–ONE

DRUG USE

Numerous recent studies and reviews have highlighted the excessive number of drugs that many NH residents receive, the inappropriateness of many drugs and/or dosage regimens ordered in NHs, the susceptibility of NH residents to adverse drug reactions, and the relatively high incidence of bothersome as well as potentially serious adverse drug reactions that occur in the frail geriatric NH population.

Several surveys indicate that on average, NH residents are prescribed 6 to 8 drugs and that some are prescribed over 20 different medications simultaneously. Close to half of these prescriptions are for prn drugs, many of which are never used. Drugs are clearly necessary for many residents in order to manage chronic medical conditions. Pressure from residents, families, and NH staff to prescribe drugs often plays an important role as well. However, drug prescribing in the NH, unlike the ambulatory care unit or acute care hospital, is frequently done without direct assessment of the resident and is based on information provided by NH staff. In some situations, the prescription of a drug is a substitute for a careful assessment of the resident leading to a precise diagnosis and management plan. Thus primary care physicians and medical directors must take appropriate steps to improve their prescribing habits.

Unfortunately, because of the seriousness and pressing nature of the problems created by this excessive and inappropriate prescription of drugs in NHs, the federal government has gotten into the act. The 1987 Omnibus Reconciliation Act (OBRA), which establishes many new rules and regulations for NH care, focuses on drug use in general as well as antipsychotic drugs in particular. The Appendix contains a summary of selected aspects of OBRA that are relevant for primary care physicians. With respect to drug therapy, OBRA mandates that NH residents be "free from unnecessary drugs." Unnecessary drugs are defined as those that are given:

In excessive doses
For excessive periods of time
Without adequate monitoring
Without a documented diagnosis or reason for the drug
When monitoring data or adverse consequences indicate the drug should be reduced or discontinued
In anticipation of an adverse consequence of another prescribed drug

Rules regarding antipsychotics are much more specific and are discussed later in this chapter as well as in the Appendix. The survey process will, therefore, include specific attention to drug use, and NHs will be subject to deficiencies and possibly fines if violations are identified.

The purpose of this chapter is not to provide primary care physicians with a compendium of specifics on the prescription of various drugs for NH residents. Selected aspects of drug therapy for specific conditions common among NH residents are included in several other chapters throughout this text, and more detailed information is available in general textbooks of medicine and geriatrics. The objective of this chapter is to give primary care physicians and medical directors some general guidelines for drug use in the NH. Because of the prevalence of psychiatric conditions and behavioral disturbances in this population, the commonplace prescription of inappropriate psychotropic drugs for NH residents, and the specific focus of OBRA on antipsychotics, a separate section of this chapter discusses psychotropic drug use.

GENERAL PRINCIPLES OF DRUG PRESCRIBING

Because the involvement of consultant pharmacists is a federally mandated requirement, most NHs have a consultant pharmacist who regularly reviews drug regimens. The American Society of Consultant Pharmacists (based in Arlington, Virginia), a national organization of pharmacists, provides services to NHs. Many state and local organizations of pharmacists also include groups whose practice focuses on the NH setting. Medical directors and primary care physicians should work collaboratively with consultant pharmacists and nursing staff in order to maximize the appropriateness of drug regimens for individual NH residents as well as to develop appropriate policies and procedures for the prescription, administration, and monitoring of drug therapy. The latter activities should be accomplished in conjunction with a pharmacy and/or quality assurance committee.

Table 21-1 lists several general principles of drug prescribing for NH residents. These can be divided into two basic sets of recommendations: one focusing on general principles of drug therapy for the frail geriatric population and the other on practical considerations in writing drug orders in the NH. As in prescribing for geriatric patients who are not in NHs, drug treatment should be ordered only when a specific indication exists and the risk/benefit considerations favor drug therapy. Any time a drug is ordered, a corresponding diagnosis or specific indications should be documented in the medical record—on a problem list, in a progress note, and in the order itself if appropriate (especially for prn orders). Age- and disease-related changes in the pharmacology of various drugs are well documented. Drug doses should therefore take into account the route of elimination of the drug and the resident's ability to eliminate the drug by that route. Renal function, liver function, cardiac output, body mass, and hydration are critical factors to consider in adjusting drug dosages and dosage intervals. "Start low and

Table 21-1   General principles of drug prescribing in the nursing home

Make sure that a drug is necessary to treat the resident's condition
An appropriate diagnosis should be recorded for each drug prescribed
When a drug is ordered
   The dose should be appropriate for the resident's condition and ability to eliminate the drug
   "Start low and go slow" is an appropriate guideline for most drugs in the NH population
   Avoid significant drug-drug interactions (see Table 21-2)
   Avoid potential "drug-condition" interactions (see Table 21-3)
   Pay attention to the practical aspects of drug orders
      Order the minimum number of doses necessary
      Avoid timed orders (e.g., "every 8 h") unless absolutely necessary based on the kinetics of the drug
      Write time-limited orders (e.g., "for 7 days") whenever possible
      Include a specific indication for all prn orders
   Pay attention to the cost of the drug
      For residents on medical assistance programs (i.e., Medicaid), use drugs reimbursed by the program whenever possible
Write appropriate orders for drug monitoring (see Table 21-4)
   Avoid unnecessary "hold if" orders, which increase nursing time necessary for drug administration
      Most "hold if" orders can be discontinued after the resident's condition is stable on the drug
   Follow drug blood levels periodically for drugs with a narrow therapeutic index and when clinical efficacy correlates with blood levels
Review each drug order monthly
Discontinue all unnecessary drugs
Work collaboratively with consultant pharmacists to ensure the appropriateness of drug orders and drug monitoring
Regularly review drug prescribing, administration, and monitoring through a pharmacy and/or quality assurance committees

go slow" is a general rule of thumb that is particularly appropriate for NH residents.

Because multiple drugs are often prescribed for NH residents, the chance of adverse drug interactions is high. Many software programs are available to detect potential drug-drug interactions. However, a caveat about these programs is that they tend to spew out all possible interactions rather than just the clinically important ones. Many programs do have the capability to identify only potentially serious interactions. Table 21-2 lists some examples of potential drug-drug interactions that are important clinically. This is an area where consultant pharmacists can provide valuable assistance in identifying the interactions, determining their clinical importance, and helping to identify an alternative drug regimen if necessary. "Drug-condition" interactions may be just as important if not more so than drug-drug interactions. Most NH residents have at least one or more chronic conditions that can influence the response to drugs prescribed for other conditions. Table 21-3 lists several examples of such drug-condition interactions. Primary care physicians should therefore document each resident's chronic conditions and be aware of how the efficacy of drug therapy may be influenced by these conditions, as well as whether a newly prescribed drug may adversely affect another underlying condition.

Table 21-2   Examples of potentially clinically important drug-drug interactions

Mechanism	Example	Potential effects
Interference with drug absorption	Antacids interacting with digoxin, isoniazid, antipsychotics, histamine-2 blockers	Diminished drug effectiveness
Displacement from binding proteins	Warfarin, oral hypoglycemics, dilantin, aspirin and other nonsteroidals	Enhanced effects and increased risk of toxicity
Altered distribution	Digoxin and quinidine	Increased risk of toxicity
Altered metabolism	Cimetidine interacting with propranolol, theophylline, dilantin	Decreased drug clearance, enhanced effects, increased risk of toxicity
Altered excretion	Lithium and diuretics	Increased risk of toxicity and electrolyte imbalance
Pharmacological antagonism	Levodopa and clonidine	Decreased antiparkinsonian effects
Pharmacological synergism	Tricyclic antidepressants and antihypertensives Narcotic analgesics and psychotropics	Increased risk of hypotension Increased risk of delirium, sedation, falls

Table 21-3   Examples of potentially clinically important drug-condition interactions

Drug	Conditions	Clinical implications
Diuretics	Diabetes	Decreased glucose tolerance, especially with hypokalemia
	Poor nutritional status	Increased risk of dehydration and electrolyte imbalance
	Urinary frequency, urgency	Precipitate incontinence
Beta blockers	Diabetes	Sympathetic response to hypoglycemia masked
	Chronic obstructive lung disease	Increased bronchospasm
	Congestive heart failure	Decreased myocardial contractility
	Peripheral vascular disease	Increased claudication
Narcotic analgesics	Chronic constipation	Worsening symptoms, fecal impaction
Tricyclic antidepressants	Congestive heart failure, angina	Tachycardia, decreased myocardial contractility, postural hypotension exacerbating cardiovascular conditions
Tricyclic antidepressants, antihistamines, and other drugs with anticholinergic effects	Constipation, glaucoma and other visual impairments, prostatic hyperplasia, reflux esophagitis, xerostomia	Worsening of symptoms
Antipsychotics	Parkinsonism	Worsening of immobility
	Seizure disorder	Lower seizure threshold and may increase seizures
Psychotropics	Dementia	Further impairment of cognitive function

Several practical aspects of drug orders for NH residents are important in reducing the nursing time necessary to administer and monitor the drugs (thus lowering the cost and also allowing nursing staff to spend time in other areas) as well as in minimizing disruption to the residents' routines. The lowest possible number of drug doses should be prescribed. Many drugs that are prescribed three or four times a day may be needed only once or twice. Long-acting and slow-release preparations are becoming increasingly available and should be prescribed when appropriate. Long-acting psychotropic drugs should, however, generally be avoided (see discussion under "Psychotropic Drugs" below). When multiple doses of drugs are necessary, timed orders (e.g., every 8 h) should be avoided unless they are essential in view of the kinetics of the drug and the condition being treated. Orders for the numbers of times per day are generally sufficient. These types of orders allow the nursing staff flexibility and minimize the potential to disrupt the residents' routines (e.g., sleep, social and recreational activities). When a drug is ordered for an acute condition, the order should contain a stop date so that drugs are not continued for longer than necessary (e.g., cough/cold preparations for 7 to 10 days). All drug orders should be reviewed monthly and all unnecessary drugs discontinued. Appropriate drug-order formats can facilitate this process by listing the drug orders *separately* from other orders and by listing the original starting date of each order. Although monitoring is extremely important (see discussion under "Monitoring" below), unnecessary or excessive orders for monitoring should be avoided. For example, monitoring orders are frequently written for cardiovascular medications (e.g., "hold if systolic blood pressure <100 mmHg"). These types of orders may be necessary and appropriate for the first several days of drug therapy in order to monitor response and adjust dosages. But continuing them unnecessarily after the resident's condition is stable creates a substantial amount of time-consuming busy work for nursing staff, who are generally in short supply.

One other consideration is important in prescribing drugs for NH residents: cost. The majority of NH residents are either on Medicaid or very close to qualifying for it. State Medicaid programs vary as to what drugs they will cover. Because most NH residents cannot afford to pay out of pocket for drugs, primary physicians should be familiar with the drugs that are covered by Medicaid or other programs and only prescribe other drugs (for which the residents or their families will have to pay) when absolutely necessary.

MONITORING

Careful monitoring of drug therapy is essential in order to minimize the number of unnecessary medications, improve the appropriateness of drug orders, and document efficacy of therapy. Monitoring consists of three basic activities:

1. Assessment of the clinical effectiveness of the drug and identification of side effects
2. Periodic measurement of various clinical parameters (e.g., pulse, blood pressure, postural blood pressure changes)
3. Periodic laboratory studies

Progress notes of both primary physicians and licensed nurses should document the results of these monitoring activities. Primary physicians

should write specific orders for monitoring clinical parameters and laboratory studies. The nature of these orders depends on the drug being monitored and the condition being treated. It is important to emphasize that these
orders should be clinically reasonable and *not* result in excessive busy work
for nursing staff or overuse of laboratory tests. There are no data from clinical trials that can provide guidelines for the monitoring of specific drug
therapies in the NH setting. Table 21-4 lists several examples of guidelines
for monitoring drugs commonly prescribed in the NH. These examples are
not based on data or on the guidelines of any state or health professional
organization but represent the authors' best judgment of what is reasonable
given the current state of knowledge.

PSYCHOTROPIC DRUGS

General Principles

Psychotropic drugs—including antidepressants, antipsychotics, and seda-
tive-hypnotics—are probably the most inappropriately used drugs in the
NH. Close to half of all NH residents are given at least one psychotropic
drug and a substantial proportion receive more than one. Ironically, the vast
majority of these prescriptions are written without any input from a mental
health professional. In a small but important subgroup of NH residents, psychotropic drugs and especially antidepressants may be underused. As mentioned earlier in this chapter, the federal government, via the 1987 OBRA
legislation, has intervened to create specific rules regarding the use of antipsychotics (see the Appendix). Some states, such as California, also have
rules regarding the use of antipsychotics as well as other psychotropic drugs
in NHs.

    Table 21-5 lists several general principles of prescribing psychotropic
drugs for NH residents. Other chapters in this book discuss details of the
diagnosis and management of dementia, depression, and related behavioral
disorders (Chaps. 9 and 10). When a psychotropic drug is prescribed, a specific diagnosis should be made whenever possible. At the very least, the
nature and frequency of target symptoms and behaviors should be documented. Although an increasing number of physicians with training in geriatrics (including geropsychiatry) are becoming available, most primary care
physicians who look after NH residents have not had such training. Thus, a
consultation from an experienced psychiatrist or psychologist should be
obtained whenever possible to provide input into diagnosis and management. In some settings, clinical nurse specialists and social workers can also
provide valuable input. Because *depression* is common, often unrecognized, and treatable, it should be on the top of the differential diagnosis list.
Depression commonly accompanies chronic medical illnesses among frail,
cognitively intact NH residents and also commonly coexists with dementia.

Table 21-4 Examples of drug monitoring for nursing home residents[a]

Analgesics
Document effectiveness regularly
   If prn doses are being used regularly for chronic pain syndromes, consider switching to
      routine orders
For nonsteroidal anti-inflammatory drugs (NSAIDs)
   Regularly (e.g., monthly) check stool for occult blood and/or measure blood hemoglobin
      level
   Renal function test should be monitored (e.g., every 2 to 3 months)

Antiarrhythmics
Blood levels should be monitored regularly (e.g., every 3 months when stable)
Pulse should be taken regularly (e.g., daily) if a supraventricular tachyarrhythmia is being
   treated
   Parameters can be set to monitor effectiveness (e.g., "Notify MD if pulse >100 or <60")
Periodic 24-h electrocardiographic monitoring may be appropriate if malignant ventricular
   arrhythmias are being treated

Antibiotics
Temperature should be taken regularly (e.g., every shift)
Culture sensitivity reports should be checked to ensure appropriateness of antibiotic
Repeat cultures (e.g., urine) should be obtained to document response

Anticoagulants
Prothrombin time should be checked regularly (e.g., monthly)

Anticonvulsants
Blood levels should be checked regularly (e.g., every 3 months when stable)
For carbamazepine, complete blood count should be checked regularly (e.g., every 2 weeks
   initially, then every 3 months); liver function tests should also be monitored periodically

Antidepressants
Blood levels may be helpful, especially if there is poor response or side effects occur (e.g.,
   nortriptyline)
For tricyclics
   Postural blood pressure and pulse should be checked for the first few days after initiating
      treatment or increasing dose
   Electrocardiogram should be done periodically (e.g., every 1 to 3 months) to detect new ⸜
      onset of heart block, especially if dose is adjusted upward
For lithium
   Blood levels should be checked regularly (e.g., monthly when stable)
   Thyroid function should be measured periodically (e.g., every 6 to 12 months)
   Electrolytes should be monitored regularly (e.g., monthly) with concomitant diuretic
      therapy
Clinical response should be assessed and documented regularly (see Table 21-7)

Antihypertensives
Blood pressure should be checked regularly (e.g., weekly when stable)
   Parameters can be set to monitor effectiveness (e.g., "Notify MD if systolic BP >180 or <
      100 or if diastolic BP >100")
Postural blood pressure and pulse should be checked regularly for the first few days after
   initiating treatment or dosage increases
For drugs that affect cardiac conduction (e.g., verapamil, diltiazem), an electrocardiogram
   should be done periodically (e.g., every 3 to 6 months) to detect new onset of heart block

Table 21-4 *(Continued)*   Examples of drug monitoring for nursing home residents[a]

Antipsychotics
Clinical effectiveness should be assessed and documented regularly (e.g., weekly) by
  determining the frequency of target behaviors (see Tables 21-5, 21-6, and 21-7)

Diuretics
Electrolytes and renal function tests should be checked regularly (e.g., every 1 to 3 months,
  depending on dose and condition)
When an acute illness decreases fluid intake, diuretics should be held

Hematinics
Blood hemoglobin should be checked regularly (e.g., monthly)
    When hemoglobin becomes normal after acute blood loss, hematinics can be discontinued
      if nutritional intake is adequate

Hypoglycemics
Fasting blood sugar should be monitored regularly (e.g., monthly) in stable diabetics
For unstable diabetics, finger-stick glucose monitoring should be done more often until
  condition is stable
Parameters should be set to monitor therapy (e.g., "Notify MD if glucose >250 or <60")

Respiratory Drugs
Blood levels of theophylline should be monitored periodically (e.g., every 1 to 3 months)
Periodic pulmonary function testing and/or pulse oximetry may be appropriate for residents
  with severe or unstable chronic lung disease

Sedative/Hypnotics
Clinical effectiveness should be assessed and documented regularly (e.g., weekly) by
  reviewing frequency and severity of target symptoms and side effects (see Tables 21-5, 21-
  6, and 21-7)

Thyroid Replacement
When initiating therapy, serum thyroid stimulating hormone (TSH) should be measured
  regularly (e.g., every 2 to 4 weeks) and dose adjusted until the TSH is normal
Serum TSH should be monitored regularly (e.g., yearly when stable)
    If it is low, a supersensitive method should be used to detect overreplacement
    Measurement of other thyroid function tests (e.g., T_3, T_4) is generally unnecessary

---

[a] These recommendations are those of the authors and are not based on well-designed
clinical trials (which are lacking) or on any particular state or association guidelines.

Like those of many medical conditions, the symptoms of depression may
be nonspecific or atypical and a variety of medications may contribute to
depression in this population (see Chap. 10). NH staff frequently describe a
wide variety of behaviors ranging from wandering to yelling to physical
aggression as *agitation* (see Chap. 10). It is critical to recognize that agitation, like delirium, may be the manifestation of a variety of underlying medical conditions. Any resident who becomes agitated or whose agitated
behaviors suddenly worsen should be evaluated to rule out an underlying
treatable medical condition before a psychotropic medication is prescribed.

Table 21-5 Basic principles of prescribing psychotropic drugs for nursing home residents

Make a specific diagnosis and identify target symptoms and behaviors before prescribing a drug
    Consult an experienced psychiatrist or psychologist whenever feasible to provide input on diagnosis and treatment
    Depression is common and treatable
      It frequently coexists with dementia
      Clinical presentation may include a variety of symptoms or behaviors
    Residents who become "agitated" should be assessed to rule out delirium caused by treatable medical conditions, drugs, or depression
Consider using nonpharmacologic approaches to manage target behaviors whenever possible
If a drug is prescribed, choose the drug that is most appropriate for the specific clinical indications and condition of the resident (see Tables 21-3, 21-6)
Start with low doses
Monitor and document response of target symptoms and behaviors as well as side effects
Increase the dose gradually until
    Target symptoms and behaviors are improved
    Intolerable drug side effects occur
Continue to monitor response of target symptoms and behaviors and observe for side effects (see Table 21-7)
If symptoms and behaviors are eliminated and remain stable over several weeks (e.g., 8 to 12 weeks), consider dose reduction and eventual discontinuation of the drug

Once a diagnosis is made and specific target symptoms and behaviors are identified, consideration should be given to nonpharmacologic approaches to treatment. A variety of nonpharmacologic approaches—such as socialization, activities, environmental manipulation, altering the way staff interacts with the resident, and behavior modification techniques—may be helpful for selected residents (see Chap. 10).

If a psychotropic drug is prescribed, the same general principles outlined in Tables 21-1, 21-2, and 21-3 should be followed. In addition, it is important to choose the most appropriate drug for the specific target symptoms and behaviors in view of the condition of the resident. Table 21-6 lists several common clinical indications for psychotropic drug therapy and appropriate types of drugs for each indication. The lowest possible dose should be prescribed initially and the dose gradually increased until target symptoms and behaviors respond or intolerable drug side effects occur.

One of the major problems with the use of psychotropic drugs in NHs is the lack of adequate monitoring after the drug is prescribed. Table 21-7 lists several of the key elements of monitoring psychotropic drug use. Each of these issues should be addressed and documented on a regular basis in nursing and physician progress notes. During the initial phase of drug therapy, it may be necessary to summarize these data daily. After symptoms have stabilized, a weekly summary in the nursing notes would be an appro-

Table 21-6   Clinical considerations in prescribing psychotropic drugs

Clinical indications	Most useful drugs	Comments
Depression with psychomotor retardation Depression with psychomotor agitation	Less sedating antidepressant (e.g., desipramine, nortriptyline) More sedating antidepressant (e.g., doxepin, trazodone)	Anticholinergic effects, potential cardiovascular effects, and potential interactions with antihypertensives are important considerations
Agitation without psychosis	Short-acting sedative (e.g., alprazolam, oxazepam, lorazepam, buspirone[a])	Should generally be used on prn basis Nonpharmacologic interventions may be more appropriate Can worsen depression
Psychosis without prominent agitation (e.g., delusions and hallucinations in patients with depression or dementia)	Less sedating antipsychotic (e.g., haloperidol, thiothixene)	Extrapyramidal effects may be prominent Akathisia can make patient appear agitated
Severe agitation poorly controlled by a sedative	More sedating antipsychotic (e.g., thioridazine, molindone)	Stronger antipsychotics (haloperidol, thiothixene) sometimes needed Extrapyramidal effects may be prominent Akathisia can make patient appear more agitated
Insomnia	Chloral hydrate, temazepam, triazolam	Underlying cause(s) should be sought Nonpharmacologic interventions often helpful Benzodiazepines should be used on an intermittent rather than a nightly basis

[a] Not effective acutely; chronic dosing rather than prn use necessary.

priate method of documentation. Routine physician progress notes should also summarize these data. Facilities with computers may want to incorporate the elements listed in Table 21-7 into a data base that can be used for quality assurance purposes.

If target symptoms and behaviors are improved and the resident's condition remains stable, consideration should be given to reducing the dose and discontinuing the drug. For some psychiatric conditions, such as depres-

Table 21-7   Key elements of monitoring and documenting responses to psychotropic drugs

Specific target symptoms and/or behaviors for which drug was prescribed
Frequency of the target symptoms and/or behaviors
Number of prn doses given (if applicable)
Frequency and nature of any potential drug side effects
Plans for dosage adjustment
   Increase dose to improve symptoms or behaviors
   Keep dose stable (adequate response)
   Decrease dose
     Due to side effects
     After symptoms or behaviors have been improved for several weeks to try to minimize
      or eliminate drug use

sion and psychosis, it is appropriate to stabilize symptoms for a period of at least several weeks (e.g., 8 to 12) before beginning to withdraw the drug. For some residents, it may not be possible or clinically indicated to withdraw the drug at all (e.g., those who have failed previous attempts to withdraw drug therapy). If the drug is to be withdrawn, it is generally best to reduce the dose gradually. Ongoing monitoring, as described above, is extremely important during these attempts to reduce or discontinue psychotropic drug use.

Specific information about the use of antidepressants can be found in Chap. 10. The sections that follow briefly discuss the use of antipsychotic and sedative/hypnotic drugs.

Antipsychotics

Among the psychotropic drugs, antipsychotics are the most controversial with respect to NH residents. There is a general sense that antipsychotics are frequently used as "chemical restraints" in this population. This concern, as well as the possiblity of permanent side effects such as tardive dyskinesia, is probably responsible for the specific attention given antipsychotics in the 1987 OBRA legislation. In addition to this concern, there is a lack of data from controlled trials on the efficacy of these drugs in the NH population.

Under the rules outlined in OBRA (see Appendix for more detail) antipsychotics should no longer be used if the only indication is a nonspecific one, such as wandering, restlessness, yelling or screaming, or uncooperativeness. They can be prescribed for specific psychotic conditions as well as in organic mental syndromes (including dementia) when

1. The syndrome includes psychotic or agitated features

2. Specific behaviors are objectively and quantitatively documented that cause resident to
   a. Present a danger to themselves
   b. Present a danger to others
   c. Interfere with care
3. Psychotic symptoms cause the resident frightful distress

When dementia and/or depression is complicated by psychosis (e.g., paranoid delusions), an antipsychotic drug is generally indicated. The more common situation, however, is that a resident with dementia presents agitated behaviors that are a danger to others or significantly interfere with care. In these situations (assuming the resident is not depressed or medically ill), the choice of drug therapy is between an antipsychotic and a short-acting sedative. There are advantages and disadvantages to each, and each class of drugs has its proponents. Data from well-controlled clinical trials comparing antipsychotics to short-acting sedatives for agitated behaviors among NH residents are not available at the present time. Whichever approach is taken, careful monitoring of the target symptoms and behaviors as well as careful observation for side effects are critical.

Table 21-8 lists examples of antipsychotic drugs. The major advantage of using the more potent antipsychotics (e.g., haloperidol, thiothixene) is that they are generally not sedating and do not have significant cardiovas-

Table 21-8   Examples of antipsychotic drugs

Drug	Relative potency/ equivalent dose, mg	Approximate dosages, mg[a]	Relative sedation	Potential for side effects	
				Hypotension	Extrapyramidal effects[b]
Chlorpromazine (Thorazine, others)	50	10–300	Very high	High	Moderate
Thioridazine (Mellaril)	50	10–300	High	Moderate	Low
Loxapine (Loxitane)	7.5	10–100	Moderate	Moderate	Moderate
Molindone (Moban)	5	5–100	Moderate	Moderate	Moderate
Thiothixene (Navane)	2.5	1–5	Low	Low	Very high
Haloperidol (Haldol)	1	0.25–6	Low	Low	Very high

[a] Per day in three or four divided doses.
[b] Rigidity, bradykinesia, tremor, akathisia.

cular side effects. They are contraindicated in residents with parkinsonism. Even in very small doses (e.g., 0.5 mg of haloperidol), they can have significant extrapyramidal side effects, the most disabling of which are bradykinesia and rigidity. These side effects can result in immobility and can predispose already immobile residents to complications such as aspiration, pressure sores, and incontinence. Another important but commonly unrecognized side effect is akathisia. Manifested by motor restlessness, akathisia may be mistaken for a failure of response to the drug or even a worsening of symptoms. As a result, the dose may be increased until the resident is so bradykinetic and rigid that she/he appears less agitated. This is obviously the wrong approach to using these drugs, and primary physicians who prescribe potent antipsychotics should be very familiar with these potential side effects. Anticholinergics should *not* be routinely prescribed to prevent these extrapyramidal side effects. It is probably better to change the drug rather than add an anticholinergic agent because of the potential for anticholinergic side effects. Anticholinergic side effects may be especially bothersome in NH residents. They include dryness of the mouth, blurring of vision, constipation and fecal impaction, exacerbation of gastroesophageal reflux, and delirium. More sedating antipsychotics (e.g., thioridazine, loxapine, and molindone) may be appropriate for very agitated, psychotic residents. Low doses of thioridazine (e.g., 10 mg) may be effective, but anticholinergic and cardiovascular side effects (hypotension) may limit its usefulness. If mild sedation is the therapeutic goal, a short-acting sedative is probably a better choice.

Sedative/Hypnotics

Table 21-9 lists examples of sedative/hypnotic drugs. If the therapeutic goal is mild sedation for disabling anxiety or intermittent severe agitated behaviors, then it is appropriate to use a short-acting drug that has a relatively short onset of action (e.g., lorazepam, which can also be given intramuscularly). Antihistamines have been used for this purpose, but they probably should be avoided in NH residents with dementia because of their anticholinergic effects. Buspirone is a new sedative that appears to have a low side-effect profile, but it may take several days of chronic therapy for its therapeutic effects to become apparent. Unlike short-acting benzodiazepines, buspirone is not useful as a hypnotic.

Before a hypnotic is prescribed, a careful assessment of complaints of insomnia is essential. First, self-reports of insomnia among NH residents are often unreliable, and this complaint should be verified by nighttime nursing staff. Second, insomnia may be caused by a lack of activity and naps during the day or by the "sundowning" associated with sensory deprivation. These factors are potentially amenable to nonpharmacologic approaches such as

Table 21-9   Examples of sedatives and hypnotic drugs

	Approximate dose equivalence, mg	Relative rapidity of effect after oral administration	Half-life, h	Active metabolites
Benzodiazepines				
Longer-acting				
Diazepam (Valium)	5	Very fast	20–100	Yes
Clorazepate (Tranxene)	7.5	Fast	30–200	Yes
Flurazepam[a,b] (Dalmane)	15	Fast	40–200	Yes
Clonazepam (Klonopin)	0.5	Intermediate	18–50	Yes
Shorter-acting				
Triazolam[a] (Halcion)	0.25	Fast	2–5	No
Lorazepam (Ativan)	1	Intermediate	10–20	No
Oxazepam (Serax)	15	Intermediate	5–15	No
Temazepam[a] (Restoril)	15	Intermediate	5–15	No
Alprazolam (Xanax)	0.25	Fast	6–20	No
Antihistamines[c]				
Diphenhydramine[a] (Benadryl, others)	25	Fast	4–7	No
Hydroxyzine (Vistaril, Atarax)	10	Very fast	Unknown[d]	Unknown
Other				
Chloral hydrate[a] (Noctec, others)	500	Fast	7–10	Yes
Buspirone (BuSpar)[e]	10	Fast	2–3	Yes

[a] More commonly used as hypnotics.
[b] When used as a hypnotic in dosages of more than 15 mg, daytime drowsiness, confusion, and ataxia commonly occur in the elderly.
[c] Anticholinergic side effects may be problematic.
[d] Duration of action: 4 to 6 h.
[e] Must be used chronically to be an effective antianxiety agent.

activity programming during the day and the use of night lights to diminish sensory deprivation. Finally, insomnia may be caused by medical conditions such as nocturia, orthopnea, gastroesophageal reflux, and nocturnal myoclonus. A careful history may be necessary to detect these symptoms, and specific therapy should be initiated when appropriate.

Whenever sedative/hypnotic drugs are prescribed, it is best to use them intermittently rather than chronically (with the possible exception of buspirone). Intermittent use may lead to less tolerance to drug effects. In addition, withdrawal syndromes—with increased insomnia, anxiety, or agitation—can occur when chronic treatment is discontinued.

SUGGESTED READINGS

Beers M, Avorn J, Soumerai SB, et al: Psychoactive medication use in intermediate-care facility residents. *JAMA* 260:3016–3020, 1988.

Dement WC: Rational basis for the use of sleeping pills. *Pharmacology* 27(suppl 2):3–38, 1983.

Greenblatt JK, Sellers EM, and Shader RI: Drug disposition in old age. *N Engl J Med* 306:1081–1088, 1982.

Greenblatt DJ, Shader RI, and Abernethy DR: Current status of benzodiazepines. *N Engl J Med* 309:354–415, 1983.

Gurwitz JH, Soumerai SB, and Avorn J: Improving medication prescribing and utilization in the nursing home. *J Am Geriatr Soc* 38:542–552, 1990.

Helms PM: Efficacy of antipsychotics in the treatment of the behavioral complications of dementia: A review of the literature. *J Am Geriatr Soc* 33:206–209, 1985.

Larson EB, Kukull WA, Buchner D, and Reifler BV: Adverse drug reactions associated with global cognitive impairment in elderly persons. *Ann Intern Med* 107:169–173, 1987.

Montamat SC, Cusack BJ, and Vestel RE: Management of drug therapy in the elderly. *N Engl J Med* 321:303–310, 1989.

Ouslander JG: Drug therapy in the elderly. *Ann Intern Med* 95:711–722, 1981.

Ray WA, Federspeil CF, and Schaffner W: A study of antipsychotic drug use in nursing homes: Epidemiologic evidence suggesting misuse. *Am J Pub Health* 70:485–491, 1980.

Schneider LS, Pollock VE, and Lyness SA: A meta-analysis of controlled trials of neuroleptic treatment in dementia. *J Am Geriatr Soc* 38:553–563, 1990.

Thompson TL, Moran MG, and Niles AS: Psychotropic drug use in the elderly (two parts). *N Engl J Med* 308:134–138, 194–199, 1983.

TWENTY-TWO

REHABILITATION IN THE NURSING HOME

Rehabilitation is the continuing and comprehensive team effort to restore an individual to his or her former functional status or to maintain or maximize remaining function. In the care of nursing home (NH) residents, rehabilitation should not necessarily be viewed as an episodic intervention for a definite period of time or as being appropriate only after the onset of a major disabling illness (e.g., stroke, hip fracture). Rather, rehabilitation involves a plan of care that may need to be continuous and an ongoing team effort. The concept of restoring functioning and/or maximizing remaining function is critical to providing a plan of care to any disabled or potentially disabled older person. Viewed in this way, rehabilitation becomes a *process of delivering the minimal services which help maintain the highest possible level of function.* On the other hand, it should be stressed that for short-stay residents, intensive rehabilitation services may be indicated to allow a rapid return to the home environment.

Table 22–1 describes the principles of rehabilitation in the NH setting. The potential benefits from rehabilitation include improvements in physical and psychological status and quality of life. Successful rehabilitation will lessen perceived dependency as well as reduce the burdens of existing disabilities. The process of rehabilitation follows the same principles outlined in Table 22–1. In order to carry out these principles and achieve the benefits of rehabilitation, a multidisciplinary team must evaluate the resident; establish a problem list with measurable goals; and work out a clear, realistic plan of rehabilitation to achieve these goals.

Table 22-1 Basic principles of rehabilitation in the nursing home

---

Treatment of the underlying disease(s)
Prevention of a secondary disability
Treatment of primary disabilities
Enhancement of residual function
Realistic goals
Emphasis on functional independence
Attention to motivation and other psychological factors
Provision of adaptive tools
Alteration of the environment to maximize function
Team approach

REHABILITATION TEAM

Central to the concept of rehabilitation is the rehabilitation team. This team must be multidisciplinary in membership and interdisciplinary in process. Members of the team traditionally represent the disciplines of physical therapy (PT), occupational therapy (OT), speech therapy (ST), medicine (physician trained in geriatrics or physiatry), social work, nursing, nutrition, and recreational therapy. Table 22–2 describes the role of each member. Chapter 8 discusses the role of teams in NH care in greater detail.

THE PHYSICIAN'S ROLE

The physician's role is to review the assessment and impressions of all team members and to prescribe interventions. The clarity and accuracy of his/her orders is critical for proper compliance and appropriate reimbursement for rehabilitative interventions. The prescribing physician should adhere to the principle of defining a problem (which relates to an ICD diagnosis) and have preferentially a measurable outcome in terms of time line and function. For example, for a resident with a poststroke contracture with measured limitation of range of motion, the physician must document the limitations and functional disability as well as set a goal to improve range of motion by set degrees, with the ability to perform a certain function (e.g., combing) to be attained within a given time (e.g., 7 days). The prescription should include the diagnosis, the treatment modality, and the treatment's frequency and duration. Keep in mind that in the NH setting the intensity of intervention for a given dysfunction should be realistic and geared toward achieving the measurable goals; otherwise payment may be denied because of an inappropriate intervention. For example, a resident with the new onset of hemiplegia should have at least three rehabilitation treatments per week, using several physical modalities, for 4 to 5 weeks. One therapy session per

Table 22-2   Rehabilitation team members in the nursing home

Physical therapist	Focuses on improvement of range of motion, strength, endurance, balance, and mobility through exercise and training with assistive devices
Occupational therapist	Focuses on activities of daily living (ADL) such as eating, grooming, dressing, and bathing as well as improving upper extremity function; may also help to compensate for visual perceptual or sensory deficits
Speech therapist	Evaluates and treats disorders of communication, speech, and swallowing
Nurse/restorative nurse's aid	Reinforces the techniques learned in physical and occupational therapy and helps to develop bowel and bladder training programs
Geriatrician/physiatrist	Provides comprehensive medical and functional evaluation and prescribes the program of therapy
Nutritionist	Provides nutritional assessment, makes recommendations for interventions, and implements interventions as prescribed
Social worker	Provides a psychosocial evaluation and assessment of mood and motivation, maintains liaison with family members; provides family support, and coordinates discharge planning
Recreation therapist	Provides evaluation for leisure-time activities; assists resident in ajusting to new situation and learning new recreational activities; utilizes music, exercise, arts and crafts

week for a NH resident may be determined by a Medicare Part B intermediary as too little therapy for the level of function expected. In contrast, therapy daily may be disallowed because the resident is too impaired and should be a candidate for an acute care hospital rehabilitation center. Issues surrounding reimbursement for rehabilitation are discussed at the end of this chapter.

TYPES OF REHABILITATION

Rehabilitation can involve either *restorative* or *maintenance* therapy. In *restorative* therapy, the goal is to reverse disability and improve function. Restorative therapy is exemplified by the NH resident disabled by a hip fracture or stroke with hemiplegia who needs rehabilitation in order to regain function and/or compensate for functional impairments. This therapy is usually quite intense, taking at least $1\frac{1}{2}$ h per day for a determined period of time (e.g., 4 to 12 weeks). *Maintenance* therapy has the goal of preserving the present level of function and preventing secondary complications (see Table 22–3). It may be less intense and of longer duration than restorative therapy. For example, ongoing bi-weekly therapy may be given to a resident who had a stroke 4 months earlier and has already had a restorative therapy program but for whom continuing therapy can prevent contractures and a "frozen" shoulder. Similarly, maintenance therapy for the acutely ill bed-ridden resident might include bedside range-of-motion exercises, frequent changes of position to prevent pressure sores, and progressive active assistance and exercise to provide easy ambulation and prevent severe deconditioning. These tasks are frequently delegated to restorative nurse's aides (RNA) and certified nurse's aids (CNA). Table 22–4 lists some examples of specific orders for common conditions requiring rehabilitation in the NH.

REHABILITATION POTENTIAL

While cure or complete restoration of function may sometimes be an unrealistic goal in the geriatric population, most NH residents may achieve benefits from the rehabilitation process. The resident and family may gain psychological benefit because they perceive that something can be done to improve function. This may also result in increased self-esteem for the resident. Quality of life may be enhanced as the resident regains control over bodily functions and interacts with therapists or other caregivers. The burden of disability may be diminished by small improvements in the ability to perform activities of daily living. For example, even an improvement in the ability to transfer from bed to chair can greatly affect quality of life and the

Table 22-3 Secondary complications preventable by rehabilitation in the nursing home

Anorexia
Confusion/delirium
Contractures
Deconditioning
Depression
Falls
Fecal impaction/incontinence
Pneumonia
Pressure sores
Psychological dependency
Urinary incontinence
Urinary tract infection
Venous thrombosis

Table 22-4 Examples of specific physician orders for conditions commonly requiring rehabilitation in the nursing home

Condition	Speech therapy orders
Swallowing disorder due to Parkinson's disease (ICD9-787.2)	Dysphagia (swallowing) evaluation by speech therapy Dysphagia treatment by speech therapy five times weekly (twice per day) for 30 days to increase oral motor strength and control and safety of swallow
Aphasia due to stroke (ICD9-784.3)	Speech therapy evaluation Speech and language therapy five times weekly for 30 days to increase functional receptive and expressive language, cognition, and memory
Dysarthria (slurred speech) due to stroke (ICD9-784.5)	Speech evaluation and follow-up treatment as indicated Speech therapy five times weekly for 30 days to increase oral motor strength/control and functional speech intelligibility
Hearing loss (ICD9-388.01)	Speech and language evaluation Speech and language therapy three times weekly for 30 days to increase use of amplification device and improve lip-reading and functional communication skills

Condition/problem	Physical therapy order
Acute vertebral fracture (ICD9-805.0)	Physical therapy evaluation Hot packs, massage, ultrasound, electrical stimulation three times a week for 30 days for diagnosis of acute vertebral fracture
Proximal muscle weakness due to arthritis (ICD9-726.5)	Physical therapy for gait and transfer exercises three times a week for 30 days for diagnosis of right hip arthritis
Right femur fracture, status post ORIF (ICD9-820.0)	Transfer and gait training and exercise five times a week for 30 days for diagnosis of right hip fracture
CVA with right hemiplegia (ICD9-346.0)	Gait training and transfer exercises five times a week for 30 days
Lumbosacral spondylosis without radiculopathy (ICD9-721.3)	Hot packs, massage, ultrasound, exercise three times a week for 30 days
Gait disturbance due to weakness after acute hospitalization (ICD9-780.7)	Gait training and exercise three times week for 30 days
Parkinson's disease (ICD9-332.0)	Gait training and exercise three times a week for 30 days

	Occupational therapy
Acute flareup of left shoulder arthritis with acute decreased ADLs (ICD9-716.91)	Compensatory ADL training Use of adaptive equipment as needed Upper extremity therapeutic activities three times a week for 30 days

Table 22-4 (*Continued*)   Examples of specific physician orders for conditions commonly requiring rehabilitation in the nursing home

Condition/problem	Occupational therapy
Acute decreased ADLs and weakness due to acute hospitalization (ICD9-799.3)	Therapeutic activities to increase functional endurance Feeding program Compensatory ADL training three times a week for 30 days Use of adaptive equipment as needed
Left hip fracture (ICD9-820.8)	Compensatory ADL training Use of adaptive equipment as needed to assist with ADL performance
Acute decreased ADLs due to acute vertebral compression fractures	Compensatory ADL training with safety instruction three times a week for 30 days Instruction in use of adaptive equipment as needed

burden of care. Subjective feelings of dependency may be alleviated by increased self-confidence and reduced perceived dependency. Some studies have alluded to the fact that individuals who undergo rehabilitation live longer than those who have not attempted rehabilitation. While data are limited, a rehabilitation program may also reduce the future costs of institutionalized care. Accordingly, the prospect of long-term institutionalization should not exclude NH residents from rehabilitation services.

Because of the possibility of benefiting from either restorative or maintenance rehabilitation therapy, all residents should be assessed for their rehabilitation potential. The most common impairments in older NH residents that may benefit from rehabilitation therapy are best quantified by a comprehensive functional assessment. Rehabilitation is most useful in trying to restore and/or maintain independence in basic ADLs, including (1) mobility, (2) transferring, (3) feeding, and (4) grooming and dressing. These functions are critical in determining the resident's degree of independence and need for assistance. The rehabilitation potential for each resident should be assessed within 7 days of admission by the physician and a note to this effect should be placed in the medical record.

Coexisting medical conditions such as peripheral vascular disease, significant arthritis, and neurologic disease (e.g., peripheral neuropathy) may adversely affect rehabilitation potential. Dementia may also have a significant adverse effect on the potential to benefit from rehabilitation, especially restorative forms of therapy. Nursing home residents with dementia should not, however, automatically be excluded from restorative therapy (e.g., gait training after hip fracture), because many residents with moderately or even severely advanced dementia may benefit. Virtually all NH residents, regardless of how cognitively impaired, can benefit from an ongoing maintenance rehabilitation program.

The following sections will briefly discuss principles of rehabilitation for common impairments of basic ADL function in the NH population.

CHAIR-BOUND RESIDENTS

The resident most often forgotten in a rehabilitation program is the bedfast or chair-bound person. The first goal of rehabilitation in these residents is to prevent contractures. These residents should have their upper and lower limbs moved through a complete range of motion on a twice-daily basis. To maintain functionality, the upper limbs should be actively or passively moved so that the hand touches the back of the head and the chest. For the lower limbs, it is important that the resident lie on his/her stomach and that the leg be lifted backward, at least 10°. This maintains adequate hip movements for walking. If pain occurs during range-of-motion exercises, an evaluation to determine the cause of the pain should be undertaken. This may require a consultation by a physiatrist or rheumatologist. If the resident already has contractures, passive stretching or the use of weights and/or splints may be helpful. In some of these residents, surgery may restore some function and prevent complications.

For chair-bound residents, a 15 to 20 min group exercise program should be provided four to five times a week. For some of these residents, supervised aerobic exercises in a swimming pool may be especially helpful. Recently it was reported that a strength-training program (lower extremity weight lifting) had a major impact on gait and balance in 90-year-old NH residents. In a program carried out by one of us, we found highly positive responses to a once-a-week walking program among residents who had been chair-bound for 3 months or longer. This program resulted in an improvement in gait and balance, an increase in morale, and a decrease in use of restraints.

IMPAIRMENT OF GAIT AND MOBILITY

Normal gait is characterized by smooth, symmetrical movement of arms, trunk, and legs. A normal gait requires coordination of weight shifts and pelvic rotation to achieve elongation of the weight-bearing side and flexion of the non-weight-bearing side. Pelvic mobility, balance, and adequate base of support are important factors influencing gait. Normal gait is composed of two phases. The *stance phase* occurs when the foot contacts the floor and bears weight. It begins when the heel strikes the floor, the midfoot and forefoot bear weight, and the heel and midfoot leave the floor as hip and knee flexion begin and the foot pushes off. This phase comprises 60 percent of normal gait. The *swing phase* of gait is the time during which the foot swings through and is clearing the floor. This phase begins when the forefoot leaves the floor and ends when the heel strikes the floor. During this phase the pelvis remains level and the hip and knee sweep through flexion and extension.

An important problem in NH residents is backward leaning. This often develops when a resident spends a period of time in a chair, with resulting contractures in the back muscles. These contractures can, in turn, result in backward leaning and poor standing balance. Having the resident move objects around on a table in front of the chair for 15 to 20 min per day will help to prevent and treat back contractures.

Table 22–5 describes common conditions leading to functional impairments of gait in NH residents. Interventions to improve ambulation consist of physical and occupational therapy, both utilizing assistive devices. Table 22–6 summarizes the most commonly used devices and their indications. Figure 22–1 depicts examples of some devices. The assessment of gait and balance is discussed further in Chap. 14.

BALANCE TRAINING

Balance is important for stability in chair-bound residents during transfers, while standing, and while walking. Physical therapy techniques are now available to improve balance in all of these residents. Catching a beach ball while in a chair improves balance for the chair-bound. Stability devices that fit around the waist and allow residents to stand safely while they catch a ball or work on a pegboard in front of them can improve standing balance, as can exercises done with the assistance of parallel bars. Walking between parallel bars can lead to marked improvement of balance and confidence.

Table 22-5 Common conditions leading to functional impairment among nursing home residents

	Functional impairment
Right hemispheric stroke	Visual loss, sensory loss, distortion of spatial relations, lack of motivation, hemiplegia
Left hemispheric stroke	Disturbances of communication (e.g., aphasia), hemiplegia
Hip fracture	Gait instability
Spinal stenosis	Gait instability, proximal muscle weakness
Peripheral neuropathy	Loss of perception, hand-grip weakness
Arthritis (pain, contractures)	Gait instability, muscle weakness
Peripheral vascular disease	Limited mobility, muscle weakness
Parkinsonism	Rigidity, impaired coordination, gait instability, muscle weakness

Table 22-6 Examples of assistive devices for impaired mobility

Assistive devices	Characteristics	Indications	Advantages/disadvantages	Caveats
Single-pronged cane	Simplest device for ambulation Minimal support (25% of body weight is supported)	Unilateral deficits such as arthritis, fracture, or hemiplegia	Light, socially acceptable	Should be held on the unaffected side
Tripod/quad cane	Significantly more support	Same as single-pronged cane	Clumsy to maneuver; physically unattractive	Length of cane should allow 30° of elbow flexion
Pickup walker or hemiwalker	Provides substantial balance	More than localized impairment of function	Energy-consuming; requires upper extremity strength to coordinate a step forward with lifting the walker	Environmental hazards become obstacles; resident must be trained
Front-wheeled roller walker	Provides slightly less balance than pickup walker	For more impaired individuals	Requires less energy, strength, and standing balance	Environmental hazards become obstacles; resident must be trained
Walker with forearm troughs or handles; crutches	Good support	For individuals with painful and deformed hand, wrist, or elbow joint (e.g., rheumatoid arthritis)		Same as for other walkers

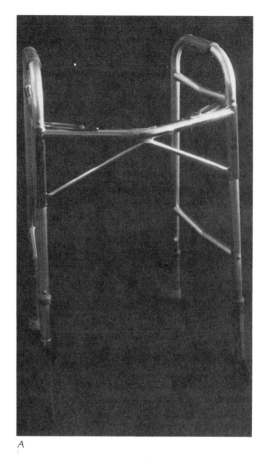

A

Figure 22-1 Examples of assistive devices for ambulation A. Front-wheeled walker.

Abnormalities of posture can also lead to balance problems. These abnormalities can be detected using a plumb line suspended from the ceiling. Specific exercise programs can help correct defects in posture. Muscle weakness can also contribute to instability, and this is responsive to strength-building exercises.

TRANSFERRING

As mentioned earlier, the ability to transfer may be critical to a NH resident's quality of life, his/her need for institutional care, and the burden of that care.

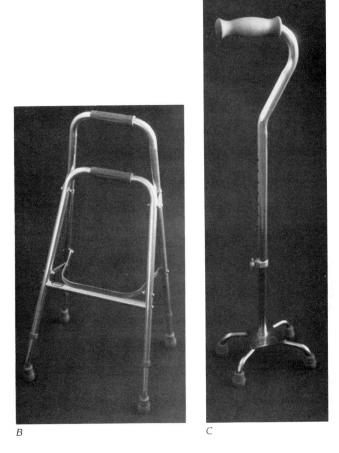

Figure 22-1 (Continued) B. hemi-walker, C. quad cane.

A transfer is a movement by which the resident goes from one surface to another. Safe and efficient transfers require a combination of physical and perceptual capabilities, proper equipment, and training techniques that are suitable for the resident's abilities. Sitting balance is also an important prerequisite for safe transfers. To transfer safely, the resident must be free of or have only minimal orthostatic hypotension and be capable of maintaining the hip and knee in a position of extension. Strong shoulder adduction and abduction, elbow flexion and extension, and hand or wrist function on one side are also required. Table 22–7 summarizes the most common transfers that the NH resident may need to learn and techniques for training for such transfers.

Table 22-7   Transfer techniques

	Process	Aids	Barriers
Bed to wheelchair (stand-pivot transfer)	Sitting position: Lock brakes Grasp side rails of bed Standing position: Grasp to wheelchair with unaffected side and sit down	Sliding board; person with belt	Dementia, obesity Neglect of affected side Upper- or lower-extremity disability Orthostatic hypotension
Wheelchair to toilet	Rise from wheelchair Stand Pivot onto toilet Must be able to manage clothing and undergarments	Toilet seat 20 in. from floor or raised toilet seat Hand rails on unaffected side	Dementia, depression, obesity Neglect of affected side Upper- or lower-extremity disability Orthostatic hypotension
Tub transfer (rarely required in NH because supervision is mandated)	Transfer from wheelchair to bench Move lower extremity with normal hand into tub	Tub transfer bench	Dementia, obesity Neglect of affected side Upper- or lower-extremity disability Orthostatic hypotension

FEEDING, BATHING, AND DRESSING

The evaluation of a resident for feeding, grooming, and dressing rehabilitation should determine whether weakness, limited range of motion, incoordination, spasticity, or perceptual loss is the primary or sole impairment. This evaluation is usually conducted by the physician and the occupational therapist. Interventions generally consist of exploiting the preserved functions and enhancing the affected functions as much as possible.

Awareness of subtle deficits such as visual and perceptual spatial distortions or lack of motivation associated with right hemispheric stroke may guide the rehabilitation program by exploiting the unaffected side and providing assistance for those with impaired judgment and safety awareness. Left hemispheric stroke victims usually have preserved perceptual functions but may suffer from aphasia and communication problems that can affect their rehabilitation. In these cases, use of communication boards, picture books, and gestures may be necessary.

Impaired feeding, grooming, and dressing can also result from rigidity and lack of coordination, as seen in Parkinson's disease. Therapy consists of gradual resistive exercise to increase the strength of muscles governing gross motor activity as well as mobility. Energy-saving techniques are also an important component of rehabilitation in these areas, since fatigue aggravates incoordination. Foods that eliminate the need for cutting, chopping, or mixing may be a useful consideration. Weighted utensils and items with double handles that can easily be gripped will also partially counteract the effects of incoordination. Stabilization can be achieved by using a spike board, rubber mat, or sponges. Oversized bowls can be used to avoid spillage by extension movements or tremor. Figure 22–2 depicts examples of eating utensils that may be beneficial in helping functionally impaired individuals regain independence in feeding.

For cognitively impaired residents who have difficulty with eating, feeding programs may be very valuable. Initiation of a feeding program should be preceded by a thorough swallowing and nutritional history as well as feeding trials to ascertain the resident's food preferences and the optimal food textures. This type of approach may prevent irreversible malnutrition in NH residents. Speech therapists are often well trained to assess and participate in the management of NH residents with feeding problems. Impairment in grooming and dressing (i.e., ADL impairment) often results from limited range of motion related to a frozen shoulder, arthritis or spasticity, or contracture from a previous stroke. The act of reaching as well as manual dexterity may be impaired, so that functions such as buttoning clothes are a problem. The goal of rehabilitation in these situations is to enhance the ability to reach and to enhance manual dexterity. Environmental alteration and devices may be helpful. Velcro closures in lieu of buttons, slip-on dressing aids (especially for socks), and long-reach zipper pulls are examples of

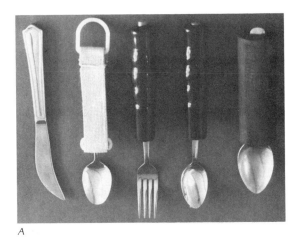

A

Figure 22–2 Examples of utensils for handicapped individuals. *A.* Utensils including a rocking knife for use by a single hand and spoons and forks for individuals with difficulty grasping.

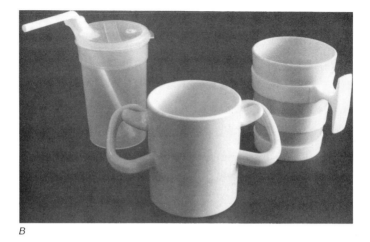

B

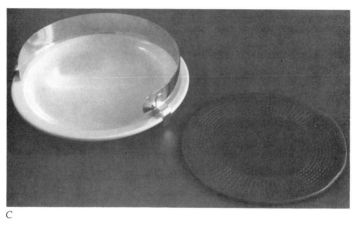

C

Figure 22-2 (Continued) B. Drinking cups for individuals with difficulty holding a cup. C. Plate with guard to facilitate cutting and skidless mat to prevent plate from moving, used mainly for individuals with hemiparesis.

devices that may help some residents regain independence in these functions.

HEAT AND COLD MODALITIES

Heat and cold modalities can play an important role in alleviating pain while undergoing physical therapy. Ultrasound can be particularly useful for pain associated with movement of the hip or shoulders. Local heat is used to allow immediate movement and to decrease pain following movement, while cold is applied for some time (10 to 15 min) before movement to anesthetize the area to be moved.

ORTHOTICS

An orthotic is an externally applied device used to modify structural and functional characteristics of the musculoskeletal system. The goals of orthotics are to

- Relieve pain
- Immobilize and protect weak, painful, or healing musculoskeletal structures
- Reduce axial load
- Prevent and correct deformity
- Improve function

A nomenclature has been devised for orthotics consisting of a series of letters that are the first letters of the English anatomic name of the joints that are crossed by the device, ending with the letter "o." Tables 22–8 and 22–9 describe various types of orthotics that may be useful in the NH.

Table 22-8   Lower limb orthotics

Orthotics	Indication	Purpose/comments
Ankle/foot orthosis (AFO)	Limited weight bearing Alignment	Limb weakness due to stroke
Knee/ankle/foot orthosis (KAFO)	Essentially an AFO with additional joint surrounding the knee Provides more stability	Severe weakness of lower extremity (e.g., hemiplegia); resident needs to be able to lock/unlock a simple hinge
Cervico-thoracic lumbosacral orthosis (CTLSO; Milwaukee Brace)	Worn 23 h a day to correct vertebral compression fracture, cervical disk disease	Pain relief Maintain adequate posture
Simple corset	Vertebral compression fracture	Pain relief Should be fitted Sold over the counter
Rigid brace	Multiple vertebral fractures	Stability Pain relief Reduce deconditioning by early mobilization Not well suited for older patients
Cervical collar (may include occipital and mandibular projections)	Cervical disk disease	Limit range of motion Should be fitted to prevent ischemia

Table 22-9   Upper extremity orthotics

Orthosis	Indication	Purpose
Wrist/hand orthosis	Stroke, carpal tunnel syndrome	Immobilize Improve alignment Assist in restoring function
Splint	Stroke Lower motor lesions Rheumatoid arthritis	Maintain position of flaccid or paretic extremity
Cockup splint	Carpal tunnel syndrome	Reduce nerve entrapment at night
Heat-moldable plastic orthosis	Interphalangeal joint immobilizer	Reduce tendency to subluxation and prevent ulnar deviation
Static interphalangeal joint orthosis	Proximal interphalangeal joint involvement	Prevent "swan neck" deformities

PROSTHETICS

The most common cause of amputation in the geriatric population is peripheral vascular disease. Thus, the majority of prostheses are prescribed for the lower extremities. The site of anatomic amputation is an important consideration. Preserving the knee joint decreases the energy required for walking and preserves proprioception.

The decision to perform a lower extremity amputation in an older individual is a major issue that requires careful weighing of risks and benefits. It involves a thorough preoperative assessment and interventions to stabilize any active medical problems. Postoperative care should be discussed before the operation, and potential problems such as pain and phantom-limb sensation should be mentioned.

Fitting protheses in the elderly in general, and in NH residents in particular, calls for some special considerations. In below-knee amputations, a prosthesis decreases energy requirements but still requires one-third more energy than before the amputation. Proprioception is more likely to be preserved with below-knee amputation, which helps to maintain balance. Above-knee amputations should be avoided, because thereafter ambulation requires two-thirds more energy than before the amputation. Table 22–10 outlines some general principles of postoperative care of amputees. Adequate nutrition, controlling blood sugar in diabetics, and meticulous local care to the suture site are important for fitting a prothesis successfully. Intensive physical therapy should begin even before the prosthesis is fitted, because it may take weeks for the edema to subside to the point where the prosthesis can be fitted. Some NH residents with moderate to severe dementia may not be candidates for a prosthesis if the eventual goal of ambulation is unrealistic due to impaired cognitive function.

Table 22-10   Basic principles of postoperative rehabilitation for amputees

Prevent contractures by range-of-motion exercises
Use compression bandages to prevent hemorrhage and decrease edema (be cautious not to obliterate arterial flow)
Meticulous local care to suture site to keep stump clear of infection
Provide adequate nutrition
Control concomitant medical conditions (e.g., diabetes, heart failure)
Mobilize stump as soon as possible
Socket of prosthesis should evenly contact the entire skin surface and fit snugly
Observe stump carefully for breakdown when ambulation with prosthesis begins

MEASURING REHABILITATION

Measuring progress toward the goal or goals of a restorative rehabilitation program is critical to planning subsequent therapy as well as to reimbursement. While progress can be measured in a semistructured manner, some of the standardized instruments used to assess function are suitable for measuring baseline function and change with time during the rehabilitation process. Some of these instruments are discussed throughout this text and will be mentioned only briefly here in the context of rehabilitation.

The Barthel Index (Table 22–11) assesses self-care and ambulation in

Table 22-11   The Barthel Index

Activities rated by examiner	Points for performance[a]	
	Independently	With help
Feeding (if food needs to be cut = help)	10	5
Moving from wheelchair to bed (includes sitting up in bed)	15	10–5
Personal toilet (wash face, comb hair, shave, clean teeth)	5	0
Getting on and off toilet (handling clothes, wipe, flush)	10	5
Bathing self	5	0
Walking on level surface	15	10
Propel wheelchair (score only if unable to walk)	5	0
Ascend and descend stairs	10	5
Dressing (includes tying shoes, fastening fasteners)	10	5
Controlling bowels	10	5
Controlling bladder	10	5

[a] Total possible points = 100.

slightly broader ranges than Katz ADL scale (Table 22–12). It includes stair climbing and wheelchair use, is administered by an interviewer on the basis of judgment or observation, and is particularly useful in the rehabilitation setting. It is not as useful as scales such as the Katz for detecting and following progress of minor impairments. The Minimum Data Set, created by the Health Care Financing Administration for use in all NHs, also contains items that may be useful for following the functional status of a resident undergoing rehabilitation (Table 22–13). Other comprehensive instruments are complex and time-consuming, and some have limited use in cognitively impaired individuals.

Because dementia can influence the outcomes of rehabilitation and cognitive function can change during rehabilitation, some type of cognitive assessment should be performed. Cognitive function can be screened by using the Folstein Mini-Mental State Examination (MMSE), which has a fairly broad range of sensitivity and will detect moderate—but not mild or subtle—impairment (see Chap. 9). This test is fairly quick to administer and is helpful for detecting changes over time. Other tests are either insensitive to change over time or able to detect only gross cognitive dysfunction (e.g., Short Portable Mental Status Questionnaire) or are too long to administer repeatedly to NH residents (e.g., Wechsler Memory Scale). For a geriatric rehabilitation center or skilled nursing facility, the MMSE is a reasonable choice. More in-depth mental function assessments should be reserved for selected residents with disabilities who score well on the MMSE.

Assessment of mood or emotional state may be important because of the prevalence of depression after major medical illnesses (e.g., stroke) and the importance of motivation to the rehabilitation process. The Geriatric Depression Scale (GDS) can be either self-administered or administered by an interviewer, is quick and reliable, and avoids somatic questions. It is good for establishing a baseline description and for monitoring progress (see Chap. 10). Although the GDS has not been evaluated among medically ill elderly in NHs, it is probably the best scale available for use in a NH rehabilitation program.

REIMBURSEMENT FOR REHABILITATION

Rehabilitation services are reimbursed predominantly by Medicare and to a lesser degree by other programs. Familiarity with the basic principles that govern these programs is essential for the primary physician and the medical director. Knowledge of Medicare guidelines will facilitate appropriate and realistic care planning.

Rehabilitative services after an acute hospitalization for conditions such as stroke, hip fracture, major abdominal surgery, or infection requiring ongoing parenteral antibiotics (e.g., osteomyelitis) are usually covered by Part A

Table 22-12   Katz Index of independence in activities of daily living

The index of independence in activities of daily living is based on an evaluation of the functional independence or dependence of patients in bathing, dressing, going to the toilet, transferring, continence, and feeding. Specific definitions of functional independence and dependence appear below the index.

A. Independent in feeding, continence, transferring, toileting, dressing, and bathing.
B. Independent in all but one of these functions.
C. Independent in all but bathing and one additional function.
D. Independent in all but bathing, dressing, and one additional function.
E. Independent in all but bathing, dressing, toileting, and one additional function.
F. Independent in all but bathing, dressing, toileting, transferring, and one additional function.
G. Dependent in all six functions.

Other Dependent in at least two functions but not classifiable as C, D, E, or F. Independence means without supervision, direction, or active personal assistance except as specifically noted below. This is based on actual status and not on ability. Patients who refuse to perform a function are considered as not performing the function, even though they are deemed able.

Bathing (sponge, shower, or tub)
Independent: needs assistance only in bathing a single part (as back or disabled extremity) or bathes self completely

Dependent: needs assistance in bathing more than one part of body and in getting in or out of tub or does not bathe self

Dressing
Independent: gets clothes from closets and drawers; puts on clothes, outer garments, braces; manages fasteners; act of tying shoes is excluded
Dependent: does not dress self or remains partly undressed

Toileting
Independent: gets to toilet; gets on and off toilet; arranges clothes, cleans organs of excretion (may manage own bedpan used at night only and may not be using mechanical supports)
Dependent: uses bedpan or commode or receives assistance in getting to and using toilet

Transfer
Independent: moves in and out of bed independently and moves in and out of chair independently (may or may not be using mechanical supports)

Dependent: assistance in moving in or out of bed and/or chair; does not perform one or more transfers

Continence
Independent: urination and defecation entirely self-controlled
Dependent: partial or total incontinence in urination or defecation, partial or total control by enemas, catheters, or regulated use of urinals and/or bedpans

Feeding
Independent: gets food from plate or its equivalent into mouth (precutting of meat and preparation of food, as buttering bread, are excluded from evaluation)
Dependent: assistance in act of feeding (see above); does not eat at all or receives parenteral feeding

Table 22-13 Selected items from the Minimum Data Set relating to functional status and rehabilitation

Customary routines
1. Cycle of daily events
    _____ Stays up late at night (e.g., after 9 p.m.)
    _____ Goes out 1 or more days a week
    _____ Stays busy with hobbies, reading, or fixed daily routine
    _____ Spends most time alone or watching TV
    _____ Moves independently indoors (with appliances, if used)
    _____ None of above
2. Eating patterns
    _____ Distinct food preferences
    _____ Eats between meals all or most days
    _____ Use of alcoholic beverage(s) at least weekly
    _____ None of above
3. ADL patterns
    _____ In bedclothes much of day
    _____ Wakens to toilet all or most nights
    _____ Has irregular bowel movement pattern
    _____ Prefers showers for bathing
    _____ None of above
4. Involvement patterns
    _____ Daily contact with relatives/close friends
    _____ Usually attends church, temple, synagogue (etc.)
    _____ Finds strength in faith
    _____ Daily animal companion/presence
    _____ Involved in group activities
    _____ None of above
    _____ Unknown—resident/family unable to provide information

Cognitive patterns
1. Comatose (no discernible consciousness/persistent vegetative state)
    0. No   1. Yes
2. Memory (recall of what was learned or known)
    a. Short-term (seems/appears to recall after 5 min)
        0. Memory OK   1. Memory problem
    b. Long-term (seems/appears to recall long past)
        0. Memory OK   1. Memory problem
3. Memory/recall ability (check all that resident normally able to recall during last 7 days)
    _____ Current season
    _____ That he/she is in a nursing home
    _____ Location of own room/facility
    _____ Staff names/faces
    _____ None of above are recalled
4. Cognitive skills for daily decision making (decisions regarding tasks of daily life)
    0. Independent—decisions consistent/reasonable
    1. Modified independence—some difficulty in new situations only
    2. Moderately impaired—decisions poor; cues/supervision required
    3. Severely impaired—never/rarely makes decisions
5. Indicators of delirium (periodic disordered thinking/awareness)
    _____ Less alert, easily distracted
    _____ Changing awareness of environment
    _____ Episodes of incoherent speech
    _____ Judgment less reliable
    _____ None of above
6. Change in cognitive status
    0. No change   1. Improved   2. Deteriorated

Table 22-13 (*Continued*)   Selected items from the Minimum Data Set relating to functional status and rehabilitation

Communication/hearing patterns
1. Hearing (with hearing appliance, if used)
   - 0. Hears adequately—normal talk, TV, phone
   - 1. Minimal difficulty when not in quiet listening conditions
   - 2. Hears in special situation only—speaker has to adjust tonal quality and speak distinctly
   - 3. Highly impaired/absence of useful hearing
2. Communication devices/techniques
   - _____ Hearing aid, present and used
   - _____ Hearing aid, present and not used
   - _____ Other receptive communication technique used (e.g., lip reading)
   - _____ None of above
3. Modes of expression

_____ Speech	_____ Signs/gestures/sounds
_____ Writing messages to express or clarify needs	_____ Communication board
	_____ Other
	_____ None of above

4. Making self understood (express information content—however able)
   - 0. Understood
   - 1. Usually understood
   - 2. Sometimes understood
   - 3. Rare/never understood
5. Ability to understand others (understanding verbal information content, however able)
   - 0. Understood
   - 1. Usually understood
   - 2. Sometimes understood
   - 3. Rare/never understood
6. Change in communication
   - 0. No change   1. Improved   2. Deteriorated

Vision patterns
1. Vision (ability to see in adequate light and with glasses if used)
   - 0. Adequate—sees fine detail, including regular print in newspapers/books
   - 1. Impaired—sees large print but not regular print in newspapers/books
   - 2. Highly impaired—limited vision, not able to see newspaper headlines, appears to follow objects with eyes
   - 3. Severely impaired—no vision—e.g., may/appears to see light, color, or shapes
2. Visual limitations/difficulties
   - _____ Side vision problems—decreased peripheral vision; e.g., leaves food on one side of tray, difficulty traveling, bumps into people and objects, misjudges placement of chair when seating self
   - _____ Experiences any of following: see halos or rings around lights, sees flashes of light, sees "curtains" over eyes
   - _____ None of above
3. Visual appliances (glasses, contact lenses, lens implant)
   - 0. No   1. Yes

ADL
1. Basic ADL (code for most support provided)
   - 0. No setup or physical help from staff
   - 1. Setup help only
   - 2. One-person physical assist
   - 3. Physical assist from two or more persons
   - a. Bed mobility: How resident moves to and from lying position, turns from side to side, and positions body while in bed
   - b. Transfer: How resident moves between surfaces—to/from bed, chair, wheelchair, standing position (*exclude* to/from bath/toilet)
   - c. Locomotion: How resident moves between locations in his/her room and adjacent corridor on same floor. If in wheelchair, self-sufficiency once in chair
   - d. Dressing: How resident puts on, fastens, and takes off all items of street clothing, including donning/removing prosthesis

Table 22-13 (*Continued*) Selected items from the Minimum Data Set relating to functional status and rehabilitation

ADL (*continued*)

    e. Eating: How resident eats and drinks (regardless of skill)

    f. Toilet use: How resident uses the toilet room (or commode, bedpan, urinal); transfers on/off toilet, cleanses, changes pad, manages ostomy or catheter, adjusts clothes

    g. Personal hygiene: How resident maintains personal hygiene, including combing hair, brushing teeth, shaving, applying makeup, washing/drying face, hands, and perineum (exclude baths and showers)

2. Bathing (how resident takes full-body bath, sponge bath, and transfers in/out of tub/shower)

    0. Independent—no help provided

    1. Supervision—oversight help only

    2. Physical help limited to transfer only

    3. Physical help in part of bathing activity

    4. Total dependence

3. Body-control problems

    _____ Balance—partial or total loss of ability to balance self while standing

    _____ Bedfast all or most of the time

    _____ Contracture to arms, legs, shoulders, or hands

    _____ Hemiplegia/hemiparesis

    _____ Quadriplegia

    _____ Arm—partial or total loss of voluntary movement

    _____ Hand—lack of dexterity (e.g., problem using toothbrush or adjusting hearing aid)

    _____ Leg—partial or total loss of voluntary movement

    _____ Leg—unsteady gait

    _____ Trunk—partial or total loss of ability to position, balance, or turn body

    _____ None of above

4. Mobility appliances/devices

    _____ Cane/walker   _____ Other person wheeled

    _____ Brace/prosthesis   _____ Lifted (manually/mechanically)

    _____ Wheels self   _____ None of above

5. ADL functional potential (check all that apply during last 7 days)

    _____ Resident believes he/she capable of increased independence in at least some ADLs

    _____ Direct-care staff believe resident capable of increased independence in at least some ADLs

    _____ Resident able to perform tasks/activity but is very slow

    _____ Major difference in ADL self-performance or ADL support in mornings and evenings (at least a one-category change in self-performance or support in any ADL)

    _____ None of above

6. Change in ADL function

    0. No change   1. Improved   2. Deteriorated

Continence in last 14 days (code as follows):

    0. Continent—complete control

    1. Usually continent—bladder, incontinent episodes once a week or less; bowel, less than weekly

Table 22-13 (*Continued*)   Selected items from the Minimum Data Set relating to functional status and rehabilitation

Continence in last 14 days (*continued*)
  2. Occasionally incontinent—bladder, two or more times a week but not daily; bowel, once a week
  3. Frequently incontinent—bladder, tended to be incontinent daily, but some control present (e.g., on day shfit); bowel, two to three times a week
  4. Incontinent—Had inadequate control. For bladder, multiple daily episodes; for bowel, all (or almost) of the time
1. Bowel continence (control of bowel movement, with appliance or bowel continence program if employed)
2. Bladder continence (control of urinary bladder function (if dribbles, volume insufficient to soak through underpants), with appliances (e.g., Foley) or continence porgrams if employed)
3. If incontinence of bladder (skip if resident's bladder continence code equals 0 or 1 and no catheter is employed)
  _____ Resident has been tested for a urinary tract infection
  _____ Resident has been checked for presence of a fecal impaction, or there is adequate bowel elimination
  _____ None of above
4. Appliances and programs
  _____ Any scheduled toileting plan
  _____ External (condom) catheter
  _____ Indwelling catheter
  _____ Intermittent catheter
  _____ Did not use toilet room/commode/urinal
  _____ Pads/briefs used
  _____ Enemas/irrigation
  _____ Ostomy
  _____ None of above
5. Change in urinary continence
  0. No change   1. Improved   2. Deteriorated

Oral/nutritional status
1. Oral status
  _____ Chewing problem
  _____ Swallowing problem
  _____ Mouth pain
  _____ None of above
2. Height and weight _____
3. Nutritional problems
  _____ Complains about the taste of many foods
  _____ Insufficient fluid; dehydrated
  _____ Has not consumed all liquids provided at/between meals during last 3 days
  _____ Regular complaint of hunger
  _____ Leaves 25% or more food uneaten at most meals
  _____ None of above
4. Nutritional approaches
  _____ Parenteral/IV
  _____ Feeding tubes
  _____ Mechanically altered diet

Table 22-13 (*Continued*)   Selected items from the Minimum Data Set relating to functional status and rehabilitation

---

Oral/nutritional status (*continued*)
_____ Therapeutic diet
_____ Supplement between meals
_____ None of above

Activity pursuit patterns
1. Average time involved in activities
    0. Most   2. Little
    1. Some   4. None of above
2. Preferred activity settings
    _____ Own room   _____ Outside facility
    _____ Day/activity room   _____ Inside NH/off unit
    _____ None of above
3. General activities preference
    _____ Cards/other games   _____ Crafts/arts
    _____ Spiritual/religious   _____ Trips/shopping
    _____ Exercise   _____ Music
    _____ Read/write   _____ Walking/wheeling outdoors
    _____ Watch TV   _____ None of above

---

of the Medicare program. Table 22–14 describes the criteria currently used by Medicare to determine eligibility for reimbursement for skilled nursing care. Table 22–15 describes requirements for rehabilitation services under Medicare. Rehabilitation for residents who do not qualify for Part A coverage can be provided under Medicare Part B. Most diagnoses can, however, be treated for only a limited time (e.g., 12 to 30 sessions) under Part B.

Appropriate documentation by all team members is critical for a successful rehabilitation program as well as for reimbursement. Physician must write appropriate orders for rehabilitation (see Table 22–4). Ongoing communication by all team members about the progress of therapy and function of the resident are essential. This communication can be carried on by way of legible notes as well as by regular team conferences. Medicare as well as other third-party payers require frequent reevaluations, at least monthly. These reevaluations are generally accomplished by the NH's utilization review committee. This committee usually includes the director of nursing, the medical director and two other physicians, the administrator, and a medical records staff person. In hospital-based skilled nursing facilities—usually referred to as transitional care units (TCU) or facilities with a "distinct part"—the review meeting takes place weekly. These meetings determine the resident's progress and therefore eligibility for ongoing program benefits. The success of any rehabilitation program in a NH depends on the Util-

Table 22-14   Criteria for Medicare reimbursement for skilled nursing care[a]

Patients admitted for rehabilitation should be alert enough to participate and benefit from a program or require skilled nursing procedures/observation at least on a daily basis.
Intravenous feedings, fluids or medication
Enteral tube feedings
Fractures of femur, pelvis, pubic ramus, vertebrae, or multiple fractures
Injectables (e.g., intramuscular antibiotics)
Wound care
Ostomy care and teaching
Skilled ostomy care
Acute diabetic observation (e.g., unstable blood sugars, sliding-scale insulin coverage)
Dialysis in unstable patient
Radiation therapy
Pain management with parenteral medications
Blood transfusions
Respiratory services
Frequent laboratory studies
Frequent diagnostic testing
Physical, occupational, and/or speech therapy (less than 3 h/day)
Chest tubes (no wall suction)
Postoperative supervision
Traction
Skilled nursing observation for an unresolved medical condition
Procedures that cannot be done on an outpatient basis or at a lower level of care
Bowel and bladder training

[a] Based on criteria for admission to a hospital-based skilled nursing unit.

ization Review Committee's familiarity with Medicare guidelines. Lack of this knowledge may deprive many NH residents of their legitimate right to a trial of rehabilitation.

In the next decade, the NH may become the center for rehabilitation of most geriatric patients, replacing other in-patient rehabilitation programs.

Table 22-15   Basic criteria for Medicare coverage of rehabilitation services[a]

Services that require registered therapists
Services must be required daily
The resident must require an in-patient treatment program
The treatment modalities, frequency, and duration must be specifically ordered by the physician
The resident must have a reasonable restorative potential and make significant improvement in a reasonable, generally predictable time period

[a] Physical therapist, occupational therapist, speech therapist.

The NH is conducive for geriatric rehabilitation by providing the option of graded interventions, as opposed to the rigid 3-hour-per-day therapy required in acute rehabilitation units. The cost-effectiveness of rehabilitation in the NH should be measured in terms of the reduction in the burden of care achieved by improved self-care and improved quality of life for residents and families.

SUGGESTED READINGS

Department of Health and Human Services, Health Care Financing Administration: *Outpatient Physical Therapy and Comprehensive Outpatient Rehabilitation Facility Manual.* Revised Material, Chapter 5, Sec. 501, Transmittal No. 79, Washington, D.C., August 1988.

Erickson RV: Principles of rehabilitation, in *Geriatrics Review Syllabus.* New York, American Geriatrics Society, 1988.

Osterweil D: Geriatric rehabilitation in the long term care institutional setting, in Kemp B, Brummel-Smith K, Ramsdell JW (eds): *Geriatric Rehabilitation.* Boston, Little, Brown & Co, 1990.

Yew E, Kropsky B, Neufeld R, Libow L: The Clinical utility of a comprehensive periodic assessment form for the geriatric rehabilitation patient. *Gerontologist* 29:263–267, 1989.

TWENTY-THREE

HOSPICE CARE AND PAIN MANAGEMENT

The appropriate care of the dying is one of the most difficult tasks for the staff in a nursing home (NH). Societal concerns, regulations, and the problems of the staff in dealing with their own mortality can all interfere with allowing the NH resident a "good death." The purpose of this chapter is to delineate management techniques that can improve the quality of the dying process. In addition, this chapter discusses the vexing problem of pain management in NH residents.

HOSPICE CARE

Treatment decisions concerning a dying NH resident require the consensus of the staff as well as that of the resident and his or her family. This often necessitates people of different spiritual and philosophical backgrounds to find a common meeting place. Thus, the first rule of caring for the terminally ill should be that anyone who finds the consensus management plan unacceptable should be allowed to withdraw from the care of that resident. Unfortunately, in most NHs many staff do not accept such an approach in reality. In these situations the staff member should be required to carry out comfort and palliative care but not to actively administer therapies that seem objectionable. Careful education of the interdisciplinary team in the philosophies and principles of hospice care can obviate the development of some of these unpleasant situations.

Hospice care is a concept of helping the dying person and his or her family cope with the dying process in the least painful way possible. The central concept of hospice care is to relieve physical and psychological suffering and to alleviate unwanted symptoms. The objectives of hospice care are outlined in Table 23-1.

Identification of NH residents who should receive hospice care can be extremely difficult. The resident with end-stage untreatable cancer is easily identifiable as a candidate for hospice care. In other cases, however, the need for hospice care is often less apparent. Residents with end-stage dementia, severe weight loss, and recurrent infections are possible candidates for hospice care, as are those with amyotrophic lateral sclerosis, Huntington's disease, or end-stage heart, lung, kidney, or liver failure. A specific group of patients with a subset of unique problems comprises those suffering from acquired immune deficiency syndrome (AIDS). When an individual

Table 23-1 Objectives of hospice care

Objective	Providers
For the resident	
Provide high-quality care	Physician, nurse[a]
Provide adequate pain relief	Physician, nurse
Provide maximum comfort[b]	Nurse, family, physical therapist
Provide psychological support[b]	Physician, nurse, family, psychologist, pastoral case worker, social worker, clergy
Provide appropriate individualized understanding of the dying process	Physician, nurse, social worker
Provide appropriate spiritual support[b]	Clergy, pastoral case worker
Provide assistance with social and financial problems	Social worker
Respect wishes regarding terminal care	Physician, nurse
For the family	
Provide psychological support[b]	Physician, nurse, family, social worker, psychologist, pastoral case worker, clergy
Provide understanding of dying process	Physician, nurse, social worker
Help with interpersonal problems (i.e., resident-family; family-family)	Physician, nurse, social worker
Provide assistance with social and financial problems[b]	Social worker
Provide appropriate spiritual support[b]	Clergy, pastoral care worker
Provide support in the period immediately following death[b]	Physician, nurse, family, psychologist, pastoral care worker, social worker, clergy

[a] Includes nurse assistants.
[b] Volunteers may also play a role in these areas.

with AIDS is admitted to a NH, he or she is generally much younger than the other residents and thus may have greater problems accepting the situation.

Table 23-2 lists the major physical symptoms that may require management in order to maintain comfort among the dying. Treatment of weakness requires appropriate attention to passive and active physical therapy and nutritional status. Among those with a relatively long-term prognosis, testosterone enanthate, 200 mg intramuscularly every 2 weeks, may be useful. Short-term use of prednisone (15 mg daily) may produce euphoric effects.

Treatment of anorexia is difficult. The use of supplements, milk shakes, and favored foods may be helpful. Small meals and snacks should be offered on multiple occasions throughout the day. Antidepressants (except fluoxetine), in particular monoamine oxidase inhibitors, may enhance food intake. Medroxyprogesterone acetate may also increase food intake. Dry mouth can be alleviated by sucking dry ice or candies. Glycerine and citric acid mouthwashes as well as artificial saliva (e.g., Salivart) may also help.

Table 23-2 Physical symptoms requiring management in order to maintain comfort among the dying

Pain	Central nervous system symptoms
Constitutional symptoms	Depression
Weakness	Anxiety/panic
Anorexia	Insomnia
Thirst/dehydration/dry mouth	Delirium
Hypercalcemia	Dementia
Bleeding	Paralysis
Fever	Seizures
Gastrointestinal symptoms	Urinary tract symptoms
Xerostomia	Incontinence
Nausea and vomiting	Urinary retention
Dysgeusia	Bladder spasms
Dysphagia	Urinary tract infection
Diarrhea/constipation	Skin and cosmetic problems
Ascites	Pressure Sores
Abdominal pain	Pruritus
Fecal incontinence	Alopecia
Cardiopulmonary symptoms	Draining fistulas
Halitosis	Fungating growths
Cough	Colostomy
Shortness of breath	
Moist, noisy respirations	
Hiccups	
Thrombosis	
Edema	

Fever should be treated with aspirin or acetaminophen. If these agents are ineffective, indomethacin may be useful. A recent study has suggested that palliative management of fever among male NH residents with end-stage Alzheimer's disease yields the same mortality as when such individuals also receive antibiotics.

If hypercalcemia occurs late in the course of a disease, it may allow a relatively painless death. However, when hypercalcemia occurs early, it may be debilitating. Fluids, corticosteroids, and phosphates will generally control hypercalcemia. Mithramycin in low dosages (1 to 2 mg intravenously twice per week) may produce the best effects in those with terminal cancer.

For the treatment of nausea and vomiting, prochlorperazine syrup (5 mg every 4 h or 25 mg suppositories three times per day) is the treatment of choice. This drug may improve nausea but can have central nervous system side effects. Pain on swallowing due to radiation-induced esophagitis is best treated with oral viscous lidocaine. While nystatin (suspension or troches) remains the treatment of choice for oral candidiasis, clotrimazole troches or ketoconazole may be necessary to obtain symptomatic relief.

Cough can be treated with guaifenesin, hydrocodeine syrup, or benzonatate (tessalon). Use of a vaporizer in order to provide humidification of the air may be useful. Hiccups can be treated by inducing a Valsalva maneuver (this can be done by getting the resident to drink water from the opposite side of a glass). If this fails, chlorpromazine (25 mg three times per day) is the appropriate treatment. Residents with moist, noisy respirations ("death rattle") may respond to transdermal scopolamine or atropine to dry secretions. Severe air hunger during the last few hours of life is best treated with morphine. Sedation is an acceptable method of decreasing awareness of terminal suffocation.

Depression is best treated with low doses of desipramine (25 to 50 mg a day) or trazadone (50 to 100 mg at night) if the resident is agitated. Methylphenidate (Ritalin) can be utilized when short-term arousal from a depressive episode may be beneficial, as when a relative the person has not seen for a while comes to visit.

Hydroxyzine or short-acting benzodiazepines are used for anxiety. Haloperidol (0.5 to 1 mg once or twice per day) is useful for the treatment of hallucinations, delusions, or agitated behaviors that are interfering with care or comfort. An indwelling bladder catheter may be appropriate for the management of incontinence among the terminally ill. Painful bladder spasms due to irritation from the catheter may respond to oxybutynin (2.5 mg three times per day). Pruritus may respond to diphenhydramine, hydroxyzine, or topical triamcinolone cream. A wig should be used for the treatment of hair loss if the resident is upset about his or her appearance. Hydrogen peroxide may decrease the smell associated with fungating lesions, and topical application of epinephrine (1 : 1000 dilution) may decrease capillary bleeding associated with such lesions. Radiation therapy may produce symptomatic relief either by relieving pain or obstruction or shrinking cosmetically the unacceptable tumor.

Table 23-3 lists the most useful orders for NH residents receiving terminal care. For all concerned, adequate hospice care demands that the resident's appearance be maintained throughout the dying process. At all times staff should put comfort measures ahead of medical treatment. Care should be taken not to talk about the resident in a derogatory manner. Finally, the role of the care team does not end with the resident's death. Allowing the family to view the body for a sufficient period of time helps with the "letting go" process. Attendance at the funeral by members of the health care team can also be helpful for both family and caregivers if the dying process is prolonged. The health care team needs to help the family through the bereavement process. This is particularly important when the spouse has no close relatives.

PAIN MANAGEMENT

Little is known about pain among elderly NH residents, although anecdotally it would seem fair to assume that pain is undertreated in NHs. The reasons for this include fear of addiction, fear of side effects of narcotics, problems associated with multiple medications and drug-drug interactions, and a failure to take complaints of pain seriously. Pain has been reported to occur in

Table 23-3   Example of orders for terminal care

Do not transfer to hospital
Do not resuscitate
No routine blood work or radiographs
Foley catheter for relief of urinary retention or incontinence
Turn every 2 h
Do not record intake/output or weights
Activity as tolerated
Ice cubes prn
Analgesics: _____
   Analgesics must be given on schedule and prns as requested.
   (Do *not* make judgments that the resident does not need analgesic or is overreacting)

Antidepressant _____
Anxiolytic _____
Oxygen _____ liters/minute
Antiemetic _____
Allow family visits at all times
Do not restrain unless necessary for comfort

71 percent to 83 percent of NH residents, while the National Nursing Home Survey of 1977 found that only 37 percent were given analgesic medications. In one study of long-term-care residents with an average age of 88.4 years, pain was considered constant in approximately one-third. Fifty-two percent described their pain as severe, horrible, or excruciating. The most common causes of pain in older individuals in the NH are listed in Table 23-4. Pain has been shown to impair involvement in recreational activities and to limit walking; impair posture; cause insomnia; produce anxiety, depression, and constipation; cause anorexia; and interfere with the ability to carry out basic activities of daily living.

Assessment of pain starts with the physician believing the complaint of pain. Older individuals are less likely to complain than younger individuals, yet their complaints are less likely to be taken seriously. Any NH resident with a complaint of pain is entitled to a careful history and examination and appropriate diagnostic tests. In addition, residents with pain should be carefully assessed for depression as well as for their level of anxiety. Although most pain complaints in older individuals are due to organic pathology rather than to psychological causes, identification and treatment of these psychological conditions may be important in the overall management of the pain.

In the geriatric population, several specific pain syndromes need to be considered (Table 23-5). Temporal headaches, with or without pain over the temporal arteries, should prompt consideration of the diagnosis of temporal (cranial) arteritis. Temporal artery biopsy is indicated, as this condition can lead to blindness. Treatment is with high-dose steroids (e.g., 60 mg of prednisone per day). Herpes zoster can be associated with severe pain. Shooting pains may respond to carbamazepine, while deep burning or aching pains respond better to desipramine. Topical capsaicin, a substance-P depleting agent, or transcutaneous electrical nerve stimulation (TENS) may be useful in some cases of post-herpetic neuralgia. Postamputation phantom limb

Table 23-4   Common types and causes of pain in the nursing home

Low back pain	Arthritis
Osteoporosis	knee
Vertebral fractures	hip
Disk disease	shoulder
Lumbar stenosis	Pain from fractures
Myeloma	Neuropathies
Metastatic bone tumors	Leg cramps
Epidural abscess	Claudication
Referred visceral pain	Foot pain
	Neck pain

Table 23-5   Specific pain syndromes common among nursing home residents

Syndrome	Management options
Temporal arteritis	Prednisone 60 mg daily
Herpes zoster	Analgesics Carbamazepine Desipramine Topical capsaicin TENS
Postamputation phantom limb pain	Local anesthetic blocks Narcotics TENS
Degenerative back pain	Analgesics Limited period of bed rest Topical ice or heat Local anesthetic injection Chymopapain injection TENS Surgery
Leg cramps	Potassium and magnesium supplementation (if indicated) Quinine Baclofen Short-acting benzodiazepines
Claudication	Exercise (graded) Lower blood sugar Pentoxifylline Consider evaluation for surgery
Osteoporosis	Flexion exercises Short-term back bracing (1 week maximum) Nonsteroidal anti-inflammatory agents Analgesics Calcitonin

pain is often very difficult to treat. TENS and local anesthetic blocks can be tried, but often narcotics are necessary. Degenerative changes in the spine (osteophyte formation, bulging intervertebral disks, and ligamentum flavum hypertrophy) can cause back pain and pain radiating down the buttocks. Diagnosis is made by computed tomography or magnetic resonance scanning. Treatment involves short periods of bed rest (no more than 4 days at a time), topical ice or heat, and injection of local anesthetics into "trigger points." Chymopapain injections into the disk space may be used. Surgery should be reserved for those with intractable pain or objective weakness due to nerve compression.

Management of leg cramps involves checking that the resident has adequate potassium and magnesium levels. Quinine may be very helpful, but its use should be limited to 3 months at a time because of side effects, such as deafness and dizziness. Some residents with severe cramps respond well to muscle relaxants, such as short-acting benzodiazepines or baclofen. Claudication can be treated by normalizing glucose levels in diabetics and by the use of pertoxifylline. If there is no response, revascularization surgery may be useful in appropriately selected candidates. Osteoporosis associated with vertebral fractures can cause severe pain. Treatment consists of flexion exercises, short-term bracing of the back, and use of nonsteroidal anti-inflammatory agents. Fear of addiction should not lead to the withholding of narcotics for the short-term relief of pain associated with an acute vertebral fracture. Calcitonin may be effective in some instances for relief of pain related to osteoporosis. However, calcitonin therapy may cause hypocalcemia and/or anorexia among NH residents.

A useful strategy for the general management of pain is to have residents who are able to do so record the degree of pain using the Present Pain Intensity Scale of the McGill Pain Questionnaire (Table 23-6). The scale can be repeated just before each dose of pain medication. Where possible, pain should be treated by physical therapy methods such as splinting, exercise (active or passive), application of heat or cold, TENS, or ultrasound. Relaxation therapy and distracting techniques may also be helpful. When pain causes insomnia, the temporary use of short-acting benzodiazepines is appropriate.

Mild to moderate pain that is not inflammatory in nature is best treated first by acetaminophen. If it is inflammatory, it is best treated by enteric-coated aspirin. Nonsteroidal anti-inflammatory agents (ibuprofen, naproxen, etc.) are excellent for arthritic pain. Residents on nonsteroidal anti-inflammatory agents should be checked regularly (e.g., every 1 to 2 months) to exclude gastrointestinal tract bleeding by examining the stool for occult blood and/or by measuring the blood hemoglobin value. Among those who have had a bleed on these agents, the addition of misoprostol should be

Table 23-6   Present pain intensity scale of the McGill Pain Questionnaire[a]

1 = Mild
2 = Discomfort
3 = Severe
4 = Horrible
5 = Excruciating

[a] This scale may be helpful in evaluating the need for or response to analgesics.

considered, but diarrhea often develops at doses that provide adequate cytoprotection.

Codeine is an excellent second-tier analgesic. It is best used in combination with aspirin or acetaminophen. The major side effect of codeine is constipation, which responds well to lactulose therapy. Propoxyphene hydrochloride has a high addiction potential. It provides only weak pain relief and should rarely if ever be used in NH residents.

For severe pain, morphine is the drug of choice. Morphine can be given orally at six times the intramuscular dose. Methadone, which can be given once a day because of its long half-life, is a useful drug for relief of chronic pain. The addition of a nonsteroidal anti-inflammatory drug to morphine or methadone therapy may increase the potency of these drugs. Medication for severe pain should be given regularly rather than on an as-needed basis. In residents undergoing hospice care, the use of diluted intravenous morphine every 2 h until pain relief is obtained is a reasonable approach and can result in reduced narcotic dosages. In the NH this can be accomplished by placing a heplock rather than administering a continuous intravenous infusion. Sometimes switching from one narcotic to another improves pain relief, as one-to-one cross-tolerance does not occur with narcotics. Tables 23-7 and 23-8 summarize drugs that are available to treat pain.

Finally, it should not be forgotten that radiation therapy can produce dramatic pain relief in some individuals with pain syndrome related to cancer. Corticosteroids may also produce pain relief when the tumor is compressing a nerve in a confined space.

Table 23-7 Examples of analgesic drugs for mild to moderate pain

	Equianalgesic dose, mg	Duration of action, h
Aspirin	650	4–6
Acetaminophen	650	4–6
Propoxyphene	65[a]	4–6[b]
Meperidine	50	4–6
Pentazocene	30	4–6
Codeine[c]	32	3

[a] Potentially transformed to toxic metabolite norpropoxyphene and has high addiction potential—should be avoided in older persons.

[b] Plasma half-life is 12 h compared to 4 or less for all other drugs. This increases chances of toxic accumulation in older persons.

[c] Codeine is biotransformed to morphine and 130 mg intramuscularly is equivalent to 10 mg of morphine.

Table 23-8   Narcotic analgesics available for treatment of severe pain

Drug	Route of administration	Equianalgesic dose, mg	Duration of action, h	Sedation	Addiction	Respiratory depression
Morphine	IM	10	4–6	+ +	+ +	+ +
	PO	60	4–7			
Meperidine[a]	IM	75	3–4	+	+ +	+ +
	PO	300	3–4			
Methadone[b]	IM	10	4–6	+	+	+ +
	PO	20	4–24 + +			
Oxycodone[c] (Percodan)	IM	15	3–5	+ +	+ +	+ +
	PO	30				
Hydro-morphone[d]	IM	1.5	2–3	+	+ +	+ +
(Dilaudid)	PO	7.5	2–3			
Butorphanol[e] (Stadol)	IM	2	4–6	+	0	0

[a] Not for use in renal disease; metabolite normeperidine produces agitation.
[b] Duration increases with repeated administration due to long half-life of 15 to 30 h.
[c] May be used in combination with aspirin or Tylenol.
[d] Also available in rectal suppository.
[e] May precipitate withdrawal in physically dependent patients; no oral form available.
Note: Different number of + 's or 0's refers to the intensity of the effect.

SUGGESTED READINGS

Hospice

Cobbs E, Lynn J: The care of the dying patient, in Hazzard WR, Andres R, Burman EL, Blass JP (eds), *Principles of Geriatric Medicine and Gerontology.* New York, McGraw-Hill, 1990, pp 354–361.

Fabiszewski KJ, Volicer B, Volicer L: Effect of antibiotic treatment on outcome of fevers in institutionalized Alzheimer patients. *JAMA* 263:3168–3172, 1990.

Levy MM, Catalano RB: Control of common physical symptoms other than pain in patients with terminal disease. *Semin Oncol* 12:411, 1985.

Zimmerman JM: *Hospice: Complete Care for the Terminally Ill.* Baltimore, Urban & Schwarzenberg, 1986.

Pain Management

Ferrell BA, Ferrell BR, Osterweil D: Pain in the nursing home. *J Am Geriatr Soc* 38:409–414, 1990.

Foley KM: Pain management in the elderly, in Hazzard WR, Andres R, Bierman EL, Blass JP (eds), *Principles of Geriatric Medicine and Gerontology.* New York, McGraw-Hill, 1990, pp 281–295.

Morley GK, Erickson DL, Morley JE: The neurology of pain, in Jognt RJ (ed), *Clinical Neurology* (Vol 2). New York, Hoeber-Harper, Chap. 18, pp. 1–95.

Payne R, Pasternak GV: Pain and pain management, in Cassel CK, Riesenberg D, Sorensen LB, Walsh JR (eds), *Geriatric Medicine.* New York, Springer-Verlag, 1990, pp 583–601.

TWENTY-FOUR

COMPUTERS AND OTHER TECHNOLOGIES

THE NEED FOR AND ROLE OF COMPUTERS IN THE NURSING HOME ENVIRONMENT

In the last two decades, the nursing home (NH) industry has been characterized by increasing complexity of its operation and increasing regulatory requirements for documentation. As a result, the need for proper documentation, recording of changes, cost tracking, and cost reporting has grown considerably. The purpose of introducing computers into the NH environment is to meet the challenge raised by these requirements and at the same time improve the information flow in the long-term-care setting. Since the introduction of the prospective payment system, there has been a shift toward care outside of hospitals; it is predicted that in the next decade, transitional care units and community-based skilled nursing facilities will play a major role in the health delivery system. Accurate and expeditious flow of information from acute care hospitals to these settings and vice versa will add significantly to the quality of care delivered. The upcoming implementation of the Minimal Data Set across the nation will add to the challenges of organizing, communicating, and documenting a large amount of information.

The physician in the NH setting receives, reviews, and provides information via the NH medical record. The NH medical record is a combination of an acute care and ambulatory record. The NH environment has elements of both settings, and the requirements for information management bridge the gap between the two. Current NH records are significantly handicapped by factors which are "people dependent," such as handwritten, illegible, inaccurate, and unreliable notes. Much information is recorded, but the retrieval process is difficult and the information is frequently not usable. Clinical decisions may therefore be based on inaccurate and incomplete information. An inefficient information system also handicaps efforts to carry out quality assurance in a timely and cost-effective manner. In addition, lack of access to good data from the NH record interferes with the ability to perform clinical research.

In this chapter, we will describe basic principles of the flow of information in the NH setting, briefly review the design of an integrated computerized information system applicable to a NH, and address ways of selecting and implementing a computer system in a NH. Other uses of technology will be reviewed briefly. The Suggested Readings contain more detailed information regarding the use of computers in the NH.

INFORMATION AND THE FLOW OF INFORMATION IN THE NURSING HOME SETTING

The information used in a NH is basically similar to the information used in the acute hospital. It includes demographic information, clinical data, and information related to the resident's resources and financial status. In contrast to the acute care hospital, much of the information in the NH relates to functional status and daily care routines, and there is more of a multidisciplinary focus. Table 24-1 describes the basic flow of information in a NH setting. Computers can provide an information center that can efficiently integrate the diverse inputs and help make data flow in an organized and efficient manner. Figure 24-1 describes the desired flow of information in a NH with a computerized information system. In a typical NH, there are three major functions: (1) *clinical*, (2) *administrative*, and (3) *business* or *accounting*. An optimal information system integrates and creates an effective flow of information among all three functions.

Table 24-2 lists some basic terminology and definitions related to information and its flow in the NH. All information pertaining to the resident is considered the database. Different people use the database for different purposes and in different ways. Traditionally, health care institutions have

Table 24-1   The basic flow of information in a nursing home

Third-party payers to institution and vice versa
Regulatory agency to institution and vice versa
Regulatory agency to physician and vice versa
Physician to resident and vice versa
Physician to nurses and other health professionals and vice versa

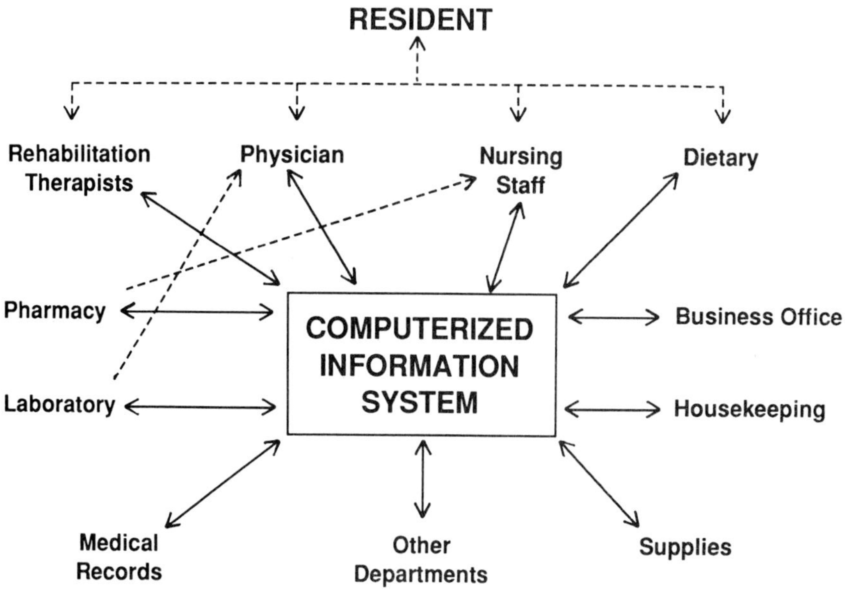

RESIDENT

Figure 24-1 Basic flow of information in a NH with a computerized information system. Dotted lines indicate verbal/written communications which are not directly incorporated into the computer database.

Table 24-2 Terminology and definitions related to information systems and computers in the nursing home

Terminology	Definition
Database	Contains specific elements of information—demographic, financial, clinical, functional status, resources utilized
Clinical information system	A coordinated approach to the systematic collection, storage, and use of information concerning residents—their health and associated needs and problems
Medical record	A sequential chart that records the timing of events and all relevant clinical and administrative data related to a resident's care
Computerized information system	The use of computers to collect, store, organize, analyze, and generate reports for clinical, administrative, or financial purposes
Report	A computer-generated document that organizes and presents information in a predetermined format based on the user's objectives; it can become a part of the medical record

relied primarily on a financial database. A financially oriented database, however, may not provide and integrate clinical information in an efficient and effective manner. Thus, clinical information should be the centerpiece of a system that determines utilization of personnel and other types of financial information essential to the operations of a facility, rather than vice versa. Clinical information can be used to generate financial data relatively easily, but the opposite does not hold true. A clinical information system that collects and organizes clinical data in a usable fashion is therefore needed.

Computer databases can help in standardizing data collection and in avoiding multiple entries of the same data. In a NH, for example, much of the clinical and functional status information is collected by more than one discipline. The computerized information system can make this process more efficient by allowing the clinical information to be input only once; at the same time, it can integrate that clinical information into multiple reports. Reports can be used for clinical purposes (by incorporating them into the medical record) as well as for administrative and financial purposes. Table 24-3 lists examples of clinical data categories that could be included into a computerized information system. Such data categories can allow for the generation of standardized reports—(e.g., a Medical Face Sheet (see Appendix), a structured progress note, an administrative face sheet—the storage of data to monitor progress and changes over time, and the organization of information in a manner that is helpful for quality assurance purposes. Standard coding systems (e.g., ICD-9, DRG) are not as applicable in NH settings as they are in acute care hospitals. Thus, a list of diagnoses for use specifically in the NH must be developed. Where applicable, these diagnoses can then be linked to a standard code, such as ICD-9.

A computerized information system in a NH setting must also be a dynamic system. After the information is collected the first time, it must be continuously revised and updated by health professionals as new information related to the resident's progress is collected and entered into the database for ongoing review. Because much of the information is redundant, the

Table 24-3 Examples of clinical data categories

- Demographic information
- Age, sex, socioeconomic data, insurance status
- Functional status
- Diagnoses
- Progress notes
- Diagnostic studies and results
- Therapeutic interventions and results
- Medical problem list or face sheet

computer can make this process much more efficient. In addition, the computer may help identify when significant changes occur that should, in turn, trigger revision of the care plan and new goals and approaches.

GENERAL PHILOSOPHY OF DESIGNING A COMPUTERIZED INFORMATION SYSTEM

A computerized information system should satisfy administrators, nursing staff, medical staff, and other health professionals. The system should integrate clinical, functional status, demographic, and financial data. It should be capable of generating reports that can be either incorporated into the medical record or used for administrative and financial purposes. A variety of quality assurance activities, discussed below, can be enhanced by properly managed computer-generated data.

Although sophisticated in its internal mechanism, the computer system must be user-friendly. It should be designed to allow the nurse, physician, physical therapist, occupational therapist, pharmacist, and social worker to enter and obtain data about the resident in a simple manner. The computer should encourage entry of data according to the true meaning (i.e., "raw data"), rather than storing it in an interpreted form. The data can then be structured and interpreted by one of several output programs to meet the focused needs of the user. Such an approach increases the variety of users who can be supported by the database and, to a degree, insulates the database from biases about the ways in which residents are classified.

Interactive terminals need to be available throughout a NH in order to facilitate data entry and retrieval. The system response time should be rapid and, to prevent loss, data must be simultaneously recorded on more than one device. Nursing home staff must come to view the system as providing enough payback to justify the time to learn the system.

It must be recognized that, realistically, all potential users will not be willing to interact directly with the terminal. Therefore, a system must be designed to work equally well in interactive and noninteractive modes. Thus, different forms of input that feed into the computer database are needed. Work sheets to be used by personnel who do not work at the terminal may be necessary. These work sheets must be user-friendly and at the same time easily coded into the computer. For personnel who do use the terminal, data entry screens must be complemented by systems that simplify the process of data entry.

Many standard software packages are available for a variety of uses in the NH. Although NHs may find many of these standard packages useful, they need to be able to tailor the software to meet different and changing needs in information content and practice over time. The more sophisticated systems can be user-defined to incorporate the rules under which a given institution must operate. Inflexible programs that focus on financial data will not be useful for clinical and quality assurance purposes.

EXAMPLES OF COMPUTER APPLICATIONS IN THE NURSING HOME

The potential applications of computers in NHs range from the generation of reports and progress notes to quality assurance. In this section we briefly review some applications that have particular relevance to primary care physicians and medical directors.

Resident Care Plan

The resident care plan is theoretically the pillar of the NH medical record. It is intended to guide the care that the individual resident receives. It consists of a synthesis of entries made by all members of the interdisciplinary team. Computer-based resident care planning can be a time saver by allowing almost instantaneous updating as the resident's condition changes and/or when goals of care are achieved and problems are resolved. Many commercially available software programs can generate NH resident care plans. Some are designed so that, once a problem has been identified and entered, the system generates a list of potential goals and approaches from a predetermined dictionary. The dictionary also facilitates the association of a problem with a diagnosis and can suggest language for the goals and approaches—enforcing, when possible, the requirement of measurability. The resident care plan thus generated can be designed in accordance with regulations and, by its simple structure and legibility, facilitate its use by the multidisciplinary team. For each problem and nursing diagnosis, there may be multiple goals (objectives); for each goal, one or more approaches. For each approach, one or more disciplines are identified and a reassessment date is determined. (A sample format of a standard care plan, which could be computer-generated, is illustrated in Chap. 8, Table 8-2.)

Higher-quality software programs have the ability to review and update the resident care plan in an interactive mode. When a resident is selected, his or her problem list is displayed in a brief form. The operator selects an existing problem category for review or adds a new one. The most recent history is automatically displayed. The operator may scroll through the complete history of the problem or any part of it. In addition to facilitating immediate updating of the care plan, many programs provided well-developed dictionaries of problems, goals, and approaches that can serve as a valuable training tool for the staff.

Utilization Review

Computers are easily used to retrieve information on various utilization patterns. One of the most important examples is the utilization of drugs. The computer can list drugs by type, frequency, potential interactions, and appropriateness in relation to diagnosis. This information may be utilized for quality assurance purposes, as discussed in the next section. Utilization of special diets and dietary supplements is another example. Utilization of resources and self-monitoring of case mix are important in states where case-mix reimbursement of NH care [e.g., Resource Utilization Groups (RUGS)] has already been implemented. The national Minimal Data Set for NHs lends itself to computerization, and assessments incorporated in this data set may serve many purposes, including care planning, monitoring trends in case mix, and clinical research. Selected elements from the Minimum Data Set are described in Chap. 22, Table 22-12. Software that includes the Minimum Data Set is currently under development.

Quality Assurance

Computers can be an invaluable resource in a quality assurance program. The computer can help to monitor trends in critical clinical areas, such as pharmacy services and medication use, accidents, infections, and adherence to various clinical protocols. In order for the computer to be helpful in these areas, it is critical that key data elements for quality assurance purposes be incorporated into the database. Thus, when one is designing a database, it is helpful to think of the types of quality assurance reports that will be desirable (e.g., monthly trends in falls, medication use, infections, cultures, antibiotic use), so that required data can be output. One of the potential advantages of the computer for quality assurance is the ability to link various trends to resident outcomes. Although using a computer for these quality assurance purposes requires some up-front time to input relevant data, the capability to generate various reports will be worth this time if the database and report format are carefully planned.

SELECTING A COMPUTER SYSTEM

Selecting hardware and software for a NH computer system may be an intimidating experience, especially for physicians, nurses, and administrators who are not versed in computer terminology and use. A computer for a NH needs must be a flexible system that serves multiple users. Clinical staff should have input into the decision-making process as it relates to the resident care components of the system. The choice of size, configuration, and sophistication of a system depends on the size of the facility and financial considerations as well as the stability and sophistication of the staff. The market offers a spectrum of systems for a broad range of needs—from personal-computer-based single-station systems that have single-module software (as for resident care planning and accounting) to microcomputer, integrated, multiple-module, and multiple-user systems. It is beyond the scope of this chapter to go into details about the various systems that are available. Systems that allow the most flexibility and are vertically integrated are the most suitable for facilities of 150 beds or larger, while the less complicated systems are better suited for smaller institutions with very specific needs (e.g., accounting, care planning).

FUTURE USES OF COMPUTERS IN THE NURSING HOME

As computers begin the transition to a "paperless" record, staff behavior will become a critical issue in successfully incorporating computers into NH care. As it stands now, nurses' aides provide most of the care and a significant portion of charting in a NH setting. Charting consists of reporting on several critical aspects of resident care, including food intake, toileting, and exercise. Staff observe and report verbally on residents' behavior, which is later recorded by either the aide or licensed staff. Computer technology can be used to enhance supervision and accountability for such resident care procedures and their documentation. Nurses' aides could carry hand-held computers, scan a resident's bar-coded band, and log in their observations and treatments in real time, very much as supermarket cashiers or package handlers do today. The resident-related information could then be entered electronically into the computer system. This type of approach could improve performance efficiency and reliability without compromising resource utilization.

Another potential use for computer technology may be direct monitoring of residents with behavioral problems such as wandering. Monitoring systems have been developed that report resident wandering patterns to a computer. This information can be utilized in care planning via adjustments in the environment, staffing, or medications. A similar approach may be used for monitoring recurrent fallers, whose beds or wheelchairs can be monitored with a fall-management sensor (see Chap. 14).

In summary, computerized information systems will be increasingly important to the future of NH care. Many benefits can be derived, including improved documentation, increased accountability, better utilization of resources, quality assurance, education, research, and potential cost savings. With limited resources, NHs may be reluctant to get involved in any activity that cannot have a favorable effect on their bottom line and on resident care. Studies and demonstration projects that focus on human resource management, quality assurance, and the fiscal aspects of NH care

are needed in order to introduce computer technology into the NH on a scale similar to that of the introduction of computerization to business and industry in the last two decades.

OTHER TECHNOLOGIES

The NH is a low-technology, high-touch industry. This has made it difficult for many NH staff to accept the possibility that technological innovations may improve the humanistic care of the resident. One example of technology that has great potential to improve the quality of that care is a voice-activated robotic arm, which can pick up objects and move them into an appropriate position in response to the resident's voice. Robots may also be particularly useful for helping dependent residents do passive exercises or for assisting nurses' aides in critical repetitive tasks, such as positioning residents or offering them water.

The introduction of high-tech environmental control systems may lead to significant improvements in NH residents' quality of life. A series of simple environmental control systems for persons with quadriplegia and poliomyelitis were first developed in Britain in 1960. A sophisticated environmental control system developed in a Canadian NH has given residents a heightened sense of independence, reduced frustration levels among both residents and nursing staff, and produced a saving of 1 h of nursing time per resident per day. These systems allow the resident to control the room lights, radio, and television set from a bed or chair and can be adapted to allow the resident to have control of any simple on/off system. Many hospital beds are now fitted with these systems, but their introduction into NHs has not been generalized. These innovative approaches can permit the resident to reestablish a level of control while allowing nursing staff more time to engage in meaningful dialogue with the resident. The science-fiction potential of such environmental control systems and robotics is suggested in Fig. 24-2.

Improvements in communication technology are also beginning to have an impact on the NH environment. Fax machines may produce a major advance in the way in which information is communicated between NHs, hospitals, and laboratories as well as between physicians and nurses. Predetermined "panic" values for laboratory tests can be established; when such results are obtained, they can be faxed immediately back to the NH or directly to the physician. Fax transmissions may become viable substitutes for many telephone calls between physicians and nurses. These calls are time-consuming and a major source of frustration for all concerned. Nurses can use fax transmissions to inform physicians of subacute changes that do not require immediate notification, to report abnormal lab results, and to request changes in orders. Physicians could fax responses back to the NH.

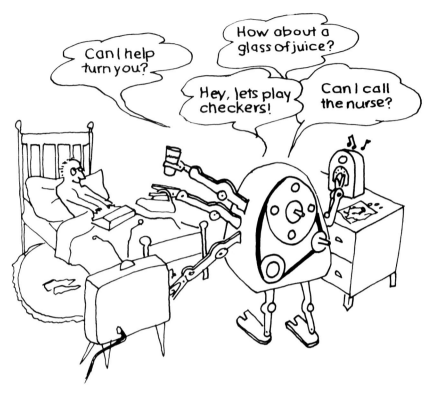

Figure 24-2 The future of NHs. Robotics could help improve the environment and quality of life for NH residents. They could reduce the nursing time needed for selected repetitive tasks—thereby freeing their time to interact with residents on a more social basis—and help restore a locus of control to dependent NH residents. (After Morley JE: New concepts of medical management of nursing home patients. *Ann Intern Med* 108:728, 1988.)

Administrative and legal issues surrounding the use of fax machines for such purposes will have to be worked out. The Mayo Clinic has already reported the successful and cost-effective use of fax machines in its relationship with several community NHs.

Finally, improvements in communication technology could lead to exciting opportunities for educational programs involving NH staff. Computer-assisted learning techniques, interactive videotapes, and teleconferences with opportunities for NH staff to ask questions of experts at different locations all hold significant potential for making the NH a more interesting and stimulating environment for staff. One hopes that these educational technologies will result in improvements in resident care and outcomes.

SUGGESTED READINGS

Bluin BI (ed): *Information Systems for Patient Care.* New York, Springer-Verlag, 1984.

Haber PAL: Technology in aging. *Gerontologist* 36:350, 1986.

Levenson SA: *Medical Directions in Long-Term Care.* Owings Mills, Maryland, National Health Publishing, 1988, 235–276.

Morley JE: New concepts of medical management of nursing home patients. *Ann Intern Med* 108:727, 1988.

Symington DC, Lywood DW, Lawson JS, MacLean J: Environmental control systems in chronic care hospitals and nursing homes. *Arch Phys Med Rehabil* 67:321, 1986.

Weiler GP, Thorpe L, Walters R, Chiziboga D: An automated medical record system for a skilled nursing facility. *J Med Systems* 11:367, 1987.

TWENTY-FIVE

ETHICAL AND LEGAL ISSUES

A myriad of ethical issues are confronted on a daily basis in the nursing home (NH), ranging from the allocation of resources and access to care, to the individual rights of NH residents, to decisions involving the withholding or withdrawal of life-sustaining treatment. These issues have recently gained widespread attention in the medical literature as well as in the lay press. Unfortunately, much of this attention has derived from several cases in which ethical dilemmas could not be resolved by residents, their loved ones, and their health care providers. As a result, the decision-making process was deferred to the court system. Concerns about the process of making difficult ethical decisions are, in fact, frequently couched in terms of fear of litigation. Medical-ethical issues and the law therefore frequently become muddled.

In this chapter we focus on important ethical issues faced by physicians who care for NH residents and suggest strategies to deal with them. A brief section has been included at the end of the chapter to discuss some of the basic legal issues that are relevant to health care professionals in the NH. But it is our contention, as well as that of most physicians and lawyers, that ethical decisions about the care of NH residents should remain at the bedside and not be made in court. By resorting to the courts to make such decisions, which involve many complex and highly individual medical and personal preference factors, we usurp the right of residents and their loved ones to decide for themselves and compromise the ability of health care professionals to serve the best interests of their patients. We hope the principles and strategies outlined in this chapter will be helpful in this regard.

OVERVIEW OF MEDICAL-ETHICAL ISSUES

Table 25-1 lists the major principles of medical ethics. These form the basic foundation of medical practice and should be considered when ethical dilemmas in the care of NH residents are being faced.

The most discussed and debated medical-ethical issues in the care of NH residents involve decisions about the intensity of treatment provided to frail, dependent, usually cognitively impaired elderly NH residents in the end stages of life. To be sure, these are critical issues that must be addressed in a careful, ethical manner in light of growing concerns over the costs of health care. Many "cost-benefit" analyses now use quality-adjusted-life years (QALYs) as an important measure of the utility of various diagnostic and therapeutic procedures. QALYs generally discriminate against the frail elderly, because for them the calculated quantitative benefits are not as great as for younger individuals. Daniel Callahan, one of America's most prominent medical ethicists, has suggested that the most practical and fair approach to the containment of skyrocketing health care costs is to limit the use of intensive, expensive treatments by age. Many other ethicists, geriatricians, and gerontologists are concerned that any limitations on treatment options will result in a "slippery slope" and facilitate the inappropriate withholding of potentially beneficial treatments from some individuals because of their age or their functional or mental status. On the other hand, most would also agree that it is not always in an individual's best interest to provide all treatments that might theoretically be beneficial.

Before discussing these "life and death" ethical dilemmas further, it is important to take a step back and emphasize that there are many other, more fundamental ethical issues that must be addressed in the care of NH residents. Table 25-2 lists common ethical issues confronted in the NH.

Table 25-1 Major principles of medical ethics

Beneficence
The obligation to do good and act in the best interests of others

Nonmaleficence
The obligation to avoid harm

Autonomy
Respect for a person's right of self-determination regarding his/her life, body, mind, and medical care

Justice
Duty to treat individuals fairly and without discrimination and to distribute resources in a nonarbitrary and fair manner

Fidelity
Duty to keep promises

Table 25-2   Common ethical issues in the nursing home

Ethical issues	Examples
Preservation of autonomy	Choices in many areas are limited in most nursing homes (see Table 25-3)
	Families, physicians, and NH staff tend to become paternalistic
Quality of life	This concept is often entered into decision making, but it is difficult to measure, especially among those with dementia
	Ageist biases can influence perceptions of NH residents' quality of life
Decision-making capacity	Many NH residents are incapable or questionably capable of participating in decisions about their care
	There are no standard methods of assessing decision-making capacity in this population
Surrogate decision making	Many NH residents have not clearly stated their preferences or appointed a surrogate before becoming unable to decide for themselves
	Family members may be in conflict, have hidden agendas, or be unable or unwilling to make decisions
Intensity of treatment	A range of options must be considered, including cardiopulmonary resuscitation and mechanical ventilation, hospitalization, treatment of specific conditions (e.g., infection) in the NH without hospitalization, enteral feeding, comfort and supportive care only

Because the vast majority of NH residents are admitted with diminished functional capacities and/or cognitive impairment, they are especially vulnerable and susceptible to having their decisions made by others (paternalism). The limits imposed by generally inflexible care routines in NHs reinforces this tendency toward paternalism. Thus, one of the most difficult challenges in caring for NH residents is to attempt to preserve their autonomy and maintain their personhood and rights as individuals. Many of the recommendations made in the Institute of Medicine's 1986 report on improving the quality of care in NHs focus on this issue, and residents' rights are a fundamental component of the new rules for NH care defined in OBRA 1987 (a summary of portions of the OBRA legislation relevant to primary physicians is included in the Appendix). A recent book edited by Rosalie Kane and Arthur Kaplan (*Everyday Ethics: Resolving Dilemmas in Nursing Home Life.* New York, Springer, 1990) describes a study and uses case examples to highlight the importance of these more fundamental and mundane ethical issues to the lives of NH residents. Table 25-3 lists examples of these basic ethical issues. Although most of these issues are more dependent upon institutional policies and care routines than on medical care, it is

Table 25-3 Basic ethical issues in daily care: the rights of nursing home residents

---

Access to and choice of medical and other health-related care
Opportunity to participate in resident and family groups (e.g., a resident council)
The right to nondisruptive care routines that account for individual preferences, such as
    Bed and awakening times
    Avoidance of routines that disrupt sleep
    Choice of when to get dressed and what to wear
    Freedom from unnecessary medications and physical restraints
Choices about eating
    Freedom from unnecessarily restrictive diets
    Opportunity to eat noninstitutional foods of preference when available
    Right to eat at other than mealtimes (e.g., bedtime snacks)
Opportunity for and freedom to participate in activities, including activities outside the
  facility
The right to have visitors
The right to manage finances when able
The right to security of personal property
The right to voice complaints and grievances
The right to privacy
    Mail
    Use of telephone
    Bathroom and bathing
    Nonintrusive roommate or roommates
    Confidentiality of medical and other records

---

important for primary physicians to consider them when writing orders, and to work with the NH to maximize the individual rights of the residents under their care. The primary physician may, in fact, be in the best position to serve as an advocate for residents in maximizing their individual rights and should take advantage of the opportunity to do so whenever possible.

DECISION-MAKING CAPACITY AND INFORMED CONSENT

A fundamental premise of the practice of medicine is that each individual who is capable of making decisions for himself or herself regarding his or her medical care has the right to do so. This right is no different for NH residents than for any other population, but—for a variety of reasons—it is more difficult to uphold in the NH setting.

Table 25-4 outlines several key principles relevant to decision-making capacity and informed consent among NH residents. The right to make decisions regarding medical care is implemented by the process of informed consent. The requirements for informed consent are outlined in Table 25-4.

Table 25-4   Key principles of decision making among nursing home residents

Informed consent requires
  The communication of relevant, understandable, and unbiased information about the
    potential risks and benefits of a given intervention
  Freedom from coercion and other factors that might unduly influence a decision
  The ability to
    Understand the information
    Weigh the risks and benefits
    Make a reasoned decision based on the given information and on individual values and
      preferences
Decision making should be done *prospectively*
  Written documentation, via an advance directive or other format, is critical (see Table 25-7)
  Because many NH residents are incapable of decision making at the time of NH admission,
    prospective decision making should be discussed *before* NH admission whenever feasible
  Specificity regarding all possible medical interventions in an advance directive is often
    impractical
    More general statements about various levels of intensity of care and common
      treatment decisions may be more appropriate
Decision-making capacity relates to the ability to make specific decisions
  Dementia and other causes of cognitive impairment do *not* necessarily render NH residents
    incapable of making decisions regarding their care
  Legal competence (or incompetence) is *not* the equivalent of being incapable of
    participating in care decisions
There is no standardized test to determine if NH residents are capable of making specific
  decisions about their care
  Scores on standard mental function tests do *not* predict a resident's ability to participate
    in care decisions
A variety of factors, some of which fluctuate over time and are reversible, can have an
  important influence on the ability to make decisions. Examples include
  Delirium and other reversible acute confusional states
  Depression
  Pain
  Medication side effects
  Perceived quality of life
  Perceived wishes of family and other loved ones
  Economic considerations
When a resident is found to be incapable of making a particular decision
  His/her prior expressed wishes relevant to the decision should be taken into account
    whenever they are known
  A surrogate or proxy decision maker, preferably assigned by the resident and who is
    known to be acting in the best interests of the resident, should be consulted

It is often difficult to fulfill these requirements among NH residents because

1. Impaired vision, hearing, and cognitive function often make it difficult
   to communicate the information the resident needs in order to make an
   informed decision.

2. Dependent NH residents may be afraid that their decisions will result in unfair treatment in the NH.
3. Impaired cognitive functioning and other factors (such as depression, pain, medical illness) may interfere with the resident's ability to make an informed decision based on his or her preferences and best interests.

Thus, an absolutely critical determination that must be made is whether or not residents are capable of playing a meaningful role in making decisions about their care. This turns out to be very tricky business. Much of the literature refers to *competence*—a legal term that may only confuse the issue. *Decision-making capacity* is a better way of describing what needs to be determined. Some of the key principles relevant to determining decision-making capacity are outlined in Table 25-4. Several of these principles are worthy of special emphasis.

First, unlike legal competence (or incompetence), the ability to make a decision about one's health care should be considered *specific to the situation at hand*. For example, a NH resident may be legally declared to lack testamentary competence (the ability to execute a will). This, however, has nothing to do with determining whether that same resident is capable of deciding if she or he should have a surgical procedure. Decision-making capacity must be determined in relation to the resident's ability to meet the criteria for informed consent about a specific diagnostic or therapeutic procedure.

Second, *there is no standardized test that determines the capacity of a NH resident to make a specific decision*. Scores on standardized mental status tests have been shown *not* to be predictive of decision-making capacity and should not be used in this manner.

Third, the fact that a NH resident is known to have a dementia syndrome *does not* automatically imply that he or she is incapable of participating meaningfully in decisions about his or her care. Even NH residents with moderate or severe dementia are capable of expressing preferences, and an attempt should be made to elicit these preferences whenever feasible.

Fourth, a variety of factors, many of which fluctuate over time and are reversible, may influence a NH resident's decision-making capacity. These factors include delirium due to acute medical conditions, depression, pain, and medication side effects. These factors must be identified and managed in order to optimize the resident's ability to express preferences and participate in making decisions.

In the final analysis, the determination of a NH resident's decision-making capacity must rest on a careful clinical judgment that takes into account all the factors discussed above. Psychiatrists are often consulted to make this determination. While they may provide helpful information, there is no scientific or legal reason to depend on a psychiatrist to make this determi-

nation. In most situations, a primary care physician can make this determination in conjunction with others who know the resident well—including
family and other loved ones, nursing staff, and the resident's social worker
and representative of the clergy. When there is disagreement about the resident's ability to participate in a specific decision, consultation with a psychiatrist or another qualified health professional is often helpful.

If the resident is found to lack the capacity to make a specific decision,
then a proxy or surrogate decision maker must be identified. As discussed
below, the surrogate is preferably chosen in advance by the resident. Generally the surrogate is a relative; even if the relative has not been legally
identified as the attorney-in-fact or conservator, his or her input is generally
sought. Whether or not the surrogate is a relative or is legally identified, it
is important to ensure that he or she is accounting for the resident's preferences if known and acting in the best interests of the resident. Only in
situations where a legally identified surrogate is not available, there is disagreement among potential surrogates, or the physician suspects that the
surrogate is not acting in the best interests of the resident should consideration be given to going to court.

One other critical aspect of decision making among NH residents is timing. Under optimal circumstances important treatment decisions should not
be made at a time of crisis. The decision to place a resident on a respirator
should not be made on the spur of the moment, as when a physician is
called in the middle of the night about acute respiratory distress, nor should
the decision about surgery for a gangrenous extremity be delayed until the
resident is septic and delirious. Prospective decision making is discussed
further in subsequent sections of this chapter.

DECISIONS ON INTENSITY OF TREATMENT

When one is helping NH residents and their surrogate decision makers to
arrive at decisions on medical care, it is generally helpful to categorize various treatment options systematically. Table 25-5 lists examples of levels of
intensity of medical care. Decisions about desired intensity of care should
preferably be made *prospectively*, when residents are still capable of
expressing their preferences and before a crisis occurs. The mechanisms to
accomplish this—advance directives—are discussed further in the following
section of this chapter.

Categorizing treatment options as illustrated in Table 25-5 is helpful in
giving relatively specific guidance to health care providers and may be helpful in meeting legal requirements for clearly documenting an individual's
preferences. But it is not absolutely necessary, and it may be problematic
in certain situations. Many individuals may find it difficult to understand all
the potential risks and benefits of the specific treatments, especially when

Table 25-5 Examples of levels of intensity of medical care that might be included in advance directives of nursing home residents

Cardiopulmonary resuscitation (CPR)
Mechanical ventilation (respirator care)
Care in intensive care unit (ICU)
Care in an acute care hospital but without CPR, respirator, or ICU care
Care in the NH only, including specific treatments when indicated (e.g., antibiotics, blood
  transfusions)
Comfort and supportive care only, with enteral ("tube") feeding if necessary for nutrition
  and/or hydration
Comfort and supportive care only, without enteral feeding

they are being asked to decide about them under hypothetical future conditions. Precluding specific types of care may not always be in the best interests of a resident, even if he or she is severely impaired or terminally ill. For example, acute care hospitalization may be necessary under certain circumstances to provide maximum comfort (e.g., pain control, management of respiratory distress). Similarly, antibiotics may be necessary to provide maximum comfort when a resident has a painful urinary tract infection, cellulitis, or other infection.

In making decisions about the intensity of medical treatments, several basic principles in addition to those outlined in Table 25-4, should be considered:

1. In addition to any decisions about specific interventions, a more general statement should be included that (a) alludes to the resident's condition (e.g., irreversible illness, coma) and (b) allows for treatment when the potential benefits outweigh the risks, especially with regard to comfort (e.g., hospitalization, antibiotics).
2. When decisions about specific treatments are made, they must be consistent (e.g., deciding for CPR but against a respirator and the ICU is not reasonable).
3. Decisions to forego the specific treatments *do not* imply that other forms of care should be withheld (e.g., a "No CPR" order does not preclude hospitalization for pneumonia).
4. In many situations, a time-limited therapeutic trial may be helpful in determining the benefits and risks of a specific treatment (this is especially true for enteral feeding; see below).

Many studies and articles have focused on decisions about CPR. Although CPR provides a good model for decision making, it has become clear that decisions about CPR for NH residents are less important than decisions about the other categories of treatment listed in Table 25-4. This is because CPR has been shown to be an ineffective procedure in the vast majority of NH residents. Its ineffectiveness relates to the overall medical condition of the residents, the survivability of CPR in this population (which is between 0 percent and 5 percent), and the ability—generally limited—of NH staff to provide effective CPR. Many geriatricians have discussed reversing the standing order in NHs (i.e., a NH resident should be on "No CPR" status unless there is an order to perform CPR). It should be emphasized , however, that a "No CPR" order may be inappropriate for some NH residents, such as those who are generally healthy and are in the NH for rehabilitation after an acute illness.

Decisions to forego acute hospitalization and specific treatments such as antibiotics and blood transfusions may be appropriate for some NH residents. These decisions, however, imply that the NH staff is able and willing to provide the care that is necessary to ensure the comfort of such residents if they become subacutely ill. Residents for whom these decisions have been made often require substantial nursing time to monitor their comfort and to provide care such as suctioning, hydration, nutrition, and prevention of skin breakdown. In addition, such decisions should not compromise appropriate medical care. If, for example, a NH resident develops pneumonia that is complicated by dehydration, congestive heart failure, or other conditions, optimal medical treatment generally requires care in a "subacute" unit or in an acute care hospital (see Chap. 17). Treating such complicated conditions in the NH without intravenous fluids and medications and close nursing monitoring is rarely effective and serves no real purpose. Thus, if a specific medical condition such as pneumonia is to be treated, treatment should be provided in an optimal manner—not compromised by limitations that preclude appropriate care.

The most difficult and controversial decisions about intensity of care center around nutrition and hydration. It is beyond the scope of this book to discuss this very complex issue in great detail. Readers are encouraged to review the suggested readings at the end of this chapter, which provide detailed analyses of the complex issues involved. A book edited by Joanne Lynn (*By No Extraordinary Means: The Choice to Forego Life-Sustaining Food and Water*, Indianapolis, Indiana University Press, 1986) is probably the most comprehensive work on this topic.

Several general principles related to decisions about withholding or withdrawing nutrition and hydration are outlined in Table 25-6. It should be emphasized that these decisions must be made at an appropriate time, before the resident becomes so malnourished that artificial feeding will not be of any benefit. Because several cases have been ruled on in the courts, physicians must be aware of federal and state rules that bear on these decisions. The Appendix contains a map that indicates how various states have

Table 25-6   Important considerations about artificial nutrition and hydration

---

Sound decision-making practices are critical when the withholding or withdrawal of artificial nutrition and hydration is being considered (see Table 25-4)

Although such a step is generally considered a medical intervention, a myriad of emotional, religious, and legal issues are involved

   Physicians should become familiar with relevant federal and state rules

Decisions about artificial nutrition should be made before a resident becomes so malnourished that artificial feeding will be of no benefit

If artificial nutrition and hydration are begun, proper techniques should be employed (see Chap. 11)

It may be appropriate to withhold or withdraw artificial feeding and hydration from carefully selected residents who

   Are severely or terminally ill with a limited life expectancy

   Have clearly expressed a preference not to have this type of intervention, given their condition

   Have no reversible causes of inability to obtain adequate oral hydration and nutrition (e.g., depression, pain)

   Are unlikely to derive significant benefit compared to the risks

NH staff who provide day-to-day care must be comfortable in providing supportive care without artificial hydrating and nutrition when such decisions are made

When there is any ambivalence about the decision

   A time-limited therapeutic trial may be appropriate

   It may be more appropriate to provide the artificial hydration and nutrition and withhold other types of treatment (e.g., antibiotics for pneumonia or sepsis)

---

viewed these decisions. We believe that it is appropriate to withhold artificial feeding and hydration only for a highly selected group of NH residents (see Table 25-6). When such a decision is made, the NH staff must be comfortable in providing the necessary supportive measures without instituting artificial feeding or hydration. When there is *any* ambivalence, however, we recommend that artificial feeding and hydration be implemented. It may be appropriate to do so on a *time-limited* basis as a therapeutic trial, so that the benefits and risks can be assessed objectively. This might involve providing fluids, nutrition, and medications through a small-caliber nasogastric tube for 1 to 2 weeks in order to determine whether the resident can benefit from and tolerate enteral feeding. Of course, proper techniques for providing artificial feeding and hydration should be employed (see Chap. 11). In many situations involving severely impaired residents, it may be most appropriate to use artificial feeding and hydration (because of the complex medical, emotional, religious, and legal issues involved) and to forego other life-sustaining treatments when acute conditions develop (e.g., withhold antibiotics if sepsis occurs and use supportive and comfort measures only).

POLICY AND PROCEDURAL CONSIDERATIONS

Policies and Guidelines

Nursing homes should develop policies and/or guidelines about common ethical dilemmas. This may be accomplished by a joint effort among administrative staff, the medical director, the director of nursing, other disciplines (e.g., social work, clergy), and residents or by a biomedical ethics committee (see below). Such policies and guidelines should, at a minimum, address resident rights and autonomy, informed consent and decision-making capacity, the use of advance directives and surrogate decision makers, procedures for resolving conflicts, and appropriate documentation practices. Examples of guidelines for foregoing life-sustaining treatment and a policy on artificial nutrition and hydration are included in the Appendix.

Advance Directives

The importance of attempting to make health care decisions in advance, when an individual still has the capacity to express preferences and before a medical crisis occurs, cannot be overemphasized. There is now available, in most states, a potentially useful instrument for prospective decision making: an *advance directive*. Advance directives include living wills, which are generally limited to situations involving terminal illness, and the durable power of attorney for health care (DPA), which is a more general document. (The Appendix contains a map of the United States that illustrates which states have adopted these advance directives through 1990.)

The DPA is a legal document executed when an individual is still capable of making decisions. It allows the individual to document two important items: (1) an attorney-in-fact whom the resident trusts as his or her surrogate decision maker in the event that the resident becomes unable to make his or her own health care decisions and (2) the types of decisions the resident would want to have made on his or her behalf. Although the DPA is a potentially powerful tool for ascertaining an individual's treatment preferences before he or she becomes incapable of expressing them, it is by no means a panacea. There are some practical problems with the use of a DPA. First, as already mentioned, it may be very difficult for an individual to think about, no less specifically identify, various treatment options under a given set of abstract circumstances and to choose among them. Some people do not want to deal with these issues and may not be able to understand all the implications of opting for or against specific treatments that are generally not relevant to their present state of health. On the other hand, several surveys suggest that elderly people are willing to take part and interested in such discussions, and they do not find them emotionally upsetting.

The biggest practical problem with the DPA or any other written advance directive is that most NH residents have not executed such a directive before entering a NH and becoming incapable of doing so. This situation is unlikely to change for several years. The basic ethical principles outlined earlier in this chapter as well as several legal precedents (which require *clear and convincing* evidence of an individual's preferences in order to withhold or withdraw life-sustaining treatment) demand that primary care physicians take a proactive stance in this area. Discussions about advance directives must become a routine component of the practice of geriatric medicine and should occur, when possible, before or shortly after an individual enters a NH.

The Appendix contains examples of advance directives. Physicians should become familiar with laws about advance directives in their state and encourage their geriatric patients to execute one if available. Even if the patient does not sign a legal advance directive, the physician should *carefully* document in the patient's medical records any discussions regarding future treatment decisions and the patient's preferences. This documentation may later be of critical importance in helping to preserve the autonomy of that patient, whether or not he or she enters a NH.

Documentation

Many of the dilemmas and conflicts about decisions to withhold or withdraw life-sustaining treatment arise from inadequate documentation procedures. Although it is impossible to eliminate the fear of litigation and to prevent lawsuits, adequate documentation is critical in order to convince whoever needs to be convinced that thorough and appropriate procedures were followed in making these decisions. Table 25-7 lists some of the key aspects of documenting decisions to withhold or withdraw life-sustaining treatment. It is essential that such documentation be clear, kept in a specific location in the medical record, and transferred with the resident when he or she leaves the NH to enter another health care institution (i.e., an acute care hospital or another NH). Various procedures can be developed to accomplish these goals. We have developed a Treatment Status Sheet that is used for all such documentation; it is kept next to the Medical Face Sheet and not thinned from the medical record. The Appendix contains the Medical Face Sheet and an example of a specific form developed for documentation purposes by the California Medical Association. In addition to the documentation, it is critical to develop strategies to communicate these decisions to the interdisciplinary team that cares for the resident.

Biomedical Ethics Committees

Many NHs have developed biomedical ethics committees, although most facilities are still without them. Many NHs do not have the resources or

Table 25-7   Medical record documentation of decisions to withhold or withdraw life-sustaining treatment

All official documents (e.g., durable power of attorney for health care or DPA) and other written documentation relevant to treatment decisions should
Be kept in a defined area of the chart
Not be thinned from the chart if, for example, the resident is hospitalized and readmitted to the nursing home
Be copied and sent with the resident if she/he is transferred to another health care institution
When a decision has been made to withhold a specific form of treatment (e.g., "No CPR"), this information should be clearly identified by
An order in the physician's orders
Appropriate labeling of the medical record
Keeping a list readily accessible to nursing staff, so that paramedics or ambulances are not called for residents who have decided against CPR or hospitalization
A physician's note, placed in a specified location in the medical record (and not thinned) should clearly and concisely address several issues
Clinical data relevant to the treatment decision, including diagnosis and prognosis
The treatment decision made
Who was involved with the treatment decision
If the resident, the note should include a statement about the resident's ability to make the decision
If a surrogate decision maker, the note should state
Who the surrogate is
His or her legal status (e.g., attorney-in-fact, conservator)
That the surrogate is acting in the best interests of the resident
The basis for the decision
Any written or verbal expression of the resident's prior known wishes should be mentioned (e.g., statements made in DPA)
The treatment plan to be implemented
Discussion of the decisions and treatment plan with NH staff and other family members

expertise to form such a committee. Options for these NHs might be to join with other local NHs to form a committee, utilize the committee of a nearby larger institution, develop a city or countywide committee, encourage a corporate owner of several facilities to form a committee, or adopt the guidelines of local medical and legal societies.

A biomedical ethics committee should include representatives from the NH's administration as well as its medical, nursing, and social service departments. It should also include a member of the clergy, a lawyer, and someone representing the community the NH serves. The NH biomedical ethics committee should devote itself to

1. Self-education about medical ethical principles and common ethical dilemmas
2. Education of NH staff, residents, and families

3. Development of policies, guidelines, and procedures to handle ethical dilemmas
4. Quality assurance activities to ensure that policies, guidelines, and procedures are implemented and are being followed

A question frequently arises as to whether such a committee should be involved in reviewing individual cases. While the committee may often be helpful in clarifying difficult issues, there are several problems with expecting the committee to help resolve conflicts and make specific recommendations about an individual case. First, many committees do not have enough expertise to do this. Second, even if the committee does have members with sufficient expertise, they may not be available to meet at the time a conflict must be resolved. Third and most important, a committee, like a court, should not be used in a manner that removes the decision-making process from its proper place: with the resident, his or her loved ones, and the health professionals responsible for his or her care. For these reasons, it is more appropriate and practical for NH biomedical ethics committees to confine their activities to those listed above and not become involved in individual cases. Only in the rare circumstance when conflicts arise that cannot be resolved any other way should a committee be involved in an individual case. In such situations, it is better for a committee to become involved than to resort to the court system.

LEGAL CONSIDERATIONS

It is beyond the scope of this book to discuss the many varied legal issues that are relevant to NH care. Readers who are interested in this area should review the suggested readings for further sources of information. The most comprehensive reference on legal issues in geriatrics is a text edited by Marshall Kapp and Arthur Bigot (*Geriatrics and the Law*, New York, Springer, 1985). A few brief comments about legal considerations are worthy of special emphasis.

The need to adhere to federal and state laws and the risk of lawsuits are facts of life. But they should not usurp the medical profession's ability to provide optimal, humane, and compassionate care or an individual's right to make decisions about his or her own health care. Medical care in the NH should not be practiced on the basis of fear of litigation. We believe that the strategies outlined in this chapter are ethically sound and in compliance with the law. Development of clear, specific, and appropriate policies and procedures, adequate documentation, and quality assurance activities to ensure that policies and procedures are being adhered to are the best protection against litigation.

There will always be test cases that reach the courts and are highly publicized. But test cases and federal and state laws should not be overinterpreted. Much of the fear of litigation stems from ignorance of what, in fact, is the relevant law. Physicians who practice in NHs should become familiar with federal and state laws, especially as they relate to decisions to forego life-sustaining treatment. Many medical journals regularly publish articles relevant to health care law, including briefs presented to the courts by professional societies and interest groups on specific cases. Federal and state laws should be reviewed when necessary, as should interpretive guidelines. It should be emphasized, however, that the latter are *not* the law but only an interpretation of it, which may or may not be appropriate in an individual case. The Appendix contains a summary of OBRA 1987, which contains new federal rules relevant to NH care.

The role of the legal system should optimally be to set up and oversee an environment in which appropriate procedures can be followed that uphold the rights of individuals and their loved ones to make decisions about their care and to enable health professionals to act in their patients' best interests given the patients' preferences. If health professionals who work in NHs work diligently to develop appropriate policies and procedures, we can avoid the unnecessary intrusion of the legal system in decisions that belong in the clinical arena, not the courts.

SUGGESTED READINGS

Applebaum GE, King JE, and Finucane TE: The outcome of CPR initiated in nursing homes. *J Am Geriatr Soc* 38:197–200, 1990.

Besdine RW: Decisions to withhold treatment from nursing home residents. *J Am Geriatr Soc* 31:602–606, 1983.

Cassel CK, Meier DE, and Traines ML: Selected bibliography of recent articles in ethics and geriatrics. *J Am Geriatr Soc* 34:399–409, 1986.

Fabiszewski KJ, Volicer B, and Volicer L: Effect of antibiotic treatment on outcome of fevers in institutionalized Alzheimer patients. *JAMA* 263:3168–3172, 1990.

Glasser G, Zweibel NR, and Cassel CK: The ethics committee in the nursing home: Results of a national survey. *J Am Geriatr Soc* 36:150–156, 1988.

Hilfiker D: Allowing the debilitated to die. *N Engl J Med* 309:716–719, 1983.

Kane RA and Caplan AL (eds): *Everyday Ethics: Resolving Dilemmas in Nursing Home Life.* New York, Springer, 1990.

Kapp MB and Bigot A: *Geriatrics and the Law.* New York, Springer, 1985.

Kapp MB, Pies HE, and Doudera AE: *Legal and Ethical Aspects of Health Care for the Elderly.* Ann Arbor, Michigan, Health Administration Press, 1985. (In cooperation with the American Society of Law and Medicine.)

Lo B and Dornbrand L: Guiding the hand that feeds: Caring for the demented elderly. *N Engl J Med* 311:402–404, 1984.

Lo B and Dornbrand L: The case of Claire Conroy: Will administration review safeguard incompetent patients? *Ann Intern Med* 104:869–873, 1986.

Lynn J: Dying and dementia. *JAMA* 256:2244–2245, 1986.

Lynn, Joanne (ed): *By No Extraordinary Means: The Choice to Forego Life-Sustaining Food and Water.* Indianapolis, Indiana University Press, 1986.

Mott PD and Barker WH: Hospital and medical care use by nursing home patients: The effect of patient care plans. *J Am Geriatr Soc* 36:47–53, 1988.

Murphy DJ: Do-not-resuscitate order: Time for reappraisal in long-term-care institutions. *JAMA* 260:2089–2101, 1988.

Murphy DJ, Murray AM, Robinson BE, and Campion EW: Outcomes of cardiopulmonary resuscitation in the elderly. *Ann Intern Med* 111:199–205, 1989.

President's Commission for the Study of Ethical Problems in Medicare and Biomedical and Behavioral Research: *Deciding to Forego Life Sustaining Treatment.* Washington, DC, U.S. Government Printing Office, publication no. 0-402-884, 1983.

Rango H: The nursing home resident with dementia: Clinical care, ethics and policy implications. *Ann Intern Med* 102:835–841, 1985.

Steinbrook R and Lo B: Artificial feeding—Solid ground, not a slippery slope. *N Engl J Med* 318:286–290, 1988.

Uhlman RF, Clark H, Pearlman RA, et al: Medical management decisions in nursing home patients: Principles and policy recommendations. *Ann Intern Med* 106:879–885, 1987.

Volicer L, Rheaume Y, Brown J, et al: Hospice approach to the treatment of patients with advanced dementia of the Alzheimer type. *JAMA* 256:2210–2213, 1986.

Wanzer SH, Federman DD, Adelstein SJ, et al: The physician's responsibility toward hopelessly ill patients: A second look. *N Engl J Med* 320:844–849, 1989.

TWENTY-SIX

EDUCATION AND RESEARCH

The continued growth of multidisciplinary educational programs in nursing homes (NHs) and of research studies that target the management of conditions common in the NH are of vital importance to improving NH care. The purpose of this chapter is to provide primary care physicians and medical directors with a brief overview of key issues involved in educational and research programs in the NH setting. Although most primary care physicians and medical directors are only indirectly involved in them, it is critical that they understand the importance and objectives of such programs so that the programs will be accepted by NHs and have a chance to be successful in meeting their goals.

EDUCATION

In this chapter we focus on medical education in the NH. We want to emphasize, however, the importance of undergraduate and postgraduate educational programs for all health professionals who work in or relate to NHs. NHs with qualified staff should be encouraged to participate in the training of nurse's aides (now mandated under OBRA 1987), licensed nurses, social workers, rehabilitation therapists, pharmacists, and administrators. Multidisciplinary rounds and conferences highlighting common clinical conditions and management issues are an effective method of involving such trainees. Participation in undergraduate and graduate education offers the NH an excellent opportunity to improve its image in the community, enhance the education of its own staff, and make the NH a more vital and stimulating environment. NHs may also benefit by attracting interested and well-trained students to jobs in the facility.

The need to educate medical students and postgraduate physician trainees in long-term care has been increasingly recognized over the last several years. The vast majority of medical schools now have at least some opportunity for medical students, internal medicine residents, and family practice residents to have an educational experience in NHs. To date, most of these programs are elective, quite limited in scope, and infrequently subscribed compared to other elective activities. Relatively few programs require rotations for medical students or house staff in a NH. Training opportunities at the fellowship level have increased dramatically over the last several years. There are now close to 70 geriatric medicine fellowship training programs and close to 30 in geropsychiatry. The Veteran's Administration has played a leadership role in developing and supporting these fellowships. Medical schools and teaching hospitals have also provided substantial support, boosted by special provisions in Medicare to support training in geriatric medicine. The National Institutes of Health, other governmental agencies, some private foundations, and a small number of pharmaceutical companies also provide support for geriatric fellowship programs, especially those with a research focus. Most fellowship programs have well-established relationships with one or more NHs, and some larger NHs have supported fellowship positions. Although these fellowship programs now graduate over 100 trainees per year, they are still far behind projected needs for academic geriatricians. As is the case with most other subspecialty fellowships, at least half the trainees have pursued clinical careers outside academic institutions. Although this may lead to improved geriatric and NH care in some areas, the goal of fellowship programs is to train physicians who will serve as role models in medical schools and spend the majority of their time in teaching and research activities. Two important recent developments should serve to enhance training in geriatrics: the formal accreditation of geriatric medicine fellowship programs and the development of a joint examination by the American Board of Internal Medicine and the American Board of Family Practice for a Certificate of Added Qualification in Geriatrics.

Table 26-1 lists several general educational objectives for trainees in a NH. These objectives focus on the care of chronically ill and functionally dependent NH residents, the limitations and advantages of the NH setting, the importance of psychological and socioeconomic factors, and their role in relation to a multidisciplinary team. Most educational programs for medical students and house staff fight an uphill battle against negative attitudes toward the geriatric population that are often engendered by experiences in medical school—such as caring for frail, dependent elderly when they are acutely ill, delirious, difficult to manage, uninteresting, and a "placement problem." Educational experiences in a NH must expose trainees to atti-

Table 26-1   General educational objectives of a nursing home rotation for trainees in geriatric medicine

To enhance the ability to care for elderly, chronically ill, and dependent residents of NHs

To improve the understanding of the appropriate evaluation and management of common problems in the NH setting

To further develop perspectives on and understanding of the rehabilitative, psychological, and socioeconomic aspects of caring for elderly, chronically ill, and disabled residents in NHs

To enhance effectiveness as members of a multidisciplinary team of health professionals in providing care to the NH population

tudes and situations that are more conducive to providing humane, compassionate, and effective care to the NH population. Table 26-2 lists several attitudinal objectives for a NH experience. Trainees must come to understand that common geriatric syndromes—such as dementia, immobility, and incontinence—are not inevitable consequences of growing old. They should recognize the importance of functional assessment and rehabilitation and that even small changes in function (e.g., the ability to transfer) may have a major impact on the health and quality of life of a frail NH resident. At the same time, they must also understand that, unlike the goals of the acute care hospital and ambulatory clinic, those of NH care are generally not to cure but to manage conditions in a way that maximizes functional capabilities, prevents complications, and enhances quality of life. In working with a multidisciplinary team, trainees should also come to understand the critical importance of the nonmedical aspects of NH care, including the many ethical dilemmas that are confronted on a daily basis in the NH setting. Table 26-3 lists more specific educational objectives for trainees in a

Table 26-2   Attitudinal objectives of a nursing home rotation for trainees in geriatric medicine

Illness and disability are not an inevitable consequence of growing old; even in long-term-care settings, active and appropriate medical care of specific disease processes and chronic illnesses can optimize health, function, and overall well-being.

The goals of NH care are often different than those of care in other settings. These goals vary depending upon characteristics of individual residents and whether rehabilitation, terminal care, or maintenance and preventive care are emphasized.

Caring rather than curing is most often the appropriate overall goal for NH residents.

Assessments of cognitive and physical function are critical in caring for this population.

Even small changes in function can make major differences in the well-being of residents and their caregivers and sometimes in the need for institutional care.

A multidisciplinary approach that encompasses the psychological and socioeconomic aspects of residents' illnesses and disabilities—as well as the medical aspects—is essential for effective care of this population.

Ethical and legal issues are common and must be attended to in caring for NH residents.

Table 26-3 Specific knowledge and skills objectives of a nursing home rotation for trainees in geriatric medicine

Knowledge
  Long-term care
    Definition and demographic considerations
    Community services
    Federal and state policies
    Economics
    Nursing home administration
  Aging
    Physiological changes that affect clinical evaluation and management of NH residents
    Altered presentation of disease in the NH
  Assessment and treatment of common clinical disorders
    Cancer
    Dementia and related behavioral disturbances
    Depression
    Diabetes
    Falls/gait disorders/postural hypotension/syncope
    Hypertension
    Incontinence
    Infection (especially pneumonia and urinary tract infection)
    Nutrition/malnutrition
    Osteoporosis
    Parkinson's disease
    Pressure sores
    Rehabilitation—stroke, hip fracture, amputations, other
    Sensory impairment
    Surgical interventions—preoperative evaluation, altered risk/benefit considerations
    Terminal illness
  Pharmacology
    Geropharmacology of drugs commonly used in the NH
    Psychotropic drugs
  Role of members of the multidisciplinary care team
    Nursing—aides, LVNs, RNs
    Social work
    Physical therapy
    Occupational therapy
    Nurse practitioners
    Geriatricians
    Others
  Ethical and legal issues
    Decisions to limit care
    Decision-making capacity
    Advance directives
    Role of family caregivers
    Examples of case law relevant to NH care
    Functions of an institutional ethics committee
Skills
  Comprehensive history and physical examination of frail elderly, including chronically ill and dependent NH residents, with emphasis on in-depth assessments of mental and functional status

Table 26-3 *(Continued)*   **Specific knowledge and skills objectives of a nursing home rotation for trainees in geriatric medicine**

Diagnostic evaluation, treatment, and follow-up assessment of common clinical problems (listed above)

Appropriate interaction and cooperation with nonphysician health professionals involved in the NH

Optimal utilization of community long-term-care resources

Effective communication with residents' families

Appropriate handling of ethical and legal dilemmas

Geriatric consultation incorporating skills listed above

NH, including both knowledge and skills. While it is impossible to meet all these objectives in a single student or house staff rotation, fellowship trainees are generally expected to develop substantial expertise in these knowledge and skill areas.

One issue that frequently arises in the design of educational experiences in a NH is the complicated logistics of attempting to meet the educational objectives involved in caring for chronically ill residents over a long period of time. It is difficult to meet these objectives if the exposure of the trainee occurs over a short time span. Most medical student and house staff rotations are scheduled for blocks of 4 to 6 weeks. An alternative which many fellowship and some residency programs have developed is a longitudinal experience. Table 26-4 outlines some of the advantages and disadvantages of block versus longitudinal NH rotations. We believe that in most NHs, longitudinal rotations are preferable, especially for residents and fellows, because they afford the trainee an opportunity to meet more of the objectives, to observe the time course of various subacute and chronic conditions common in a NH, and to assume a primary-care role for a cohort of NH residents. To make a longitudinal rotation effective, several important details must be attended to:

1. A regular time must be scheduled for primary care activities and for attending rounds with a faculty member who is experienced in long-term care. The best way to accomplish this is to substitute monthly NH rounds for another regularly scheduled activity, such as a longitudinal ambulatory clinic.
2. There should be planned exposure to the major objectives of the NH rotation over the course of the longitudinal experience.
3. Trainees should have the opportunity to meet with the administrator, medical director, and the multidisciplinary team on one or more occasion.
4. If trainees assume a primary care role, they should have close supervision by a faculty attending and should have backup coverage for acute

Table 26-4   Advantages and disadvantages of block versus longitudinal rotations in the nursing home

Block Rotations
  Advantages
    Concentrated exposure
    More opportunity to observe
      Interdisciplinary process
      Management of acute problems
      Administrative issues
  Disadvantages
    Difficult to obtain exposure to all objectives
    May miss some of the course of acute/subacute problems
    Difficult to integrate into primary care
    Frequent reorientation of new trainees necessary
Longitudinal Rotations
  Advantages
    Primary care role possible
    Chance to meet more objectives
    Opportunity to observe time course of various conditions
  Disadvantages
    May miss interdisciplinary and administrative aspects
    Set time for rounds may be difficult to integrate with other responsibilities
    Availability for management of interim problems may be difficult

problems when they are busy on other rotations. The latter can be provided by the faculty, a fellow, a nurse practitioner or physician's assistant, the medical director, or an interested member of the NH medical staff.

Block rotations may offer some advantages in an academic NH with enough faculty to provide continuous on-site supervision. An intensive in-depth exposure will allow the trainee to interact with multidisciplinary staff more frequently, get an idea of the day-to-day routines in a NH, and become a functioning member of the multidisciplinary team—albeit for a short period of time. If the block rotation is chosen, faculty should make sure that the trainee receives a broad exposure to the various aspects of NH care. He or she should also be helped to gain a perspective on the overall time course of conditions and situations that commonly occur in the NH setting (of which the trainee may observe only a small portion).

RESEARCH

Research is absolutely vital if NH care is to be improved. There remains a paucity of data from well-designed studies that scientifically demonstrate the most effective methods of managing common conditions in the NH. But it is not easy to implement research in the NH successfully. Table 26-5 lists several of the major challenges faced by researchers who embark on studies in the NH setting. Many researchers, including ourselves, have encountered the pitfalls outlined in Table 26-5. Although many NHs now participate in a wide variety of research studies, most do not, and there remains a great deal of apprehension about research among NH administrators, staff, residents, and residents' families. Of particular concern to administrators, owners, and governing bodies is the potential cost of participating in research. There are, in fact, many potential costs, some of which may not be obvious either to the researchers or the NH. Table 26-6 lists these potential costs. It is incumbent upon researchers to address these costs thoroughly when planning a study and preparing a budget. NHs should be made aware of these costs and be assured that adequate resources are available to support a study before it is implemented.

More NHs must become involved in research for at least two reasons. First, the results of research that is carried out in "teaching" NHs, which often have more resources and staff than nonteaching facilities, may not be translatable to the typical American NH. Thus, research studies should include typical as well as teaching NHs, so that research findings will be generalizable to the former as well as the latter. Second, the nature of the NH population, especially its heterogeneity and high turnover rate, and the types of outcomes being sought require relatively large sample sizes in order to obtain scientifically valid data. Many studies, therefore, will require the involvement of several different NHs. As a result, an increasing number of primary care physicians and medical directors will be asked to assist in facilitating research in the their own NHs. Thus, it is important for practicing physicians to become familiar with some of the key issues that must be addressed if NH research is to be successful.

Because NH residents are an especially vulnerable population, it is essential that research in the NH setting conforms to the highest possible scientific and ethical standards. Just because NH residents are vulnerable, however, does not mean that they should be precluded from participation

Table 26-5   Major challenges faced by researchers in the nursing home setting

General apprehension among administrators, staff, residents, and families about research
Potential costs to facilitate (see Table 25-6)
Assessment of NH residents is time-consuming compared to research in other settings
Logistical difficulties in performing various tests that require specialized equipment (e.g., radiographic studies, complex urodynamics, electrophysiologic studies)
Informed consent may be problematic in the cognitively impaired
Nursing home medical records often contain scant and inaccurate data for research purposes
Sample size may be limited by informed consent, failure to meet screening criteria, and dropouts due to illness, death, or discharge

Table 26-6   Potential costs of research for nursing homes

Disruption of usual care routines
Preparing and transporting residents to research activities
Identifying surrogates and witnessing informed consent
Providing information on functional status
Answering questions of residents and families
Minor supplies, space, and telephones used by research staff
Assisting in administering treatment protocols
Assisting in assessing outcomes

in research that may benefit them as individuals while also leading to improvements in NH care in general. Table 26-7 lists several guidelines that we believe, on the basis of our experience as well as that of others, are critical if NH research is to succeed. Research in the NH, as all other settings, should be scientifically sound. It should undergo peer review and be approved by a federally sanctioned institutional review board or human subjects protection committee. Pilot studies are extremely important in developing efficient, nonintrusive methods of screening potential subjects, refining the research protocol, and determining sample sizes. In general, research that involves minimal risk to subjects (i.e., no more risk than they normally

Table 26-7   Keys to success of research in the nursing home

Plan research that is
   Scientifically sound
   Poses minimal risk
   Is of potential benefit to individual subjects
   Is clinically relevant
   Is generalizable to typical NHs (as opposed to teaching facilities affiliated with universities)
Educate and enlist the support of facility administration and staff, governing body, residents,
   and families
Address the potential costs of the research to the facility before starting the study (see Table
   26-6)
Develop explicit and detailed procedures for informed consent
   Enlisting and reimbursing a staff member (nurse or social worker) for assistance in
     determining decision-making capacity, identifying surrogates, and witnessing the consent
     process is very helpful
Develop efficient, nonintrusive screeng procedures
Perform pilot studies
   Data-collection instruments
   Assessment procedures
   Treatment protocols
   Determination of sample size
Provide feedback to facility staff
   Present progress reports and results to staff meetings

incur in the NH), is of potential benefit to individual subjects, and is gener-alizable to typical NHs is more likely to be accepted than research that does not meet these criteria. Educational and discussion sessions should be held with NH staff, residents, and families to convey the importance, objectives, and anticipated benefits of the proposed research. The potential costs of the research to the facility (see Table 26-6) should be addressed in detail with the administrator. A written list of mutual expectations is helpful in this regard. Because many NH residents are not capable of providing informed consent, procedures for obtaining informed consent must be developed. Meetings with families may be especially important, because most often one or more family members provide the informed consent required for the resi-dent's participation. We have found that enlisting and reimbursing a NH staff member to assist in determining a resident's capacity to consent, iden-tifying an appropriate surrogate, and witnessing the consent process is extremely helpful and may go a long way toward assuaging fears of exploi-tation. Finally, it is very important that the research team provide feedback about the results of the research to NH staff. A conference that describes the results and their implications for care in the NH, along with written mate-rials, will be an effective means of accomplishing this objective.

SELECTED READINGS

Education

Aiken LH, Mezey MD, Lynaugh JE, et al: Teaching nursing homes: Prospects for improving long-term care. *J Am Geriatr Soc* 33:196–201, 1985.

Breitenbacher RB and Schultz AL: Extended care in nursing homes: A program for a country teaching medical center. *Ann Intern Med* 1:96–100, 1983.

Grady MJ and Earll JM: Teaching physical diagnosis in the nursing home. *Am J Med* 88:519–521, 1990.

Kane R, Solomon D, Beck J, and Keeler E: The future need for geriatric manpower in the United States. *N Engl J Med* 302:1327–1332, 1980.

Kapp MB: Nursing homes as teaching institutions: Legal issues. *Gerontologist* 24:55–60, 1984.

Libow LS: Geriatric medicine and the nursing home: A mechanism for mutual excellence. *Ger-ontologist* 22:134–141, 1982.

McVey LJ, Davis DE, and Cohen HJ: The 'aging game': An approach to education in geriatrics. *JAMA* 262:1507–1509, 1989.

Pawlson LG: Education in the nursing home: Practical considerations. *J Am Geriatr Soc* 30:600–602, 1982.

Robbins AS, Fink A, Kosecoff J, et al: Studies in geriatric education: I. Developing education objectives. *J Am Geriatr Soc* 30:281–288, 1982.

Rosenthal MS, Mashall CE, Martin SE, et al: Nursing home rounds as a format for teaching residents and medical students. *J Med Educ* 62:975–980, 1987.

Rowe JW, Grossman E, Bond E, et al: Academic geriatrics for the year 2000: An Institute of Medicine report. *N Engl J Med* 316:1425–1428, 1987.

Schneider EL, Ory M, and Aung ML: Teaching nursing homes revisited: Survey of affiliations between American medical schools and long-term-care facilities. *JAMA* 257:2771–2775, 1987.

Vivell S, Solomon DH, and Beck JC: Medical education responds to the 20th century's success story. *J Am Geriatr Soc* 35:1107–1115, 1987.

Woolliscroft JO, Calhoun JG, Maxim BR, et al: Medical education in facilities for the elderly: Impact on medical students, facility staff, and residents. *JAMA* 252:3382–3385, 1984.

Research

Cohen-Mansfield J, Kerin P, Pawlson G, et al: Informed consent for research in a nursing home: Processes and issues. *Gerontologist* 28:355–359, 1988.

Lipsitz LA, Pluchino FC, and Wright SM: Biomedical research in the nursing home: Methodological issues and subject recruitment results. *J Am Geriatr Soc* 35:629–634, 1987.

Melnick VL and Dubler NN (eds): *Alzheimer's Dementia: Dilemmas in Clinical Research.* Clifton, New Jersey, Humana Press, 1985.

Palumbo FB, Magaziner JS, Tenney JH, et al: Recruitment of long-term care facilities for research. *J Am Geriatr Soc* 35:154–158, 1987.

Warren JW, Sobal J, Tenney JH, et al: Informed consent by proxy: An issue in research with elderly patients. *N Engl J Med* 315:1124–1128, 1986.

Zimmer AW, Calkins E, Hadley E, et al: Conducting clinical research in geriatric populations. *Ann Intern Med* 103:276–283, 1985.

APPENDIX

APPENDIX

SUMMARY OF NEW FEDERAL REGULATIONS RELEVANT TO PRIMARY PHYSICIANS AND MEDICAL DIRECTORS IN NURSING HOMES: 1987 OMNIBUS BUDGET RECONCILIATION ACT (OBRA)

The 1987 OBRA was passed into law on December 22, 1987. This law contains several new requirements, offers more detail, and has higher expectations for nursing home (NH) care than previous laws. Some of the new regulations were specified in the law, while others are the result of interpretations of the intent of the statutes by the Health Care Financing Administration (HCFA), which is the agency of the Department of Health and Human Services (HHS) responsible for Medicare and Medicaid.

The new regulations were published in the *Federal Register*, volume 54, number 21, on February 2, 1989. They combine previous regulations related to skilled and intermediate-care facilities into one set, which is contained in Title 42, Code of Federal Regulations, Part 483—Medicare and Medicaid Requirements for Long-Term-Care Facilities (abbreviated 42 CFT Part 483).

The intent of the new regulations is severalfold:

1. To implement the requirements and the survey, certification, and enforcement process contained in the 1987 OBRA
2. To revise and consolidate the requirements for long-term-care facilities to participate in both the Medicare and Medicaid programs
3. To consolidate conditions for both skilled nursing facilities (SNFs) and intermediate care facilities (ICFs; both will be referred to as *nursing facilities*)
4. To attempt to improve the quality of care in NHs in response to studies and public statements critical of the care currently provided
5. To focus more on actual performance in meeting residents' needs rather than on the capacity or potential to do so

Facilities must comply with these regulations in order to qualify for Medicare and Medicaid reimbursement. HCFA can deny payment to facilities that do not comply. Violation of Level A requirements (previously termed *conditions of participation*) can result in termination of a facility's participation in the Medicare program. Violation of Level B requirements (subsections of Level A requirements which were previously termed *standards*) can result in other sanctions.

The information presented below is a summary of several of the regulations and guidelines issued for surveyors and their implications for primary physicians and medical directors in NHs. It is based on a synopsis written by Dr. Steve Levinson for the American Medical Directors' Association and on the Interpretive Guidelines transmitted by HCFA to state agencies regarding the new regulations and survey process. Some states and organizations are considering legal challenges to the implementation of these regulations. The degree to which these regulations will be implemented is therefore currently not clear.

Resident Rights (483.10)

A. Level A requirement
   The resident has a right to a dignified existence, self-determination, and communication with and access to persons and services inside and outside of the facility. A facility must protect and promote the rights of each resident.
B. Level B requirements specify many rules related to
   1. Exercise of rights
   2. Notice of rights and services
   3. Protection of resident funds
   4. Free choice
   5. Privacy and confidentiality
   6. Grievances
   7. Examination of survey results
   8. Work
   9. Mail
   10. Access to the facility and visitation rights
   11. Telephone
   12. Personal property
   13. Married couples
   14. Self-administration of drugs
C. Implications for the medical director
   1. The medical director will have to assist in the development of policies and procedures that help meet the requirements for protecting and enhancing residents' rights.
   2. Specific policies and procedures will be needed for
      a. Decision-making capacity and the right to refuse treatment
      b. Notification of significant changes in a resident's status and the need to alter treatment or transfer the resident
      c. Self-administration of medication
   3. The medical director will have to help ensure that the resident has appropriate choice of and access to medical care.

D. Implications for the primary care physician
  1. Help ensure that resident is informed of health status in comprehensible language.
  2. Help ensure that resident is fully informed about care and treatment and participates in planning that care and treatment to the extent possible.
  3. Play a role in determining and documenting a resident's decision-making capacity and ability to self-administer medications.

Admission, Transfer, and Discharge Rights (483.12)

A. Implications for the medical director
  1. The medical director will have to participate in the development of appropriate procedures, especially documentation of the medical aspects of admissions, transfers, and discharges.
    a. This requirement covers intrafacility transfers (e.g., to and from a Medicare distinct part unit) as well as transfers out of the facility.
B. Implications for the primary care physician
  1. The primary care physician will have to certify and document the medical necessity and appropriateness of all admissions, transfers, and discharges.

Resident Behavior and Facility Practices (483.13)

A. Level B requirement: Restraints
  1. The resident has the right to be free from any physical restraints imposed or psychoactive drug administered for purposes of discipline or convenience and not required to treat the resident's medical symptoms.
  2. Physical restraints are any manual method of physical or mechanical device, material, or equipment attached or adjacent to the resident's body that the individual cannot remove easily which restricts freedom of movement or access to one's body (includes leg and arm restraints, hand mitts, soft ties or vest, wheelchair safety bars, and gerichairs).
  3. Psychoactive drugs are covered below, under "Quality of Care."
  4. There must be a trial of less restrictive measures unless the physical restraint is necessary to provide lifesaving treatment.
  5. The resident or his/her legal representative must consent to the use of restraints.
  6. Residents who are restrained should be released, exercised, toileted, and checked for skin redness every 2 h.
  7. The need for restraints should be reevaluated periodically.

B. Implications for medical directors
  1. The medical director will have to help develop policies and procedures for the appropriate use of restraints and psychoactive drugs.
C. Implications for primary care physicians
  1. Primary physicians will have to
    a. Write appropriate orders for restraints and psychoactive drugs
    b. Help ensure that restraints and/or psychoactive drugs are used appropriately for residents under their care

Resident Assessment (483.20)

A. Level A requirement:
  The facility must conduct initially and periodically a comprehensive, accurate, standardized, reproducible assessment of each resident's functional capacity.
  (*Note*: By the time this book is published, the Minimum Data Set developed by HCFA will have become a mandatory component of this assessment.)
B. Level B requirements include rules relevant to
  1. Admission orders
  2. Comprehensiveness and accuracy of assessments
  3. Care plans
  4. Discharge summaries
  5. Preadmission screening for mentally ill individuals and individuals with mental retardation
C. Implications for medical directors
  1. The medical directors will need to establish policies and procedures for appropriate documentation of admission assessments, orders, and discharge summaries.
  2. Develop a mechanism for incorporating the medical assessment into the comprehensive care plan.
D. Implications for primary care physician
  1. The primary care physician will need to
    a. Provide appropriate admission orders
    b. Participate in a comprehensive assessment
    c. Assist the staff in developing a comprehensive care plan and review it periodically
    d. Provide a pertinent and timely discharge summary

Quality of Care (483.25)

A. Level A requirement
  Each resident must receive and the facility must provide the necessary

care and services to attain or maintain the highest practicable physical, mental, and psychosocial well-being, in accordance with the comprehensive assessment and plan of care.

B. Level B requirements include rules relevant to
  1. Activities of daily living
     a. The facility must ensure that a resident's abilities in activities of daily living do not diminish unless circumstances of the resident's clinical condition demonstrate the diminution was unavoidable.
  2. Vision and hearing
  3. Pressure sores
     a. The facility must ensure that a resident who enters the facility without pressure sores does not develop pressure sores unless the individual's clinical condition demonstrates that they were unavoidable.
     b. A resident having pressure sores must receive necessary treatment and services to promote healing, prevent infection, and prevent new pressure sores from developing.
  4. Urinary incontinence
     a. A resident who is incontinent of urine must receive the appropriate treatment and services to restore as much normal bladder functioning as possible.
     b. A resident who enters the facility without an indwelling catheter is not catheterized unless the resident's clinical condition demonstrates that catheterization was necessary.
        (1) Generally, chronic use of an indwelling catheter should occur only after a restorative program to improve bladder function has been attempted and/or facility staff have tried to manage the incontinence (e.g., use of adult diapers, an external catheter, or a prompted voiding program)
        (2) Clinical conditions demonstrating that catheterization is unavoidable include
            (a) Urinary retention that
                1. Is causing persistent overflow incontinence, symptomatic infections, and/or renal dysfunction
                2. Cannot be corrected surgically
                3. Cannot be managed practically with intermittent catheter use
            (b) Skin wounds, pressure sores, or irritations that are being contaminated by incontinent urine
            (c) Care of terminally ill or severely impaired residents for whom bed and clothing changes are uncomfortable or disruptive

    c. A resident who is incontinent of urine must receive appropriate treatment and services to prevent urinary tract infections and to restore as much normal bladder function as possible.

5. Range of motion
6. Psychosocial functioning
7. Nasogastric tubes (includes gastrostomy and jejunostomy tubes)
    a. A resident who has been able to eat enough alone or with assistance is not fed by nasogastric tube unless the resident's clinical condition demonstrates that use of a nasogastric tube was unavoidable.
       (1) Clinical conditions demonstrating that nourishment via an enteral tube is unavoidable include
         (*a*) The inability to swallow without choking or aspiration, as in cases of Parkinson's disease, pseudobulbar palsy, or esophageal diverticulum
         (*b*) Lack of sufficient alertness for oral nutrition (i.e., resident comatose)
         (*c*) Malnutrition not attributable to a single cause or causes that can be isolated and reversed plus documented evidence that the facility has not been able to maintain or improve the resident's nutritional status through oral intake
    b. A resident who is fed by a nasogastric or gastrostomy tube must receive the appropriate treatment and services to prevent aspiration pneumonia, diarrhea, vomiting, dehydration, metabolic abnormalities, and nasopharyngeal ulcers and to restore, if possible, normal feeding function.

8. Accidents
    a. An *accident* is an unexpected, unintended event that can cause a resident bodily injury. It does not include adverse outcomes associated with treatment or care.

9. Nutrition
    a. Resident's care maintains acceptable parameters of nutritional status, such as body weight and protein levels, unless the resident's clinical condition demonstrates that this is not possible.
    b. Receives a therapeutic diet when there is a nutritional problem.
       (1) Unacceptable parameters of nourishment include weight loss as well as other indices such as clinical signs and symptoms of malnourishment and laboratory tests indicating malnourishment (e.g., serum albumin levels).
       (2) Suggested parameters for evaluating significance of unplanned and undesired weight loss are as follows:

Interval	Significant loss %	Severe loss %
1 month	5	> 5
3 months	7.5	> 7.5
6 months	10	>10

10. Hydration
11. Special needs (e.g., injections, colostomy care, respiratory care, podiatric care, prostheses)
12. Drug therapy
    a. Each resident's drug regimen must be free from unnecessary drugs
       (1) "Unnecessary drugs" are drugs that are given in excessive doses, for excessive periods of time, without adequate monitoring, or in the absence of a diagnosis or reason for the drug. An unnecessary drug is a drug for which monitoring data, or undue adverse consequences indicates that the drug should be reduced or discontinued entirely. An unnecessary drug is also one which is prescribed only in anticipation of an adverse consequence of another prescribed drug.
       (2) In deciding whether an unnecessary drug is being used, surveyors are instructed to be very sure that reputable literature and thorough understanding of the resident's clinical condition justifies this judgment. (HCFA is developing additional guidelines for surveyors for determining unnecessary drugs which will include specific drugs and dosages.)
    b. Antipsychotic drugs
       (1) Residents who have not used antipsychotic drugs are not given these drugs unless antipsychotic drug therapy is necessary to treat a specific condition.
          (a) Antipsychotic drugs should not be used unless the clinical record documents that the resident has one or more of the following "specific conditions":
             1. Schizophrenia
             2. Schizoaffective disorder
             3. Delusional disorder
             4. Psychotic mood disorders (including mania and depression with psychotic features)
             5. Acute psychotic episodes
             6. Brief reactive psychosis
             7. Schizophreniform disorder
             8. Atypical psychosis
             9. Tourette's disorder

10. Huntington's disease
11. Organic mental syndromes (including dementia) with associated psychotic and/or agitated features as defined by
    - Specific behaviors as quantitatively (number of episodes) and objectively (e.g., biting, kicking, and scratching) documented by the facility which causes residents to
      —Present a danger to themselves
      —Present a danger to others (including staff)
      —Actually interfere with staff's ability to provide care
    - Psychotic symptoms (hallucinations, paranoia, delusions) not exhibited as specific behaviors listed above but *which cause the resident frightful distress*
12. Short-term (7 days) symptomatic treatment of hiccups, nausea, vomiting, or pruritus

(*b*) Antipsychotics should not be used if one or more of the following is/are the *only* indication
1. Simple pacing
2. Wandering
3. Poor self-care
4. Restlessness
5. Crying out, yelling, or screaming
6. Impaired memory
7. Anxiety
8. Depression
9. Insomnia
10. Unsociability
11. Indifference to surroundings
12. Fidgeting
13. Nervousness
14. Uncooperativeness
15. Any indication for which the order is on an "as needed" basis

(2) Residents who use antipsychotic drugs must receive gradual dose reductions, drug holidays, or behavioral programming (unless clinically contraindicated) in an effort to discontinue these drugs.

(*a*) *Drug holiday* means a periodic tapering and subsequent discontinuation of a drug to test the need for its continued use.

(b) *Behavioral programming* means modification of the resident's behavior and/or the resident's environment, including staff approaches to care, to the largest degree possible to accommodate the resident's behavioral disturbances.

(c) Gradual dose reductions consist of tapering the resident's daily dose to determine if the resident's symptoms can be controlled by a lower dose or if the dose can be eliminated altogether. At a *minimum*, a resident with a stable condition should be tapered (after no more and possibly less than 6 months of therapy) at a maximum of 25 percent (approximately) of the initial dose per month.

(d) *Clinically contraindicated* means that a resident has a diagnosis as described above and has had gradual dose reductions to the lowest possible dose necessary to control symptoms.

13. Medication errors

C. Implications for medical directors

    1. The medical director will have to work with other administrative staff to develop policies and procedures that strive to optimize the quality of care, with specific reference to the areas covered under Level B requirements (Items 1 to 13 above).

D. Implications for primary care physicians

    1. Primary care physicians will have to make careful assessments and appropriately document the results of these assessments, the plan of care, and the outcomes of interventions, especially related to

        a. Changes in physical and psychosocial functional status

        b. Potentially correctable vision and hearing problems

        c. Pressure sore treatment and prevention

        d. Assessment and management of urinary incontinence

        e. The need for indwelling bladder catheters

        f. Prevention and management of contractures

        g. Nutritional and hydration status and the need for and management of enteral feeding tubes

        h. Drug therapy

        i. The use of and response to antipsychotic drugs

Physician Services (483.40)

A. Level A requirements

A physician must personally approve a recommendation that an individual be admitted to a facility. Each resident must remain under the care of a physician.

B. Level B requirements
   1. Physician supervision
   2. Physician visits
      a. The physician must review the resident's total program of care, including medications and treatments, at each required visit.
      b. At each visit, the physician must write, date, and sign a progress note and sign all orders.
   3. Frequency of physician visits
      a. The resident must be seen by a physician at least once every 30 days for the first 90 days after admission and at least once every 60 days thereafter.
         (1) A physician visit is considered timely if it occurs not later than 10 days after the date the visit was required.
         (2) Required visits after the initial visit may alternate between personal visits by the physician and visits by a physician's assistant or nurse practitioner.
   4. Availability of physicians for emergency care
   5. Physician delegation of tasks
      a. Physicians may delegate tasks to a physician's assistant or nurse practitioner who
         (1) Meets the applicable federal definition
         (2) Is acting within the scope of practice as defined by state law
         (3) Is under the supervision of a physician
      b. Tasks may not be delegated for which regulations specify that the physician must perform them personally or when delegation is prohibited by state law or the facility's own policies.
C. Implications for medical director
   1. The medical director will need to establish policies and procedures that relate to
      a. Admission
      b. Required routine and emergency care
      c. Physician's assistants and nurse practitioners
   2. The medical director will be responsible for monitoring the medical staff's compliance with required visits and availability for 24-h emergency coverage.
D. Implications for primary care physicians
   1. Primary care physicians will need to
      a. Personally approve a resident's admission to a facility
      b. Make required visits within 10 days of the scheduled date or supervise a physician's assistant or nurse practitioner in making alternate visits after the initial visit
      c. At each visit, review the resident's plan of care, sign orders, and write, date, and sign a progress note

   d. Arrange for coverage for required activities and for 24-h availability for emergencies

Specialized Rehabilitative Services (483.45)

A. Level A requirement
   A facility must provide or obtain rehabilitative services—such as physical therapy, speech-language pathology, and occupational therapy—to every resident it admits.
B. Implications for medical directors
   1. The medical director will need to
      a. Ensure the availability of adequate rehabilitative services
      b. Assist in establishing policies and procedures that arrange for assessment of rehabilitation potential and for ordering of rehabilitative services
C. Implications for primary care physicians
   1. Primary care physicians will need to
      a. Perform or request an assessment of functional abilities and rehabilitation potential
      b. Request or approve specific rehabilitative services

Infection Control (483.65)

A. Level A requirement
   The facility must establish and maintain an infection control program designed to provide a safe, sanitary, and comfortable environment in which residents may reside and to help prevent the development and transmission of disease and infection.
B. Level B requirements relate to
   1. The infection control program
   2. Preventing spread of infection
   3. Linens
C. Implications for the medical director
   1. The medical director will need to assist in the development and implementation of an infection control program, including surveillance procedures, vaccinations, isolation, and universal precautions.
D. Implications for primary care physicians
   1. Primary care physicians will need to
      a. Assist the medical director and facility in preventing, managing, and reporting significant infections and particularly outbreaks
      b. Document the occurrence of infections and the need for antimicrobial therapy (if applicable)
      c. Order isolation or other preventive measures when indicated in specific cases

Administration (483.75)

A. Level A requirement
A facility must be administered in a manner that enables it to use its resources effectively and efficiently to attain or maintain the highest practicable physical, mental, and psychosocial well-being of each resident.
B. Level B requirements relate to a broad range of administrative issues. Those of most relevance to medical care include
  1. Medical director
    a. The medical director is responsible for
      (1) The coordination of medical care in the facility
      (2) Implementation of resident care policies
        (a) Examples of "resident care policies" include admissions, transfers, and discharges; infection control; and physician privileges and practices.
        (b) The medical director is also responsible for policies related to accidents and incidents; ancillary services such as laboratory, radiology, and pharmacy; use of medications; use and release of clinical information; utilization review; and overall quality of care.
        (c) The medical director's coordination role also includes but is not limited to assuring that visits by or to medical consultants occur as needed.
  2. Laboratory, radiology, and other diagnostic services
  3. Clinical records
  4. Transfer agreement (with one or more hospitals)
  5. Quality assessment and assurance
    a. A facility must maintain a quality assessment and assurance committee consisting of
      (1) The director of nursing services
      (2) A physician designated by the facility
      (3) At least three other members of the facility's staff
    b. The committee
      (1) Meets at least quarterly to identify issues with respect to which quality assessment and assurance activities are necessary
      (2) Develops and implements appropriate plans of action to correct identified quality deficiencies
C. Implications for medical directors
  1. Medical directors will need to
    a. Establish a job description
    b. Assume responsibility for implementing resident care policies and coordinating medical care

   c. Help ensure the provision of appropriate and timely laboratory, radiology, and other diagnostic services

   d. Assist the facility in creating complete, accurate, and systematically organized medical records

   e. Establish policies and procedures for appropriate documentation by physicians in medical records

   f. Assist the facility in developing a written transfer agreement with one or more hospitals

   g. Assist the facility in establishing and implementing a quality assessment and assurance program and committee

   h. Evaluate the results of quality assurance reviews as they relate to medical services

D. Implications for primary care physicians

 1. Primary care physicians will need to

   a. Provide appropriate documentation in the medical record, including

    (1) Assessments and care plans

    (2) Progress notes

    (3) Follow-up on the results of diagnostic studies

   b. Follow up in a timely fashion on results of laboratory, radiology, and other diagnostic tests

   c. Participate in quality assessment and assurance activities

POLICIES, PROCEDURES, AND GUIDELINES

Nurse Practitioner Clinical Privileges

Professional nurses assigned as nurse practitioners shall be clinically privileged in the following:

A. Verification and transcription of the following orders on physician's order sheet, which require a physician's signature (within _____ working days):
   1. Admitting diagnosis
   2. Resident condition
   3. Resident activity level
   4. Diet order
B. Renewing of prescribed medication
C. Renewing of existing "No CPR" orders
D. Independent initiation of
   1. Nursing care orders (i.e., weights, vital signs, finger sticks for glucose, catheter/wound/skin care)
   2. Oral fluids
   3. Over-the-counter drugs (refer to facility prescription drug formulary), nonnarcotic antidiarrheals, antacids, antihistamines, decongestants, expectorants, nonnarcotic analgesics, dermatological products, and vitamins
   4. Rehabilitation evaluations (occupational, physical, speech therapies)
   5. All diagnostic studies except x-ray studies involving radiocontrast, nuclear medicine studies, echocardiography, and invasive vascular studies
   6. Oxygen therapy and respiratory therapy
E. Initiate new treatment per standardized procedure and/or after discussion with primary physician
   1. Consults
   2. All other treatment and diagnostic studies
F. Orders for intravenous fluids
G. Perform venipuncture for obtaining blood specimens
H. Perform electrocardiograms
I. Perform simple cystometry in the evaluation of urinary incontinence
J. Remove sutures
K. Debridement and packing of minor wounds and pressure sores
L. Irrigate ears and remove impacted cerumen
M. Pack anterior nares for epistaxis

N. Administration and interpretation of diagnostic skin testing according to established criteria

Jewish Homes for the Aging of Greater Los Angeles—Guidelines for Notification of Physicians and/or Nurse Practitioners of Changes in Resident Status

Policy

A. Specific signs, symptoms, and laboratory values suggestive of *acute* illness needing immediate medical assessment (as defined below) will be reported to the primary medical doctor (PMD) or nurse practitioner (NP) by the charge nurse or nursing supervisor as soon as possible after they are identified.

B. All acute changes in resident status reported to the medical staff on an immediate basis will be assessed and documented in the medical record by the nursing staff.

C. In the event of a witnessed cardiac or respiratory arrest (for residents who have full code status), "911" will be called, with later notification of PMD.

D. When contacting medical on-call coverage during night and weekend hours, nursing staff will have the following information available:
   1. Present problem with symptoms, signs, and results of physical assessment, including vital signs and mental status
   2. Active medical diagnoses
   3. Relevant information about any recent hospitalization
   4. Current medications
   5. Allergies
   6. CPR status and/or hospitalization status
   7. Family contact/DPA
   8. Date of last PMD visit

E. Specific signs, symptoms, and laboratory values suggestive of *subacute* illness (as defined below) will be reported to the PMD or NP by the charge nurse or nursing supervisor, but not on an immediate basis (e.g., the next time the PMD makes rounds).

F. All subacute changes in resident status reported to the medical staff on a nonimmediate basis will be assessed and documented in the medical record by the nursing staff.

Procedure

I. *Immediate Notification (Acute) Problems*
   The following symptoms, signs, and laboratory values should prompt *immediate* notification of the PMD or NP.

Immediate implies that the PMD or NP should be notified as soon as possible either directly or by beeper (charge nurse must always inform the clinical supervisor prior to PMD or NP notification).

Situations requiring immediate *action* (i.e., transport of the resident to the emergency room) with later notification of the physician are rare.

These situations include

1. Witnessed cardiac or respiratory arrest for residents who have full code status (*call 911*).
2. Rapid progression of signs or symptoms listed below before PMD or NP response is obtained. This applies only to residents with full code status (refer to transfer policy).

A. *Symptoms*
   1. Any complaint or apparent discomfort which is
      a. *Sudden* in onset
      b. *A marked change* (i.e., much more severe) in relation to usual complaints
      c. *Unrelieved* by measures which have already been prescribed (e.g., nitroglycerin for chest pain, antacid for abdominal pain, acetaminophen for other pain)
   2. Specific examples of symptoms (not meant to be all-inclusive)
      a. Shortness of breath
      b. Cough
      c. Chest pain, pressure, or tightness
      d. Nausea
      e. Diarrhea
      f. Musculoskeletal pain
      g. Severe headache
      h. Partial or complete loss of vision
      i. Dizziness or unsteadiness
      j. Weakness of an arm or leg
      k. Slurred speech
      l. New or worsening confusion
      m. Suicidal thoughts

B. *Signs*
   The following list of physical signs is not meant to be all inclusive. Any other sign about which you are uncertain should prompt PMD or NP notification.
   1. *Change* in vital signs
      General guidelines
      Temperature >101 degrees rectally
      Respiratory rate >28/min
      Pulse >110 or <55/min
      Blood pressure >200 systolic or <90 systolic
   2. Any loss of consciousness

3. Any seizure activity
4. Severe bleeding
   Examples
   Intractable nose bleed
   Hematemesis
   Melena
   Bright red blood in stool (not due to hemorrhoids)
   Profuse vaginal bleeding
   Gross hematuria
5. Laceration requiring sutures
6. Fall with any suspected serious injury (e.g., fracture)
7. New and/or severe gastrointestinal signs (not due to fecal impaction), including
   Nausea and vomiting
   Diarrhea
   Abdominal distention
8. Abnormal drainage, foul-smelling discharge, or wound complications
9. Sudden onset of new or severe worsening of confusion and/or agitation
10. New focal neurological sign, such as profound weakness of an extremity or slurring of speech

C. *Laboratory Results*
   1. Any lab report, normal or abnormal, which the PMD or NP requests on a "stat" or "same day" basis.
   2. In the event that "panic levels" are received from the laboratory, the PMD or NP will be notified *immediately* by phone or beeper.
   3. Any of the following, *unless values are consistently at this level and PMD or NP is aware.*

a.	Hematocrit	<30
b.	WBC	$>12,000$
c.	Sodium (Na)	<125
d.	Potassium (K)	<3.0 or >5.5
e.	Glucose	>250
		<90 in a diabetic on oral hypoglycemic or insulin <60 in anyone (diabetic or nondiabetic)
f.	BUN	>40

   g. Positive urine culture ($>10^5$ col/ml of a pathogen) only if (1) the patient has symptoms and is not on treatment; *or* (2) the pathogen is *NOT sensitive* to antibiotic which has been *prescribed*
   h. X-ray report revealing an unsuspected finding which may require immediate intervention (e.g., pneumonia, new long bone fracture)

D. *Other*
   1. Medication error (overdose or underdose)
      a. If it involves a cardiac or psychotropic drug
      b. If, in your judgment, the PMD or NP should be notified imme-diately because of the nature of the medication

II. *Nonimmediate Notification (Subacute) Problems*

The following types of problems should be reported to the PMD or NP, *but not on an immediate basis* (*nonimmediate* implies that the PMD or NP should be informed of the problem or event, but not immediately):

A. *Symptoms*
   1. **In general**
      Any *persistent* or *recurrent* complaint by a resident or family member that cannot be responded to satisfactorily with already existing understanding of the condition and/or orders for treatment.
   2. Specific examples of symptoms (not meant to be all-inclusive):
      Constipation
      Weakness or fatigue
      Diminished appetite
      Sleep difficulty
      Itching
      Headache
      Change in vision
      Hearing loss
      Dyspnea or orthopnea
      Difficulty swallowing
      Abdominal discomfort (e.g., bloating, cramps, etc.)
      Urinary hesitancy or poor stream
      Urinary incontinence
      Vaginal discharge or spotting
      Musculoskeletal pain
      Dizziness
      Difficulty walking
      Recurrent falls
      Memory loss
      Depressive thoughts

B. *Signs*
   1. Signs
      In general
      Any substantial *change* in physical condition, functional status, or *new* physical sign which does not require immediate notification should be discussed with the PMD or NP on rounds.
   2. Examples of signs and changes in condition (not meant to be all inclusive):

Progressive weakness

Diminished appetite

Weight loss or weight gain (e.g., greater than 5 lb in a month or shorter time period)

Sleep disturbance

Difficulty swallowing

Nocturia

Incontinence of urine or stool

Skin rash or pressure sore

Edema

Gait disturbances

Forgetfulness or confusion

Depressed affect

Agitation or behavioral disturbance

Personality change

C. *Other*

1. Consult reports requesting specific actions or changes in resident's management.
2. Observations in the course of routine nursing procedures that might require physician action. For example:
   (a) Poorly controlled blood pressure in a patient on antihypertensive therapy
   (b) Changes in urine or finger stick glucose values in diabetics (e.g., persistently high determinations in a patient who is normally well controlled)
   (c) Symptoms unresponsive to recently prescribed treatment
   (d) PRN medications which are never used
3. Medication errors (that do not require immediate notification)
4. Special topics concerning a resident's family
5. Annual lab and diagnostic study results

Jewish Homes for the Aging of Greater Los Angeles—Primary Care Physician Response to Calls from JHA Nursing Staff and Nurse Practitioners

Policy

Purpose of Policy

To ensure that the timing and nature of the response of primary care physicians to calls from JHA staff are appropriate.

1. This policy is meant to complement the existing policies entitled "Guidelines for Notification of Physicians and/or Nurse Practitioners of Changes in Resident Status."

2. Nursing staff and nurse practitioners (NP) will call 911 for paramedics only when in their judgment a resident (who is not on "No CPR" status) will require cardiopulmonary resuscitation before Encino Hospital can be reached by ambulance.

3. Calls to primary care physicians should be limited to those situations requiring immediate notification, as outlined in "Guidelines for Notification of Physicians and/or Nurse Practitioners of Changes in Resident Status," unless otherwise requested in the physician's orders.

4. If there is any doubt about whether the primary care physician should be called, the nursing supervisor should make the decision and in doing so generally favor making the call if there is any question.

5. Primary care physicians will be notified of situations requiring nonimmediate notification, as outlined in "Guidelines for Notification of Physicians and/or Nurse Practitioners of Changes in Resident Status," the next time they make rounds or are in clinic.

6. Primary care physicians must be available to respond to calls from JHA staff at all times during weekdays and nights.

    a. If they will not be available, they must arrange coverage by another member of the JHA primary care medical staff and inform the nursing staff of this change.

7. Weekend call schedules for each campus will be published monthly.

8. When a primary care physician is called, he or she should respond promptly, generally within 15 min.

    a. Response time should not exceed 30 min.

    b. Staff should call or page the physician again if he or she has not responded within 30 min.

9. If the primary care physician does not respond within 15 min of the second call, staff should contact, in the following order: (1) the medical director of their campus, (2) the medical director of the other campus, (3) the associate medical director.

10. Primary care physicians must be courteous and respectful when answering calls from JHA nursing staff and NPs. Verbal abuse of staff is a violation of the JHA Standards for Primary Physicians and will not be tolerated.

    a. If nursing staff or the NP feel that the primary care physician has been unnecessarily discourteous or disrespectful when responding to a call, they will convey this to the medical director of their campus in writing.

    b. If the nursing staff or NP is uncomfortable with the primary care physician's response and feel that the resident needs further attention, they will contact the medical director or associate medical director as outlined in item 9 above.

    c. Situations in which a primary care physician has difficulty respond-
ing to a call or has been called inappropriately should be reported
to the appropriate medical director.

Policy and Procedures for Sending Resident Information to Consultants and Hospitals

I. OBJECTIVES

To transfer pertinent information to health care providers caring for a
resident of the Jewish Homes for the Aging when the resident must be
evaluated outside the facility.

    This is necessary to improve understanding by consultants and
emergency room personnel of the resident's overall health and medication history and to enhance the conveyance of their findings and new
orders.

    The overall goal is to help residents obtain maximum benefit from
visits to caregivers when outside of the Jewish Homes for the Aging.

II. TRANSFER FORMS

Two different checklist forms are to be used to assemble:

1. INFORMATION PACKET FOR CONSULTANTS
2. TRANSFER PACKET FOR HOSPITALS and EMERGENCY ROOMS

    Each contains a list of necessary documents to be sent with the
resident (Figs. A-1 and A-2).

III. PROCEDURES

The nursing supervisor and charge nurse are responsible for completing
the transfer forms.

A. The LVN charge nurse will oversee
   1. The timely photocopying of pertinent parts of the medical record
   2. Initial his/her name after each part is included
B. The RN nursing supervisor will
   1. Confirm that all necessary papers are in the information packet
   2. Sign his/her name certifying that the packet has been reviewed
C. Whenever possible, clerical personnel in the medical clinic will assist
in the photocopying, collating, and completion of the above records.
D. The only occasion when the above information package would be
waived is when
   1. The resident has a life-threatening condition
   2. Completion of the forms would delay immediate transfer by emergency medical services

In such a situation, the information packet should still be assembled and
its contents faxed or delivered to the receiving facility as soon as
possible.

Acute Hospitalization
Transfer Check List

Initial

1. Copy of Medical Face Sheet and
   Treatment Status Sheet (and Forms re:
   No CPR or No Artificial Feeding and Hydration,
   if applicable)   _____

2. Copy of last 2 progress note pages   _____

3. Copy of Medicare, Social Security,
   Medi-Cal cards   _____

4. Copy of latest computer-generated MD orders,
   plus any additional orders since printout   _____

5. Copy of latest complete H & P   _____

6. Copy of original admission H & P (if available)   _____

7. Copy of recent lab test results (CBC or hemoglobin, BUN,
   Creatinine, other lab done recently)   _____

8. Copy of last chest x-ray report   _____

9. Copy of last EKG   _____

10. Copy of DPA pages   _____

11. Check list of personal belongings (including dentures, hearing aid) _____

12. Notify social worker and administration if resident is admitted _____

    (If DPA or conservatorship **not** available, let Social Worker know)

The above papers were sent with _____
                                        Name of Resident

To:_____   On:_____/_____/_____
           Name of Hospital   Date

                          By:_____
                             Name of Person Preparing Packet

Figure A–1 Example of a checklist that is transferred to the acute care hospital with the
resident.

**Consultant Information
for Initial Consult**

Initial

1. Copy of Consultation Request Form and a Progress Note page   _____

2. Blank Physician Order page   _____

3. Copy of Medical Face Sheet   _____

4. Copy of last 2 progress note pages   _____

5. Copy of Medicare, Social Security,
    Medi-Cal cards   _____

6. Copy of latest computer-generated MD orders,
    plus any additional orders since printout   _____

7. Copy of recent lab test results (CBC or hemoglobin, BUN,
    Creatinine, other lab tests done recently)   _____

8. Copy of last chest x-ray report   _____

9. Copy of last EKG   _____

10. Copy of latest complete H & P   _____

11. Copy of original admission H & P (if available)   _____

The above papers were sent with _____
                                    Name of Resident

To:_____ On:_____/_____/_____
            Name of Consultant   Date

By:_____
           Name of Person Preparing Packet

Figure A–2 Example of a checklist that is sent to consultants with the resident.

E. The original copy of the completed and signed transfer form should be sent with the documents and the resident to the receiving consultant or hospital. A photocopy of the transfer form is to be retained in the medical record.

Examples of Centers for Disease Control (CDC) Definitions for Nosocomial Infections

The definitions included below are abstracted from Garner JS, Jarvis WR, Enori TG, et al: CDC definitions for nosocomial infections, 1988. *J Infect Control* 16:128–140, 1988.

Because of the nature of nursing home (NH) residents and the typical diagnostic evaluations that are done in NHs, these definitions may need to be modified for NH infection control programs.

Urinary tract infection

Urinary tract infection (UTI) includes symptomatic UTI, asymptomatic bacteriuria, and other infections of the urinary tract.

Symptomatic UTI must meet these criteria:

1. One of the following: fever ($>38°C$), urgency, frequency, dysuria, or suprapubic tenderness *and* a urine culture of $\geq 10^5$ colonies/ml urine with no more than two species of organisms.
2. Two of the following: fever ($>38°C$), urgency, frequency, dysuria, or suprapubic tenderness *and* any of the following:
   a. Dipstick test positive for leukocyte esterase and/or nitrite
   b. Pyuria [≥ 10 white blood cells (WBC)/ml^3 or ≥ 3 WBC/high-power field of unspun urine]
   c. Organisms seen on Gram stain of unspun urine
   d. Two urine cultures with repeated isolation of the same uropathogen with $\geq 10^2$ colonies/ml urine in nonvoided specimens
   e. Urine culture with $\leq 10^5$ colonies/ml urine of single uropathogen in patient being treated with appropriate antimicrobial therapy
   f. Physician's diagnosis
   g. Physician institutes appropriate antimicrobial therapy

Asymptomatic bacteriuria must meet either of the following criteria:

1. An indwelling catheter is present within 7 days before urine is cultured *and* patient has no fever ($>38°C$), urgency, frequency, dysuria, or suprapubic tenderness *and* has urine culture of $\geq 10^5$ organisms/ml urine with no more than two species of organisms
2. No indwelling urinary catheter is present within 7 days before the first two urine cultures with $\geq 10^5$ organisms/ml urine of the same organisms with no more than two species of organisms *and* patient has no fever ($>38°C$), urgency, frequency, dysuria, or suprapubic tenderness.

Eye, ear, nose, throat, and mouth infection

Eye infection includes conjunctivitis and other eye infections. Ear infections include otitis externa, otitis media, otitis interna, and mastoiditis. Nose, throat, and mouth infections include oral cavity infections, upper respiratory infections, and sinusitis.

Conjunctivitis must meet either of the following criteria:

1. Pathogen isolated from culture of purulent exudate obtained from conjunctiva or contiguous tissues such as eyelid, cornea, meibomian glands, or lacrimal glands
2. Pain or redness of conjunctiva or around eye *and* any of the following:
   a. WBCs and organisms seen on Gram stain of exudate
   b. Purulent exudate
   c. Positive antigen test on exudate or conjunctival scraping
   d. Multinucleated giant cells seen on microscopic examination of conjunctival exudate or scrapings
   e. Positive viral culture on conjunctival exudate
   f. Diagnostic single antibody titer (IgM) or fourfold increase in paired serum samples (IgG) for pathogen

Otitis externa must meet either of the following criteria:

1. Pathogen isolated from culture of purulent drainage from ear canal
2. One of the following: fever ($>$38°C), pain, redness, or drainage from ear canal *and* organisms seen on Gram stain of purulent drainage

Sinusitis must meet either of the following criteria:

1. Organism isolated from culture of purulent material obtained from sinus cavity
2. One of the following: fever ($>$38°C), pain or tenderness over the involved sinus, headache, purulent exudate, or nasal obstruction *and* either of the following:
   a. Positive transillumination
   b. Radiographic evidence of infection

Upper respiratory tract infection (pharyngitis, laryngitis, epiglottis) must meet one of the following criteria:

1. Two of the following: fever ($>$38°C), erythema of pharynx, sore throat, cough, hoarseness, or purulent exudate in throat *and* any of the following:
   a. Organism isolated from culture of specific site
   b. Organism isolated from blood culture
   c. Positive antigen test on blood or respiratory secretions

    d. Diagnostic single antibody titer (IgM) or fourfold increase in paired serum samples (IgG) for pathogen
    e. Physician's diagnosis
2. Abscess seen on direct examination, during surgery, or by histopathologic examination

Pneumonia

Pneumonia is defined separately from other infections of the lower respiratory tract. The criteria for pneumonia involve various combinations of clinical, radiographic, and laboratory evidence of infection. In general, expectorated sputum cultures are not useful in diagnosing pneumonia but may help identify the etiologic agent and provide useful antimicrobial susceptibility data. Findings from serial chest x-ray studies may be more helpful than those from a single x-ray film.

Pneumonia must meet one of the following criteria:

1. Rales or dullness to percussion on physical examination of chest *and* any of the following:
    a. New onset of purulent sputum or change in character of sputum
    b. Organisms isolated from blood culture
    c. Isolation of pathogen from specimen obtained by transtracheal aspirate, bronchial brushing, or biopsy
2. Chest radiographic examination shows new or progressive infiltrate, consolidation, cavitation, or pleural effusion *and* any of the following:
    a. New onset of purulent sputum or change in character of sputum
    b. Organism isolated from blood culture
    c. Isolation of pathogen from specimen obtained by transtracheal aspirate, bronchial brushing, or biopsy
    d. Isolation of virus or detection of viral antigen in respiratory secretions
    e. Diagnostic single antibody titer (IgM) or fourfold increase in paired serum samples (IgG) for pathogen
    f. Histopathologic evidence of pneumonia

Lower respiratory tract infection (excluding pneumonia)

Lower respiratory tract infection (excluding pneumonia) includes infections such as bronchitis, tracheobronchitis, bronchiolitis, tracheitis, lung abscess, and empyema.

Bronchitis, tracheobronchitis, bronchiolitis, or tracheitis without evidence of pneumonia must meet either of the following criteria:

1. Patient has no clinical or radiographic evidence of pneumonia *and* has two of the following: fever (>38°C), cough, new or increased sputum production, rhonchi, wheezing, *and* either of the following:

a. Organism isolated from culture obtained by deep tracheal aspirate or bronchoscopy
b. Positive antigen test of respiratory secretions

Other infections of the lower respiratory tract must meet one of the following criteria:

1. Organisms seen on smear or isolated from culture of lung tissue or fluid, including pleural fluid
2. Lung abscess or empyema seen during surgery or by histopathologic examination
3. Abscess cavity seen on radiographic examination of lung

Skin and soft tissue infection

Skin infection must meet either of the following criteria:

1. Purulent drainage, pustules, vesicles, or boils
2. Two of the following at affected site: localized pain or tenderness, swelling, redness, or heat *and* any of the following:
   a. Organism isolated from culture of aspirate or drainage from affected site. If organism is normal skin flora, must be pure culture of single organism
   b. Organism isolated from blood culture
   c. Positive antigen test on infected tissue or blood
   d. Multinucleated giant cells seen on microscopic examination of affected tissue
   e. Diagnostic single antibody titer (IgM) or fourfold increase in paired serum samples (IgG) for pathogen

Decubitus ulcer infection, including both superficial and deep infection, must meet two of the following criteria: redness, tenderness, or swelling of wound edges *and* either of the following:

1. Organism isolated from culture of fluid obtained by needle aspiration or biopsy of tissue obtained from ulcer margin
2. Organism isolated from blood culture

Gastrointestinal system infection

Gastroenteritis must meet either of the following criteria:

1. Acute onset of diarrhea (liquid stools for more than 12 h) with or without vomiting or fever ($>38°C$) *and* no likely noninfectious cause (e.g., diagnostic tests, therapeutic regimen, acute exacerbation of a chronic condition, psychological stress)

2. Two of the following with no other recognized cause: nausea, vomiting, abdominal pain, or headache *and* any of the following:
   a. Enteric pathogen isolated from stool culture or rectal swab
   b. Enteric pathogen detected by routine or electron microscopy examination
   c. Enteric pathogen detected by antigen or antibody assay on feces or blood
   d. Evidence of enteric pathogen detected by cytopathic changes in tissue culture (toxin assay)
   e. Diagnostic single antibody titer (IgM) or fourfold increase in paired serum samples (IgG) for pathogen

Medical and Nursing Department Policy—Tuberculosis Screening and Management

Purpose

To provide optimal care for and prevent spread of tuberculosis.

General information

The age-specific case rate for tuberculosis (number of cases per 100,000 population) is known to have increased among people over 65 in the last two decades. Tuberculosis is recognized as an illness that can cause both endemic and epidemic infections in nursing homes. Routine admission screening and appropriate follow-up surveillance of patients with purified protein derivative (PPD) and anergy panel is useful to diagnose active tuberculosis, previous tuberculin infection, anergy, or recent exposure requiring treatment.

Policy

All residents of this facility will have tuberculin and anergy panel skin testing at admission as well as appropriate follow-up testing and treatment as indicated. Results of skin testing will be documented in the medical record.

Procedures

The infection control practitioner will be responsible for overseeing the surveillance program. The Tuberculosis Admission Surveillance Form (Fig. A-3) will be incorporated in the medical record of all new residents. The infection control practitioner or designee will be responsible for verifying preadmission status and giving appropriate skin tests on all new residents within 1 month of admission. The practitioner will assure that appropriate follow-up skin testing occurs and that proper documentation is made in the resident's medical record. The results of screening will be summarized for the Infection Control Committee.

I. Admission Surveillance
   A. Preadmission fulfillment of survey requirements
      An incoming resident who fulfills one of the following criteria does not need skin testing or further evaluation at admission:
      (1) Positive PPD (≥ 6 mm induration) documented in resident's records or determined through history and chest x-ray within 60 days of admission without evidence of active tuberculosis.
      (2) Negative PPD (≤ 5 mm induration) and positive simultaneous skin testing for any other antigen (e.g., mumps, *Candida*, *Trichophyton*, etc.) documented in the resident's records within 60 days before admission.
      (3) History of a previous severe reaction to skin testing with PPD (chest x-ray on admission will rule out active disease).
      (4) Residents who are on steroids or other immunosuppressants should not receive PPD but should get a chest x-ray.
      (5) Residents who have received any vaccine within 6 weeks should have the PPD given 6 weeks after admission.
   B. Admission testing and evaluation
      All residents who do not have adequate preadmission documentation must be tested by admitting nurses simultaneously with PPD and an anergy screen. These tests should be reviewed on the third day after application. The possible test results and appropriate work-up of each follow.
      (1) Positive PPD/Positive Anergy Screen
         A positive PPD is defined as ≥ 6 mm of induration and a positive anergy is defined as any amount of induration in either control. These residents may have active tuberculosis or previous infection. Most residents with these results will *not* have active tuberculosis. The attending physician will be notified when the results are known. Chest x-ray should be ordered on all such residents if none has been obtained in the previous 60 days. Further management decisions (e.g., need for cultures or isolation) will be made by the attending physician.
            Current guidelines suggest that individuals with diabetes mellitus, lymphoma, leukemia, end-stage renal disease, chronic peptic ulcer disease, or a malabsorption syndrome and those who are on chronic steroid or other immunosuppressive therapy who have a positive PPD should be treated with INH for 6 to 12 months.
      (2) Positive PPD/Negative Anergy Screen
         Follow procedures of B.1.

    (3) Negative PPD/Positive Anergy Screen

These residents have intact cellular immunity as measured by their response to the anergy screen. However, PPD should be repeated in 10 to 14 days to confirm lack of immunity to tuberculosis. The reason for the repeat testing is that some residents will have activation of their response to PPD by being given the first PPD, so that the second PPD is positive (the so-called booster phenomenon).

        If the second PPD is positive, follow the procedure outlined in B.1. If the second one is negative, no further work-up is indicated.

    (4) Negative PPD/Negative Anergy Screen

These residents are anergic (i.e., they have an abnormal immune system, by definition). Follow-up testing with 250 TU PPD should be placed within 24 h. If positive, follow procedure under B.1. If the results are negative, a chest x-ray should be obtained to rule out active tuberculosis if not documented in the past 60 days.

  C. All results will be recorded on the Admission TB Screening Form (Fig. A-3). Positive results will be noted as a problem on the Medical Face Sheet.

II. Follow-up Testing and Treatment

  A. Routine follow-up. Each resident who has a negative PPD at admission should have a follow-up evaluation using PPD and anergy screen every year. Possible outcomes and treatment for each follow.

    (1) Negative PPD/Positive Anergy Screen

No further evaluation or treatment is indicated. Repeat testing in 1 year.

    (2) Positive PPD/Positive Anergy Screen

Obtain a chest x-ray to rule out active tuberculosis. Treat active tuberculosis, if present, according to current recommendations. If there is no evidence of active infection, the attending physician should order a prophylactic antibiotic regimen for all residents with documented conversion of PPD from negative to positive, unless contraindicated, according to the current CDC recommendations (e.g., INH 300 mg qd for 9–12 months).

    (3) Negative PPD/Negative Anergy Screen

These residents are anergic. If anergy was not diagnosed at admission, a chest x-ray should be obtained, and further evaluation done as previously predetermined by the attending physician. Residents previously diagnosed as anergic need a chest x-ray and further evaluation only if clinically indicated.

  B. Emergent Skin Testing

Each resident who had a negative PPD at admission should have follow-up testing with PPD and anergy screen between 60 to 90 days

Admission TB Screening

	Date	Result	Anergy Screen	
			Candida	Mumps

**Initial
Test*** ___/___/___   Neg Pos____mm   Neg Pos   Neg Pos
                       of induration

*If not done, indicate reason below:

_____PPD done and result verified within 60 days of admission

_____History of severe reaction

_____On steroids or other immunosuppressants

_____Vaccine within 6 weeks

_____
                   Signature

Follow-up Test   <u>Date</u>   <u>Strength</u>   <u>Result</u>

              ___/___/___   5 TU   Neg Pos_____mm

              ___/___/___   250 TU   Neg Pos_____mm

_____
                   Signature

Physician notified: _____No   _____Yes

Figure A–3 Documentation for tuberculosis screening.

after a confirmed or suspected exposure to another resident with tuberculosis. All roommates of a resident who converts on routine or follow-up testing should be tested emergently. Recommendations outlined in II.A., 1 to 3, should be followed when emergent testing is done.

C. All results will be recorded in the Medical Progress Notes using a standard format. Positive results will be noted as a problem on the Medical Face Sheet.

Example of Guidelines for Foregoing Life-Sustaining Treatment*

A. Application of Guidelines
   1. These guidelines are applicable to all adult persons, no matter what type of health facility they are in.
B. Rights of Patients
   1. An adult person capable of giving informed consent has the right to make his or her own decisions regarding medical care.
   2. For adult patients who are unable to give informed consent, the legal authority to make decisions regarding life-sustaining treatments rests with a surrogate decision maker.
C. Surrogate Decision Makers
   1. The surrogate decision maker is the attorney-in-fact appointed in a Durable Power of Attorney for Health Care or, when there is none, the family or significant others.
      a. Only in rare cases should it be necessary to seek court appointment of a conservator to make these decisions.
      b. When there is no attorney-in-fact or conservator, and there is disagreement among family members or other potential surrogate decision makers
         (1) Life-sustaining treatments should be maintained until either the disagreement is resolved or a conservator is appointed and makes the decision.
   2. The surrogate should act in accordance with the patient's treatment preferences if known.
   3. If the surrogate does not know any of the patient's treatment preferences, the surrogate should act in the patient's best interest after weighing all relevant factors.
D. Role of the Physician
   1. The physician must provide sufficient information to enable patients or their surrogates to understand the medical condition and the potential risks and benefits of treatment decisions.
   2. Before withdrawing or withholding life-sustaining treatment from a competent patient, it is the responsibility of the physician to assess the patient's mental and emotional status carefully, so as to identify any factors (such as pain) that might be affecting the patient's decision.

---

* These guidelines are based on those developed by a Joint Committee on Biomedical Ethics of the Los Angeles County Medical and Bar Associations, and approved by the LACMA Council and Board of Trustees of the LACBA in 1990.

Other states and local committees and agencies may have published guidelines that are relevant in different areas.

These guidelines are consistent with those of the California Department of Health Services, and those developed by the President's Commission on these issues, as well as position statements published by various national medical organizations.

3. The physician should provide surrogates the same information he/she would provide to the patient.
   a. Recommendations by the physician are often requested, are appropriate, and may be helpful to the surrogate.
   b. The decision, however, belongs to the surrogate.
4. Should the patient or surrogate choose a course of action that violates the ethical or religious beliefs of the physician, the physician may choose, after attempting to reconcile their views, to transfer the patient's care to another physician.
5. If a surrogate's decision appears to be inconsistent with the patient's previously expressed preferences or best interests, the physician should:
   a. Thoroughly discuss the issue with the surrogate
   b. If unable to resolve the issue, consult a bioethics committee or other institutional resource

E. General Treatment Principles
1. Life-sustaining treatment need not be continued solely because it was initiated.
   a. It may be appropriate to initiate a treatment in order to
      (1) Determine whether it will be a beneficial therapeutic trial
      (2) Provide time for patients or surrogate to reach decisions
2. Dignity, hygiene, and comfort should be preserved in all circumstances, even if specific life-sustaining treatment is withheld or withdrawn.
3. Medications should be given to relieve pain or discomfort, even if they may tend to hasten death, but they should not be used with the primary intent to hasten or cause death.
4. Medically administered nutrition and hydration (enteral or intravenous feeding) should be analyzed in the same way as any other medical treatment.

F. Documentation and Institutional Policies
1. In cases in which life-sustaining treatment is withheld or withdrawn, the medical record should include appropriate documentation, and decisions should be communicated and discussed among relevant members of the caregiving team.
2. Decisions to withhold or withdraw life-sustaining treatment should be made in accordance with any applicable institutional policies and procedures.

G. Use of Ethics Committees
1. Biomedical ethics committees may be helpful in dealing with decisions to withhold or withdraw life-sustaining treatment.
   a. Development of institutional policies and procedures
   b. Discussing and clarifying issues, exploring alternative approaches, attempting to resolve conflicts

2. Such committees should not make individual treatment decisions.
    a. Treatment decisions should be made by the patient, surrogate, and physician

H. Role of the Courts

1. Most cases involving the foregoing of life-sustaining treatment can be, should be, and are resolved without the involvement of the courts.
2. When necessary, the court may be approached to resolve such legal disputes
    a. Determination of proper surrogate
    b. Surrogates who may not be acting in the patient's best interests
3. Withholding or withdrawing life-sustaining treatment at the direction of a patient or appropriate surrogate does not legally constitute encouraging or participating in suicide.
4. Physician orders to withhold or withdraw life-sustaining treatment in appropriate circumstances do not create civil or criminal liability for the physician.

Jewish Homes for the Aging of Greater Los Angeles— Cardiopulmonary Resuscitation (CPR) Policy

I. Purpose

1. The CPR policy is designed to clarify, for residents, staff, and family members, procedures for administering and withholding of CPR for residents at the Jewish Homes for the Aging.
    a. Currently this policy relates only to those residents residing in the Homes' nursing facilities, since state regulation does not currently allow a "No CPR" order in residential care facilities.
2. This policy is consistent with the homes' policy as it relates to conformity with Jewish law.

    In recommending this statement of policy it relates only to the administration of *Cardiopulmonary Resuscitation* and is not to be considered as a precedent to be used in discussion of other treatments. This policy was recommended because the literature indicates that CPR is not efficacious treatment and that the potential risks can outweigh the benefits when used on an elderly institutionalized person.
3. The policy is designed to ensure that
    a. The decision of whether or not to initiate CPR is made, whenever possible, at a time when the resident is mentally competent, not in the midst of a medical crisis, and with input from other parties when appropriate (e.g., family, friends, physician, rabbi, Homes' staff).
    b. The right of competent residents or the appointed guardian, or the

person designated in the *Durable Power of Attorney for Health Care* (DPA) to make decisions, is respected.

    c. Best interest decisions regarding CPR are made for residents not competent to decide for themselves, preferably through advance directive.

    d. Decisions regarding CPR status for each resident are carefully documented by the resident's physician and communicated by him/her to Jewish Homes' staff and health professionals from outside the Homes who may become involved in the resident's care during an acute illness, and to other parties when authorized by the resident.

  4. Upon admission to the Jewish Homes, all residents are encouraged to sign a DPA.

As part of this process, the resident should be

    a. Informed about the medical care available at the Jewish Homes, including procedures followed in emergency situations

    b. Encouraged to include in the DPA a statement that specifies what types of treatment they would or would not want, particularly regarding CPR

II. Definitions

  1. CPR is a set of emergency procedures, including chest compression and maintenance of ventilation, that are carried out by trained health professional in the event of a sudden, unexpected cardiac and/or respiratory arrest. The purpose of is to prevent sudden, unexpected death.

    a. At the Jewish Homes for the Aging, only basic life support measures can be undertaken in efforts to resuscitate residents during these kinds of medical crises. The fundamental objective of these measures is to maintain adequate oxygenation of the brain until paramedics arrive.

    b. Advanced life support measures, such as intubation, electrical cardioversion, and central venous lines are not available at the Homes. Initiation of these more advanced measures can only be carried out by either paramedics or hospital emergency room personnel.

  2. "No CPR" orders refer *only* to the measures described above under item 1. *This in no way implies that any other form of medical and nursing care should be withheld from residents. Comfort care will never be withheld.*

  3. *Competence*, as used in this policy refers *only* to the capacity of the resident to make decisions about medical care.

III. Basic Policy and Procedures

  1. Prior to admission, residents are informed that, while living in the Board and Care, CPR will be carried out in the event of cardiopulmonary arrest.

2. Unless there is a "No CPR" order signed by the physician within the past 30 days in the medical record, CPR should be carried out and paramedics called.

3. Primary physicians should, within 90 days after each new resident's admission, discuss the different types of levels of intensity of treatment that they may want in the event of serious or terminal illness, including CPR. The physician should carefully document this discussion in the resident's chart, including a detailed summary of the issues discussed and the decisions made (if any).

4. The rabbi or social worker should discuss the "No CPR" option with the residents.

5. Within 90 days after the resident becomes a permanent nursing resident, the physician should:

    a. If the resident is competent, discuss the appropriateness of a "No CPR" order with him/her.

        (1) Until more precise procedures for assessing capacity for medical decision making become available, the responsibility for assessing the capacity of an individual resident to make an informed decision regarding the appropriateness of using resuscitative measures rests with the primary care physician. He/she should solicit the opinion of the resident's social worker and other Jewish Homes' staff who know the resident well in making this determination. When there is any doubt or disagreement, a geriatric medicine or psychiatric consultation should be considered.

    b. If the resident has been evaluated and deemed not competent, but has executed a DPA

        (1) Review the resident's DPA for any statements about CPR and for other types of treatment decisions.

        (2) Clarify these statements with the resident's attorney-in-fact in relation to a "No CPR" order.

    c. If the resident is not competent and has not executed a DPA

        (1) Discuss the appropriateness of a "No CPR" order with the resident's legal guardian. The resident's attitudes and preferences about health care when they were competent if known and input from family and Jewish Homes' staff who know the resident well should enter into this discussion whenever possible.

6. After these discussions, the physician must:

    a. Document in a concise and legible progress note on the Treatment Status Sheet the discussions and reasoning that led to the decision about CPR, and mark the Medical Face Sheet accordingly.

    b. If appropriate, write a "No CPR" order. (If the "No CPR" order is written, the medical basis for the decision must be included in the progress note.)

    c. Communicate the decision to the interdisciplinary team that is directly involved in the resident's care.

        The residents should be encouraged to allow their families to be informed. They should be notified that it is impractical to maintain strict confidentiality, because a significant number of staff must be informed of their wish. (The resident should, whenever capable, be given the opportunity to decide whether he/she wants family members to be informed.)

  7. The CPR status of each resident should be reviewed when the resident is discussed at the interdisciplinary patient care planning meeting.

  8. The resident's CPR order must be discussed and reviewed with the resident annually.

  9. If a "No CPR" status is discontinued, documentation and communication procedures should be followed as above and the resident should be removed from the "No CPR" list and the medical record marked accordingly.

IV. Documentation

  1. In all instances, the decision-making process that leads to the initial writing of the "No CPR" order should be documented by the physician in a *concise, legible progress note* on the Treatment Status Sheet, and the Medical Face Sheet should be marked accordingly.

  2. The medical records of those residents who decide *against* CPR must contain:

    a. A *written physician's "No CPR" order* renewed every 30 days.

    b. Annually, or when the resident's condition changes, the CPR status must be discussed and documented in the medical record.

    c. Two copies of a "No CPR" status form in the front of the chart, one labeled "Transfer Copy," which should accompany the resident in the event he/she is hospitalized (see attached example, Fig. A-4).

    d. A *clearly visible marking* on the outside of the medical record, identifying the resident's "No CPR" status.

    e. A notation in the *interdisciplinary care plan* of the resident's "No CPR" status.

  3. A clearly visible list of "No CPR" status residents should be kept at each nurses' station near the telephone. This list should be updated at least weekly and should list the date of the last "No CPR" order.

V. Communication with Acute Care Hospitals

  1. Communication with acute care hospitals is critical in order to ensure that the resident's desires regarding CPR are carried out.

  2. All Jewish Homes nursing and medical staff are responsible for being aware of the CPR status of residents under their care.

    a. The marking on the outside of the medical record as well as the

JEWISH HOMES FOR THE AGING OF GREATER LOS ANGELES

NO CPR STATUS FORM

_____
(Resident Name)

IS NOT

to be resuscitated in the event of cardiopulmonary arrest

Refer to progress notes dated: _____

_____
(Physician's Signature)

Figure A–4 Form placed in chart and transferred to acute care hospital for residents on no-CPR status.

    list at the nurses' station should provide this information, _even in emergency situations._

    b. _Paramedics should not be called when cardiopulmonary arrest occurs in a resident with a "No CPR" status._

    c. _If CPR status has not been determined or is unavailable in an emergency, CPR should be initiated and the paramedics called._

3. In the event that paramedics are called and arrive after a resident who is on "No CPR" status has had a cardiac arrest, the nurse on duty should inform the paramedics of this status.

4. Whenever a Jewish Homes resident is transferred to the acute care hospital, the Transfer Copy of the "No CPR" Status Form should accompany him/her, as well as the Medical Face Sheet and Treatment Status Sheet.

5. It is the primary care physician's responsibility to communicate the resident's CPR status to all those involved in the resident's care at the hospital.

VI. Review of CPR Status
   1. The Jewish Homes Biomedical Ethics Committee should
      a. Maintain an updated record of the number of residents on "No CPR" status.
      b. Periodically review the adequacy and appropriateness of documentation of CPR status and the decision-making process that led to it.
      c. Periodically review deaths at the Jewish Homes, focusing on deaths of residents for whom "No CPR" orders had been written.

Jewish Homes for the Aging of Greater Los Angeles—Interim Policy on Feeding and Hydration

I. Purpose
   1. The feeding and hydration policy is designed to clarify, for residents, staff, and family members, procedures for administration of artificial feeding and hydration for residents at the Jewish Homes for the Aging.
      a. Currently this policy relates only to those residents residing in the Homes' nursing facilities, since state regulation does not currently allow a *"No Artificial Feeding or Hydration"* order in residential care facilities.
   2. This policy is consistent with the Homes' Policy as it relates to conformity with Jewish Law.
      In recommending this statement of policy it relates only to the artificial feeding and hydration and is not to be considered as a precedent to be used in discussion of other treatments.
   3. The policy is designed to ensure that
      a. The decision whether or not to initiate artificial feeding and hydration is made, whenever possible, at a time when the resident is mentally competent, not in the midst of a medical crisis, and with input from other parties when appropriate (e.g., family, friends, physician, rabbi, Homes' staff).
      b. The right of competent residents or the appointed guardian, or the person designated in the *durable power of attorney for health care* (DPA) to make decisions.
      c. Best interest decisions regarding artificial feeding and hydration are made for residents not competent to decide for themselves, preferably through advance directive.
      d. Decisions regarding artificial feeding and hydration status for each resident are carefully documented by the resident's physi-

cian and communicated by him/her to Jewish Homes' staff and health professionals from outside the Homes who may become involved in the resident's care during an acute illness, and to other parties when authorized by the resident.

4. Upon admission to the Jewish Homes, all residents should be encouraged to sign a (DPA).

As part of this process, the resident should be

a. Informed about the medical care available at the Jewish Homes, including procedures followed in emergency situations

b. Informed about the policy on artificial feeding and hydration

c. Encouraged to include in the DPA a statement that specifies what types of treatment they would or would not want, particularly artificial feeding and hydration.

II. Definitions

1. Artificial feeding and hydration may be administered orally, through a nasogastric tube, or a surgically inserted gastric tube (the latter is a procedure performed in a hospital).

2. A *"No Artificial Feeding and Hydration"* order does not in any way imply that any other form of medical and nursing care should be withheld from residents. *Comfort care will never be withheld.*

3. *Competence* as used in this policy refers *only* to the capacity of the resident to make decisions about medical care.

III. Basic Policy

1. The general standing order of the Jewish Homes for the Aging regarding treatment provided to all of its residents requires the administration of both nutrition and hydration at all times.

2. Every effort should be made to help residents obtain food and hydration orally.

3. If enteral feeding is necessary, and if, in the opinion of the attending physician, and after review of the medical director, director of nurses, and director of social services, the resident meets one or more of the criteria outlined below, *and* if there is a written directive by the resident stating that he or she does not want either life sustaining treatment or artificial feeding and hydration, enteral feeding may be withheld or withdrawn under the following circumstances:

a. Coma or persistent vegetative state from which there is no reasonable medical probability of emerging *or*

b. Irreversible illness with imminent death within a few months and when the anticipated burdens of enteral feeding exceed the benefits *and*

c. The enteral feeding poses a greater threat to the resident's life than the probable benefit of such treatment *or*

d. The enteral feeding causes tremendous, persistent, or recurrent pain

IV. Basic Procedures

1. This policy assumes artificial feeding and hydration will be ordered if appropriate unless there is a "No Artificial Feeding and Hydration" order signed by the physician within the past 30 days in the medical record.

2. Within 90 days after the resident becomes a permanent nursing resident, the physician should

   a. If the resident is competent, discuss the appropriateness of a "No Artificial Feeding and Hydration" order with him/her.

      (1) Until more precise procedures for assessing capacity for medical decision making become available, the responsibility for assessing the capacity of an individual resident to make an informed decision regarding the appropriateness of using artificial and feeding hydration rests with the primary physician. He/she should solicit the opinion of the resident's social worker and other Jewish Homes' staff who know the resident well in making this determination. When there is any doubt or disagreement, a geriatric medicine or psychiatric consultation should be considered.

   b. If the resident has been evaluated and deemed not competent, but has executed a DPA

      (1) Review the resident's DPA for any statements about artificial feeding and hydration and for other types of treatment decisions.

      (2) Clarify these statements with the resident's attorney-in-fact in relation to a "No Artificial Feeding and Hydration" order.

   c. If the resident is not competent and has not executed a DPA

      (1) Discuss the appropriateness of a "No Artificial Feeding and Hydration" order with the resident's legal guardian. The resident's attitudes and preferences about health care when he or she was competent if known, and input from family and Jewish Homes' staff that know the resident well should enter into this discussion whenever possible. The resident's prior stated preferences will take priority in decision making.

3. After these discussions, the physician must

   a. Document in a concise and legible progress note on the Treatment Status Sheet the discussions and reasoning that led to the decision about artificial feeding and hydration.

   b. If appropriate, write a "No Artificial Feeding and Hydration" order. (If the "No Artificial Feeding and Hydration" order is written, the medical basis for the decision must be included in the progress note.) The Medical Face Sheet should be marked accordingly.

   c. Communicate the decision to the interdisciplinary team that is directly involved in the resident's care.

The residents should be encouraged to allow his or her family to be informed. They should be notified that it is impractical to maintain strict confidentiality because a significant number of staff must be informed of the resident's wish. (The resident should, whenever possible, be given the opportunity to decide whether he/she wants family members to be informed.)

4. The artificial feeding and hydration status of each resident should be reviewed when the resident is discussed at the interdisciplinary patient care planning meeting.

5. The resident's "Artificial Feeding and Hydration" order must be discussed and reviewed with the resident periodically if the resident's condition permits.

6. If a "No Artificial Feeding and Hydration" status is discontinued, documentation and communication procedures should be followed as above and the resident should be removed from the "No Artificial Feeding and Hydration" list and the medical record marked accordingly.

7. Whenever conflicts arise that cannot be resolved by the parties involved, the Biomedical Ethics Committee should be consulted.

V. Documentation

1. In all instances, the decision-making process that leads to the initial writing of the "No Artificial Feeding and Hydration" order should be documented by the physician in a *concise, legible progress note*, on the Treatment Status Sheet.

2. The medical records of those residents who decide *against* artificial feeding and hydration must contain

   a. A *written physician's "No Artificial Feeding and Hydration" order* renewed every 30 days. The Medical Face Sheet should be marked accordingly.

   b. Annually, or when the resident's condition changes, the "Artificial Feeding and Hydration" status must be discussed and documented in the medical record.

   c. Two copies of a "No Artificial Feeding and Hydration" status form in the front of the chart, one labeled "Transfer Copy," which should accompany the resident in the event he/she is hospitalized (see attached example, Fig. A-5).

   d. A *clearly visible marking* on the outside of the medical record identifying the resident's "No Artificial Feeding and Hydration" status.

   e. A notation in the *interdisciplinary care plan* of the resident's "No Artificial Feeding and Hydration" status.

VI. Communication with Acute Care Hospitals

1. Communication with acute care hospitals is critical in order to ensure that the resident's desires regarding artificial feeding and hydration are carried out.

JEWISH HOMES FOR THE AGING OF GREATER LOS ANGELES

NO ARTIFICIAL FEEDING AND HYDRATION STATUS FORM

(Resident Name)

IS NOT

to be Artificially Fed or Hydrated

Refer to progress notes dated:_____

(Physician's Signature)

Figure A–5 Form placed in chart and transferred to acute care hospital for residents on no-artificial-feeding-and-hydration status.

2. All Jewish Homes nursing and medical staff are responsible for being aware of the artificial feeding and hydration status of residents under their care.
3. Whenever a Jewish Homes resident is transferred to the acute care hospital, the Transfer Copy of the "No Artificial Feeding and Hydration" status form as well as the Medical Face Sheet and Treatment Status Sheet should accompany him/her.
4. It is the primary care physician's responsibility to communicate the resident's artificial feeding and hydration status to all those involved in the resident's care at the acute hospital.
VII. Review of Artificial Feeding and Hydration Status
   1. The Jewish Homes Biomedical Ethics Committee should
      a. Maintain an updated record of the number of residents on "No Artificial Feeding and Hydration" status

    b. Periodically review the adequacy and appropriateness of documentation of artificial feeding and hydration status and the decision-making process that led to it

    c. Periodically review deaths at the Jewish Homes, focusing on deaths of residents for whom "No Artificial Feeding and Hydration" orders had been written

EXAMPLES OF DOCUMENTATION FORMATS

Admission Medical Data Bases

The medical data base outlined on the following pages is intended for the *initial* admission of a nursing home (NH) resident (as opposed to readmission after an acute hospitalization).

The acute hospital admission history and physical exam and/or the discharge summary are *not* appropriate medical data bases for an initial admission to a NH because they generally do not contain adequate information about chronic health problems, health maintenance issues, and functional and mental status.

Some of the data suggested are required by OBRA (see earlier section of Appendix) and overlap with the Minimum Data Set, which will be required on all new admissions.

For a detailed description of the Minimum Data Set, see Morris JN, Hawes C, Fries BE, et al: Designing the national resident assessment instrument for nursing homes. *Gerontologist* 30:293–307, 1990.

Medical Face Sheet

The Medical Face Sheet (Fig. A-6) is completed on each resident at the Jewish Homes for the Aging at the time they are admitted to the nursing home section. It is updated annually and whenever relevant changes occur.

Administrative information is kept on a separate administrative face sheet. The Treatment Status sheet is used to document conversations about cardiopulmonary resuscitation and other treatment issues.

Neither the Medical Face Sheet nor the Treatment Status Sheet is thinned from the chart. They are copied and sent to the acute care hospital when the resident requires hospitalization.

We are currently in the process of linking this form to a computerized data base. The eventual goal is to have the functional status data input into the computer by nursing staff and printed out onto the Medical Face Sheet (as well as for nursing documentation) to avoid duplicative efforts.

Suggested Format and Content for the Medical Data Base for an Initial Nursing Home Admission

  I. Active Medical Problems
     List all active medical problems requiring specific treatment and/or monitoring

Jewish Homes for the Aging of Greater Los Angeles
MEDICAL FACE SHEET

ACTIVE MEDICAL PROBLEMS

1._____
2._____
3._____
4._____
5._____
6._____
7._____
8._____

PAST HISTORY

A. Acute hospitalizations since admission to JHA (including surgery)

	Diagnoses	Month/Year
1.	_____	_____/_____
2.	_____	_____/_____
3.	_____	_____/_____
4.	_____	_____/_____

B. Major surgical procedures **before** admission to JHA

	Procedure	Year
1.	_____	_____
2.	_____	_____
3.	_____	_____
4.	_____	_____

C. Allergies

1._____
2._____

NEUROPSYCHIATRIC STATUS

A. Dementia _____Absent _____Present
If present:
_____Alzheimer's
_____Multi-infarct
_____Mixed
_____Uncertain/Other

B. Psychiatric/behavioral disorders
1._____
2._____

C. Usual Mental Status
_____Alert, oriented, follows simple directions
_____Alert, disoriented, but **can** follow simple directions
_____Alert, disoriented, **cannot** follow simple directions
_____Not alert (lethargic, comatose)

D. Most recent Mini Mental State Score
_____/30 (Date____/____/____)

FUNCTIONAL STATUS

A. Ambulation
_____Unassisted
_____With cane
_____Wtih walker
_____Unable If unable:
Transfers: _____Ind _____Dep

B. Continence

	Continent	Inc
Urine	_____	_____
Stool	_____	_____

C. Basic ADLS

	Ind	Dep
Bathing	_____	_____
Dressing	_____	_____
Grooming	_____	_____
Feeding	_____	_____

TREATMENT STATUS   (See Treatment Status Sheet Note Date____/____/____)

_____Full Code   _____DNR   _____ DNR, do not hospitalize

This Form Completed By _____ Date____/____/____

Resident's Name	Bldg.	Room Number	JHA Record No.

☐ **Victory Village**   ☐ **Grancell Village**

Figure A–6 Example of a Medical Face Sheet.

II. Goals of the Admission

List the overall goals of the admission, such as

Rehabilitation to regain ambulation, functional abilities, and discharge home

Complete therapy for an acute illness (e.g., prolonged parenteral antibiotic therapy)

Manage disruptive behavior and impaired functional status associated with dementia

Palliative, supportive care for terminal illness

III. Rehabilitation Potential

    A. Categorize potential for rehabilitation

        Good

        Fair

        Poor

        None (not relevant to current care plan)

    B. Specific goals for rehabilitation

IV. Present Medical History

    A. Symptoms and other data relevant to active medical problems

    B. Summarize acute care hospital course (if applicable)

V. Past Medical History

    A. Surgeries

    B. Other major illnesses/hospitalization

    C. Allergies

    D. Tuberculosis

    E. Immunizations

        1. Influenza (if during fall/winter)

        2. Pneumococcal vaccine

        3. Tetanus

    F. Results of any recent assessments (e.g., ophthalmologic, dental, audiologic)

VI. Habits

    A. Smoking

    B. Alcohol

    C. Dietary restrictions/preferences

VII. Social History

    A. Cultural background

    B. Education

    C. Work experience

    D. Family/caregiver/significant other relationships

    E. Previous living environment

VIII. Advance Directive

    A. Existence of advance directive

    B. If it exists:

        1. Identified surrogate

        2. Treatment preferences

C. If no advance directive:
1. Anything known about preferences for surrogate and treatment decisions

IX. Symptom Review
(Note: this list is not all-inclusive; it focuses on more common and important symptoms in the nursing home population.)

A. General
1. Overall perception of health
2. Level of energy/fatigue
3. Sleep habits
4. Appetite

B. Skin
1. Rash/pruritus
2. Skin lesions/pressure sores

C. Head, Ears, Eyes, Nose, Throat
1. Headaches
2. Ability to hear conversation (with or without a hearing aid)
3. Ability to read
4. Difficulty chewing/swallowing

D. Respiratory
1. Cough
2. Dyspnea

E. Cardiovascular
1. Chest pain
2. Palpitations
3. Dizziness/syncope/falling
4. Dyspnea/Orthopnea
5. Edema
6. Claudication

F. Gastrointestinal
1. Abdominal pain/heartburn
2. Bowel habit
3. Melena/hematochezia

G. Genitourinary
1. Frequency/nocturia
2. Urgency
3. Incontinence
4. Dysuria
5. Hematuria
6. Voiding difficulty (hesitancy, straining, intermittent stream)

H. Musculoskeletal
1. Pain
2. Limited range of motion

I. Neuropsychiatric
1. Transient focal neurological symptoms

    2. Paresthesias

    3. Tremor

    4. Memory

    5. Depression (suicidal ideation if depressed)

    6. Paranoia/delusions

    7. Behavioral disturbances (if dementia present)

X. Functional Status

(Note: standard scales are available; all items included in Minimum Data Set.)

    A. Instrumental Activities of Daily Living

        1. Include specific assessment of ability to take own medications

    B. Mobility

        1. Ambulation status

            a. Use of assistive device and/or human assistance

            b. Gait pattern

            c. Balance

            d. Endurance

        2. If not ambulatory

            a. Wheelchair mobility

            b. Transfer

            c. Bed mobility

    C. Basic Activities of Daily Living

        1. Bathing

        2. Dressing

        3. Grooming

        4. Continence

        5. Feeding

XI. Mental/Affective Status

(Note: it is recommended to record a score on a standardized mental status test; standardized instruments to screen for depression are also available. Each of the items listed below should be specifically addressed as well.)

    A. Alertness

    B. Speech and language

    C. Remote, recent, and immediate memory

    D. Insight and judgment

    E. High cortical functions such as

        1. Calculations

        2. Reading, writing, drawing

        3. Abstraction

    F. Mood and affect

    G. A specific statement about the resident's capacity to participate in health care decisions

XII. Physical Examination
   (Note: this list is not all-inclusive; it focuses on aspects of the examination especially important in nursing home residents.)
   A. Vital signs
      1. Weight, height
      2. Blood pressure, pulse
         a. Postural changes if indicated
         b. Check for Osler's sign if systolic hypertension present
   B. Skin
      1. Pressure sores
      2. Rash
      3. Other lesions
   C. Head, Ears, Eyes, Nose, Throat
      1. Ability to hear conversation
      2. Ear canals
      3. Visual acuity/ability to read
      4. Pupils
      5. Presence/absence of cataracts
      6. Status of teeth/dentures
      7. Oral lesions
   D. Neck
      1. Range of motion
      2. Thyromegaly, mass
   E. Chest
      1. Kyphosis
      2. Vertebral tenderness
      3. Breast masses
      4. Lung sounds
   F. Cardiovascular
      1. Heart rhythm
      2. Murmur(s), gallop(s)
      3. Pulses (carotid, dorsal pedis)
      4. Bruits (carotid, abdominal, femoral)
      5. Edema
      6. Signs of peripheral vascular insufficiency (arterial, venous)
   G. Abdominal/Rectal
      1. Mass/organomegaly
         a. Aortic aneurysm
      2. Tenderness
      3. Rectal sphincter tone
      4. Impaction, mass, painful hemorrhoid
      5. Stool occult blood
      6. Hernia

    H. Pelvic (especially if incontinent)
      1. Vaginitis
      2. Prolapse
    I. Musculoskeletal
      1. Pain/inflammation
      2. Deformity
      3. Limited range of motion/contracture
    J. Neurological
      1. Cranial nerves
      2. Sensation
      3. Motor
        a. Strength
        b. Tremor
        c. Signs of Parkinsonism
      4. Reflexes
        a. Deep tendon
        b. Pathological (e.g., Babinski, glabellar)
      5. Cerebellar
XIII. Laboratory Data
    A. Hemoglobin
    B. Electrolytes and renal function tests
    C. Blood sugar (fasting or postprandial)
    D. Thyroid function tests
    E. Albumin (transferrin if tube fed)
    F. Calcium
    G. Latest chest x-ray
    H. Latest electrocardiogram
    I. Drug blood levels (if applicable)
    J. Other laboratory data relevant to active medical problems

Annual Medical Reassessment

The annual medical reassessment outlined is recommended for all long-staying nursing home residents.

This assessment can be tailored to the resident's overall condition. All the items may not be relevant for some residents—for example, those with terminal illness or end-stage dementia.

Standardized, scored instruments are available for the assessment of activities of daily living, mobility/gait/balance, mental status, and depression which can be incorporated into the annual reassessment. Changes in performance on these standardized assessments may indicate a need for further evaluation and possibly intervention (e.g., incontinence evaluation, gait retraining, psychiatry consultation, etc.).

Components of an Annual Medical Reassessment
of a Nursing Home Resident

I. Active medical problems
   Update list of active medical problems requiring specific treatment and/or monitoring
II. Goals
   Update the goals of care
III. Rehabilitation potential
   Update assessment of rehabilitation potential or note that rehabilitation is not part of care plan at present time
IV. Medical history
   A. Describe any acute medical conditions or changes in status of active medical problems that occurred in the past year
V. Social status
   A. Describe any changes that occurred in the resident's relationships with relatives and significant others
   B. Note any major life events (e.g., death of a spouse or child)
VI. Advance directive
   A. Review status of any advance directive
      1. Surrogate decision maker
      2. Treatment preferences
   B. In absence of advance directive, document what is known about resident's preferences for surrogate and treatment status
   C. Summarize symptoms relevant to active medical problem
VII. Symptom review (see Admission Medical Data Base)
VIII. Functional status (see Admission Medical Data Base)
   A. Note changes over the year
IX. Mental/affective status (see Admission Medical Data Base)
   A. Note changes over the year
   B. Include a specific statement about the resident's decision-making capacity
X. Physical examination (see Admission Medical Data Base)
   A. Note weight change
   B. Note any major new findings
XI. Health maintenance
   A. Document any relevant information related to annual evaluation, including
      1. Auditory screening
      2. Visual screening
      3. Dental assessment
      4. Podiatric assessment
   B. Tuberculosis reactivity
   C. Weight loss/nutritional status
   D. Monitoring laboratory data relevant to chronic medical conditions

XII. Screening laboratory tests (if not done for monitoring)
   A. Stool for occult blood
   B. Complete blood cell count
   C. Fasting glucose
   D. Electrolytes
   E. Renal function tests
   F. Albumin (transferrin if tube-fed)
   G. Calcium
   H. Thyroid function
XIII. Plans
   A. List specific plans related to
      1. Changes in active medical conditions
      2. Weight loss
      3. Changes in functional status
      4. Changes in mental status
      5. Development of depression and/or behavioral disorders associated with dementia
      6. Abnormalities in screening laboratory tests

Resident Transfer Form—Nursing Home to Hospital

The form illustrated (Fig. A-7) contains information that should be transferred to the acute care hospital when a NH resident is hospitalized.

This form is modeled after Chutka DS, Freeman PI, and Tangalos EG: Convenient form for transfer of patients from nursing home to hospital. *Mayo Clin Proc* 64:1324–1325, 1989.

(See also "Policy and Procedures for Sending Resident Information to Consultants and Hospitals," contained in this Appendix.)

Medical Transfer Summary—Acute Care Hospital to Nursing Home

The form illustrated (Fig. A-8) is used by primary care medical staff at the Jewish Homes for the Aging of Greater Los Angeles.

It is completed the day before or the morning of the resident's transfer back from the acute care hospital to the Jewish Home and is accompanied by a preprinted Physician's Readmission Order Form (Fig. A-9).

This summary form does *not* replace the hospital discharge summary, which is dictated, transcribed, and subsequently sent to the Jewish Home and placed in the resident's record.

This summary does meet all the documentation requirements for readmission. When the resident arrives back at the Jewish Home, a nurse practitioner reviews the form and orders, assesses the resident, and writes a medical readmission note.

Transfer Form - Nursing Home to Hospital

Name_____
      Last   First

```
┌──────────────────────────────────────────────────────────────────┐
│                                                                    │
│  Code Status/Critical Care Plan_____   │
│                                                                    │
└──────────────────────────────────────────────────────────────────┘
```

Date of Birth_____/_____/_____ Age____ Physician_____

Sex ____Male ____Female   Nursing Home_____

Religion_____   Phone_(____)_____

Relative/Guardian_____ Family notified of transfer ____Yes ____No

       Phone_(____)_____

Social Security #_____ Medicare #_____ Medicaid #_____

Reason for Transfer_____
_____
_____
_____

Valuables accompanying patient_____

Medical Information

Diagnoses:
_____   _____
_____   _____
_____   _____
_____   _____

Medications - Dosages   **Time Last Given**
_____   _____   Diet_____
_____   _____   Alergies_____
_____   _____
_____   _____
_____   _____

Usual Mental Status ____Alert ____Wanders ____Confused
                     ____Oriented ____Combative ____Withdrawn

Vital signs   HR_____   Resp_____   Temp_____   BP_____

Figure A–7 Example of a transfer form to go with residents when they are sent to the acute care hospital.

ACTIVITIES OF DAILY LIVING

			COMMENTS
Ambulation	1. 2. 3. 4. 5.	Independence with two assistive device Walks with supervision Walks with continuous physical support Bed to chair (total help) Bedfast	
Transfer	1. 2. 3. 4. 5.	No assistance Equipment only Supervision only Requires transfer with two equipment Bedfast	
Bladder Control	1. 2. 3. 4. 5. 6.	Continent Rarely Occasional - once a week or less Frequent - up to once a day Total incontinence Catheter - indwelling	
Bowel Control	1. 2. 3. 4. 5.	Continent Rarely Frequent - once a week or more Total incontinence Ostomy	
Bathing	1. 2. 3. 4. 5.	No assistance Supervision only Assistance in shower/tub Is bathed in shower/tub Is bathed - bed bath procedure	
Dressing	1. 2. 3. 4.	Dresses self Minor assistance Partial help, completes 1/2 dressing Has to be dressed	
Feeding	1. 2. 3. 4.	No assistance Minor assistance - needs tray set up only Help in feeding/encouraging Is fed	

SENSORY/LANGUAGE IMPAIRMENTS

			AID/ PROSTHESIS
Sight	1. 2. 3. 4.	Good Vision adequate - unable to read fine print Vision limited - Gross object observation Blind	
Hearing	1. 2. 3. 4.	Good Hearing slightly impaired Limited hearing (e.g. must speak loudly) Virtually completely deaf	
Speech	1. 2. 3.	Speaks clearly with others of same language Some defect - usually gets message across Unable to speak clearly or not at all	

Figure A–7 (*Continued*)

435

MEDICAL TRANSFER SUMMARY

Encino Hospital to Jewish Homes for the Aging

Patient's name_____

Primary physician_____

Admission date_____/_____/_____   Discharge date_____/_____/_____

A.   Discharge diagnoses:

   1. _____

   2. _____

   3. _____

B.   Surgical procedures and endoscopies during admission (include results and name of
     M.D. who performed the procedure):

   1. _____Date_____/_____/_____

   2. _____Date_____/_____/_____

   3. _____Date_____/_____/_____

C.   Laboratory values - please record the latest results:

   HCT   _____   BUN   _____
   NA   _____   Creat   _____
   K   _____   Glucose   _____
   Other:

D.   Results of other pertinent studies (radiology, CT, MRI, sonography, nuclear scans,
     etc.):

   1. _____

   2. _____

   3. _____
- -For
JHA Use Only

_____   _____ _____ _____
        Resident   Bldg.   Room   JHA Record No.

Figure A–8 Brief transfer summary completed at the time of discharge and sent to the nursing
home. A complete dictated summary is sent subsequently.

436

E.   Treatment decisions

Were No CPR and/or No Hospitalization orders discussed during admission?

_____No   _____Yes   If yes,:

Orders decided: _____No CPR   _____No Hospitalization

Reason for order(s):_____

Discussed with:_____

F.   Comments on hospital course (complications, etc.):

_____

_____

G.   Re-admission diagnoses for JHA: **(Please list all diagnoses for Medical Face Sheet)**

1. _____   5. _____

2. _____   6. _____

3. _____   7. _____

4. _____   8. _____

H.   Is the patient aware of their diagnosis(es)?   _____No   _____Yes

If no, why not:

_____

I.   Is the patient a candidate for rehabilitation therapy?   _____No   _____Yes

1.   State goals of rehabilitation:

_____

2.   Estimate rehabilitation potential:

_____Good   _____Fair   _____Poor

Doctor's signature:_____Date_____/_____/_____

- -For

JHA Use Only

Resident	Bldg.	Room	JHA Record No.

Figure A–8 (*Continued*)

Re-Admission Orders to Jewish Homes for the Aging
PHYSICIAN'S ORDERS

Order Date	
	1. Readmit to ____ Board & Care ___ Nursing ___ Victory ___ Grancell
	2. Activity: ___ Up ad lib ___ Restricted; specify_____
	3. Diet:_____
	4. Vital signs: ___ TPR q _____ ___ Blood Pressure q _____
	5. Weigh q _____
	6. Other routine nursing orders: (Include catheter care, oxygen, turning, positioning, etc.)
	7. Standard orders: (Check the appropriate orders)
	_____ May participate in scheduled activities
	_____ May go out on day or overnight pass with family designee prn
	_____ Podiatry care prn for corns, calluses, fungus, nail debridement
	8. Therapies: (Check the appropriate orders)
	_____ Physical therapy for:_____
	_____ Occupational therapy for:_____
	_____ Respiratory therapy for:_____
	9. CPR Status: ___ Full Code ___ No CPR See note dated ___ / ___ / ___
	10. Laboratory tests and frequency:
	11. Skin and wound care, if any: _____
	12. Medications (routine first, followed by prns; use additional page if necessary)

Date_____ / _____ / _____   Time_____

_____ _____   _____ _____
Physician's Name   Phone #   Alt Physician's Name   Phone #

_____   _____
Diagnosis   Allergies

_____ _____ _____   _____ _____ _____
Patient Name   Patient #   Station   Room   Bed   Page

Figure A–9 Standard format for admission orders from the acute care hospital; these are completed by the primary care physician at the acute care hospital and transferred to the nursing home.

Admission Orders

The illustrated format (Fig. A-9) is used by primary care physicians at the Jewish Homes for the Aging of Greater Los Angeles to write readmission orders for residents returning from the acute care hospital.

The physician order forms are preprinted and kept at the nursing stations in the acute care hospital. Each form has multiple copies so that no reproduction or transcribing of orders is necessary when the resident is readmitted.

Infection Control Reporting Formats

The Infection Control Reporting Form (Fig. A-10) can be used by nursing staff to report infections and possible infections.

The information on the completed forms can be evaluated, along with documentation in the medical record, by the infection control practitioner. These data should be summarized monthly and reviewed at meetings of the infection control committee. When completed in a timely fashion, the form will help the infection control practitioners to identify outbreaks in the facility.

Infection control data can be recorded in a simple computer spread sheet to follow trends over time. An example of a report format is also included (Fig. A-11).

Specific definitions of infections should be developed for the infection control program. Definitions used by the Centers for Disease Control, which may need modification for most NHs, are included elsewhere in this Appendix.

Advance Directive to Physician and Caregivers

The form illustrated is one example of an advance directive for use by NH residents (Fig. A-12). It is taken from Uhlman RF, Clark H, Pearlman RA, et al: Medical management decisions in nursing home patients—Principles and policy recommendations. *Ann Intern Med* 106:879–885, 1987.

Many states have laws relating to advance directives [maps illustrating these laws as of 1990 are included (Figs. A-13 and A-14)]. Some states have developed a document constituting standardized durable power of attorney for health care. This should be used in place of the form shown in the states that have done so.

Documentation of Preferred Intensity of Care

The format illustrated was developed by the California Medical Association in 1989 to provide physicians with a method of documenting preferred intensity of treatment and related issues (Fig. A-15).

INFECTION CONTROL REPORTING FORM

Resident's Name _____

Ward/Building _____ Room_____

Primary Physician _____

Date of report _____/_____/_____

I. **Infection Symptoms and Test Results (Please check off one or more)**

Fever ____ Over 100^0 F ____ Over 102^0 F

Urinary Tract ____ Pain or burning on urination
____ Increased frequency or incontinence
____ > 10 WBC's/high power field in UA
____ > 50,000 colonies on C&S

Upper Respiratory ____ Sore throat or sinus pain
____ Dry cough

Lower Respiratory ____ Productive cough/sputum
____ New infiltrate on chest Xray

Gastrointestinal ____ Unexplained diarrhea for > 2 days
____ Positive culture for pathogens
____ Positive test for C. difficile

Wound / Skin ____ Redness ____ Pain
____ Drainage ____ Foul Odor

Other site (specify)

II. **Culture Data**

Was Culture and Sensitivity Done? _____ yes _____ no

                     Site   Organism

If yes, results: _____date___/___/___

                   _____date___/___/___

Were Antibiotics Prescribed? _____ yes _____ no

If yes, names, dose, duration, and dates:

_____date___/___/___

_____date___/___/___

Figure A–10 Example of an infection-control-reporting format for nursing staff and the infection control practitioner.

III. Disposition

____ Improved without treatment
____ Improved with treatment
____ No improvement
____ Patient Hospitalized   date___/___/___

Report filed by _____(please sign)

_____
_____

THIS SECTION TO BE COMPLETED BY INFECTION CONTROL NURSE

Classification of Infection   _____Asymptomatic bacteriuria
                                 _____UTI (symptomatic)
                                 _____Upper respiratory
                                 _____Lower respiratory
                                 _____Skin (describe)
                                 _____Conjunctivitis
                                 _____Gastroenteritis
                                 _____Other (describe)

Nature of infection   _____Nosocomial
                                 _____Infection on admission from
                                 acute hospital
                                 _____Infection on admission from
                                 Board and Care
                                 _____No Infection

Was isolation utilized? _____ yes   _____ no

If so, what type and why?_____date___/___/___

Comments:

Figure A–10 *(Continued)*

Sample Format for Infection Control Data Base

Unit/Infections	MONTH											
	Jan	Feb	Mar	Apr	May	Jun	Jul	Aug	Sept	Oct	Nov	Dec

Unit A

Urinary
Asymptomatic
bacteriuria
UTI (symptomatic)

Respiratory
Upper
Lower

Skin
Pressure sore
Cellulitis
Abscess
Surgical wound
Other
Conjunctivitis

Gastroenteritis
Culture negative
C. Difficile positive
Other

Other

Total

Nursing home acquired

Hospital/community acquired

Number of Antibiotic courses prescribed

Figure A–11 Example of a basic format for a computer data base on infection control.

-2-

Unit/Infections	MONTH											
	Jan	Feb	Mar	Apr	May	Jun	Jul	Aug	Sept	Oct	Nov	Dec

Unit B

Urinary
 Asymptomatic
 bacteriuria
 UTI (symptomatic)

Respiratory
 Upper
 Lower

Skin
 Pressure sore
 Cellulitis
 Abscess
 Surgical wound
 Other
Conjunctivitis

Gastroenteritis
 Culture negative
 C. Difficile positive
 Other

Other

Total

 Nursing home acquired

 Hospital/community acquired

Number of Antibiotic courses prescribed

Figure A–11 (*Continued*)

Directives to Physicians and Caregivers

Below you are given the opportunity to indicate your health care preferences should you become unable to communicate them in the future. You are asked to indicate your preferences for two situations, serious medical problems, and "cardiac arrest." **These decisions may be changed at any time.**

1. Approach to Medical Problems

    In most instances when medical problems arise, patients discuss the situation with their physicians and make decisions about a preferred course of action. Sometimes the need for decisions arises when patients are unable to communicate their wishes. To ensure that your wishes are followed as closely as possible under such circumstances, your guidance in the approach to serious medical problems is requested.

    Please indicate your choice below:

___ All possible measures should be taken including hospitalization, consultations, surgery, and life-support systems. (If no choice is indicated, this option will initially be followed. If you remain unable to communicate your preferences, your physician and closest relative or guardian will decide what would be in your best interest regarding further treatment.)

___ All measures considered appropriate by the individual designated below should be taken. My condition and the probable outcome of these measures should be taken into consideration.

    Designated individual:

    Name of designee:_____

    Relationship:_____

    Alternate designee:_____

    Relationship:_____

___ Measures that can return me to my usual state should be taken, but measures considered principally life-prolonging should be avoided.

___ Treat only to improve comfort and dignity

    Addition instructions: (If you wish to provide additional instructions regarding your medical care, please list them here):

    _____

    _____

2. In Case of Cardic Arrest

    Virtually all medical decisions that arise will be made with your physician, or, if you become unable to communicate the decisions will be covered in the medical measures you specified in the "Approach to Medical Problems." A separate decision needs to be made, however, regarding treatment should you experience "cardiac arrest" (heart stoppage). Cardiac arrest results in death unless promptly treated. Should cardiac arrest occur, a technique for revival called cardiopulmonary resuscitation (CRR) is available. This technique involves artificial ventilation (breathing), chest compressions and, often, drugs and electric shocks, as well.

Figure A–12 Example of an advance directive.

Directives   **Page 2**

If cardiac arrest occurs, CPR must be started immediately to optimize chances for survival. There is no time for consultations; therefore, a decision regarding CPR needs to be made in advance.

Washington State Law requires that attempts at revival must be made unless there has been a specific request not to use such efforts.

The following general information about cardiac arrest may be helpful in your decision making:

1.   Most deaths in a nursing home follow a long-term decline in the person's health. Approximately 5% to 20% of ill elderly persons who have cardiac arrest survive if they receive CPR. Survival is much less likely if resuscitation is initiated 5 or more minutes after cardiac arrest occurs. Approximately 60% of patients who survive cardiac arrest have permanent brain damage such as memory loss, coma, or paralysis.

2.   Sudden death is thought to be painless.

3.   Successful resuscitation is followed by transfer to a hospital for other measures.

Do you wish to receive CPR (cardiopulmonary resuscitation) if you should have cardiac arrest, or would you prefer to accept this event as the end of your natural life? Please indicate your choice:

___   All efforts should be made at revival in the event of cardiac arrest.

___   No efforts at revival should be made. and I will accept cardiac arrest as the end of my natural life.

Additional instructions (if any):_____

_____

_____

_____

Patient's name_____

Patient's signature_____Date___/___/___

Witness:_____   Relationship_____

Witness:_____   Relationship_____

Figure A–12 (*Continued*)

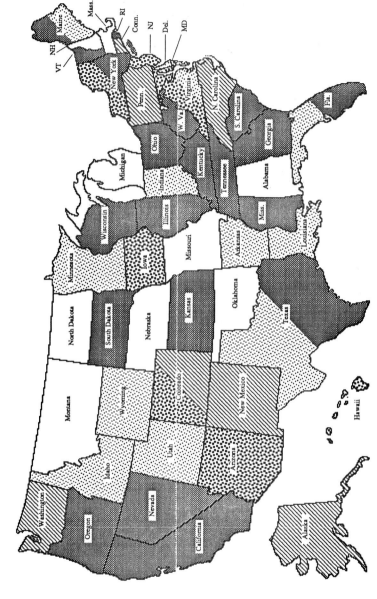

State Law Governing
Durable Power of Attorney • Health Care Agents
• Proxy Appointments •

Documents are available from the Society for states that clearly recognize an agent's power to have life support withheld or withdrawn.

 Jurisdictions with Durable Power of Attorney statutes that permit agents to make medical decisions, specifically including decisions to withhold or withdraw life support (**California, Florida, Georgia, Illinois, Kansas, Kentucky, Maine, Mississippi, Nevada, New York, Ohio, Oregon, Rhode Island, South Carolina, South Dakota, Tennessee, Texas, Vermont, West Virginia, Wisconsin and the District of Columbia**). The agent can act when the patient loses the ability to make his or her own medical decisions.

 States with Durable Power of Attorney statutes that positively authorize consent to medical treatment, but do not specifically authorize the withdrawal or withholding of life support (**Alaska, Colorado, Connecticut, New Mexico, North Carolina, Pennsylvania and Washington**).

 States with Durable Power of Attorney statutes that, through court decisions, Attorney Generals' Opinions or other statutes, have been interpreted to permit agents to make medical decisions, including those to withhold or withdraw life support (**Arizona, Colorado, Hawaii, Iowa, Maryland, New Jersey, New York and Virginia**).

 States that authorize proxy appointments through their "living will" or "natural death" acts (**Arkansas, Delaware, Florida, Idaho, Indiana, Louisiana, Maine, Minnesota, Texas, Utah, Virginia and Wyoming**). Proxies are permitted to make decisions authorized by the act when the patient is in a medical condition covered by the act (usually "terminal" as defined in the act).

 States with general Durable Power of Attorney statutes that make no mention of medical decisions.

Prepared by *Society for the Right to Die, 250 West 57th Street, New York, NY 10107, (212) 246-6973*   August 3, 1990

Figure A–13

447

Tube Feeding Law in the United States

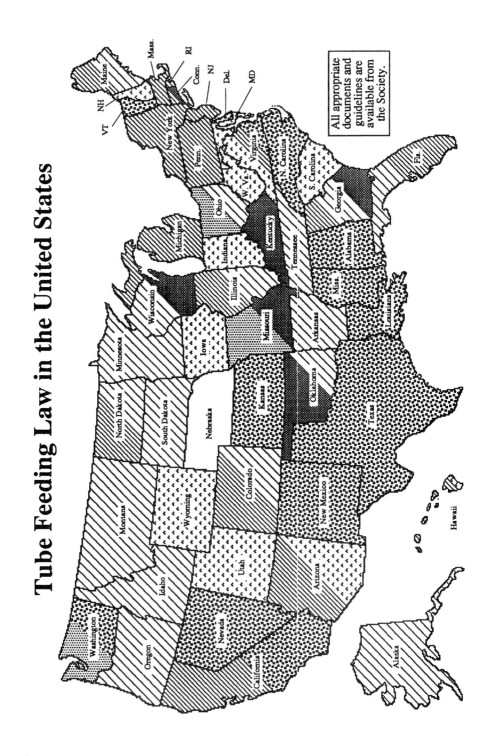

All appropriate documents and guidelines are available from the Society.

▨ States with court decisions indicating it is permissible to withhold/withdraw tube feeding (**Arizona, California,* Colorado,* Connecticut,** Florida,* Georgia,* Hawaii, Illinois, Maine, Massachusetts, Michigan, New Jersey, New York, North Dakota, Pennsylvania, Rhode Island and Virginia***).

▦ States with court decisions that prohibit withholding/withdrawing tube feeding under certain circumstances (**Missouri, Ohio and Washington**).

▧ States with "natural death," "living will," "durable power of attorney for health care" or other statutes that specifically authorize withholding/withdrawing tube feeding (**Alaska, Arkansas, Colorado,* Florida, Georgia,* Idaho, Illinois, Maine, Minnesota, Montana, North Dakota, Ohio, Oklahoma, Oregon, South Dakota, Tennessee† and Wisconsin**).

▩ States with statutes requiring tube feeding in some circumstances (**Oklahoma**) or with "natural death" legislation that permits withholding/withdrawing some forms of life support but explicitly excludes tube feeding from these (**Connecticut,** Georgia,* Kentucky, Missouri and Wisconsin**).

▨ Jurisdictions with "natural death" or "living will" statutes that authorize the removal of life support in general but make no specific mention of tube feeding (**Alabama, California,* Delaware, Kansas, Louisiana, Mississippi, Nevada, New Mexico, North Carolina, Texas,†† Vermont, Virginia,* Washington and the District of Columbia**). Withholding/withdrawing tube feeding is implicitly permissible (except in **Washington**) when the patient is in a medical condition covered by the act.

▨ States in which legislative or judicial interpretation is necessary to determine whether tube feeding may be withheld/withdrawn. "Natural death" or "living will" statutes in these states typically associate tube feeding with comfort care, suggesting that it may be withheld/withdrawn if not necessary for comfort (**Arizona, Hawaii, Indiana, Iowa, Maryland,†† New Hampshire, South Carolina, Utah, West Virginia and Wyoming**).

* Courts have held that patients in these states have constitutional or common law rights to have tube feeding withheld regardless of the terms of the "natural death" or "living will" statutes. (Georgia's durable power explicitly permits refusal of tube feeding.)

** Court decisions interpreted the act to permit withdrawing tube feeding, despite language that would seem to prohibit it.

† Both an Opinion of the attorney general and the durable power of attorney statute seem to forbid the withdrawal of tube feeding when the result would be death "by starvation or dehydration."

†† Interpreted by an Opinion of the attorney general to permit withholding/withdrawing tube feeding.

Note: The majority of "natural death" and "living will" statutes apply to patients who are in a "terminal condition" (variously defined in the statutes). Court cases are frequently concerned with patients in other conditions — e.g., those who are "permanently unconscious" but not "terminal."

Prepared by *Society for the Right to Die*, 250 West 57th Street, New York, NY 10107, (212) 246-6973   August 30, 1990

Figure A–14

DOCUMENTATION OF PREFERRED INTENSITY OF CARE
(Including Orders Concerning Life-Sustaining Treatment)

I,_____ , hereby attest that_____
　(PHYSICIAN'S NAME)　　　　　　　　　　　　(PATIENT'S NAME)

has been my patient of record since_____ /_____ /_____
　　　　　　　　　　　　　　　　(DATE)

1.　I have discussed the pertinent diagnoses and prognoses of_____

　　　　　　　　　　　　　　　　　　　　　Date_____ /_____ /_____

　　　　　　　　　　　Name　　　　　　　　　　Relationship

___Patient　　　　_____

___Patient's legally　_____　　_____
　　empowered
　　representative*　_____　　_____

___Family member/　_____　　_____
　　significant
　　other　　　　_____　　_____

*Individuals who may have legal authority to consent to health care for an incompetent patient include the parents or guardian of a minor child, a conservator, or an attorney in fact designated in a valid durable power of attorney for health care.

2.　I have attached copies of the documents checked below:

___　　Durable power of attorney for health care　　___　　Court orders

___　　Natural Death Act directive　　　　　　　　___　　Other:_____

___　　Certified letters of guardianship or　　　　　___　　Other:_____
　　　　conservatorship

3.　In my judgement, the above-named patient (__has __has not) the mental capacity to understand the nature and consequences of the diagnosis, prognosis and treatment options.

4.　The patient (___has ___has not) expressed to me (___verbally ___in writing) his or her desires concerning with withholding and removal of life-sustaining treatment. (Attach documentation if available.) The statement checked below best reflects the desires expressed to me by the patient:

___　I do not want my life to be prolonged and I do not want life-sustaining treatment to be provided or continued: 1) if I am in an irreversible coma or persistent vegetative state; or 2) if I am terminally ill and the application of life-sustaining procedures would serve only to artificially delay the moment of my death; or 3) under any other circumstances where the burdens of the treatment outweighs the expected benefits.

___　I want my life to be prolonged and I want life-sustaining treatment to be provided unless I am in a coma or vegetative state which my doctor reasonably believes to be irreversible. Once my doctor has reasonably concluded that I will remain unconscious for the rest of my life, I do not want life-sustaining treatment to be provided or continued.

Figure A–15 Example of a format for an advance directive documenting preferred intensity of care.

_____   I want my life to be prolonged to the greatest extent possible without regard to my condition, the chances I have for recovery or the cost of the procedures.

_____   Other or additional desires:_____

_____

_____

5.   In the absence of the patient's personal directives to me, the following individual has stated the wishes of the patient and/or that individual concerning intensity of treatment (attach documentation if available):

Name:_____ Relationship_____

The statement below reflects this individual's preferences regarding intensity of care:_____

_____

_____

6.   Treatment options have been discussed. A decision has been made among those named in #1 above that the intensity of care provided to the above-named patient should include:

a)   ____Maximum treatment **or**   ____Supportive care only

b)   ____CPR   **or**   ____No CPR

7.   If a "supportive care only" status is elected, the above-named patient (and/or legally empowered representative or other surrogate) understands that the principle goals of treatment will be to alleviate suffering, promote comfort and preserve dignity. The following guidelines have been agreed upon:

Therapy	**Not to be used**	**Used only to promote comfort**
Antibiotics	___	___
Intravenous fluids	___	___
Nasogastric fluids	___	___
Hospitalization	___	___
Oxygen	___	___
Other:_____	___	___
Other:_____	___	___
Other:_____	___	___

8.   The following medical conditions support the intensity of care determination made above:_____

_____

_____

_____

Physician's signature:_____ Date_____/_____/_____

Figure A–15 (*Continued*)

Although this format may not be optimal or applicable for many nursing homes, it does contain all the information that should be documented when decisions to forego life-sustaining treatment have been made.

INDEX

Page references in *italic* indicate tables and illustrations.